Advances in Surgery®
Volume 22

Advances in Surgery®

Volumes 1–16 (out of print)

Volume 17

Total Parenteral Nutrition Patients, *by Murray F. Brennan and Glenn D. Horowitz*
Management of Trauma to the Spleen, *by Roger Sherman*
Microsurgery: Replantation and Free Flaps, *by Foad Nahai and M.J. Jurkiewicz*
The Impact of Cyclosporin A on Transplantation, *by Peter J. Morris*
Hepatic Resection in Trauma, *by Dato M. Balasegaram*
Computed Tomography of the Abdomen, *by William A. Rubenstein, Yong Ho Auh, and Elias Kazam*
Arthroscopic Knee Surgery, *by Robert W. Metcalf*
Staples and Staplers, *by Mark M. Ravitch and Felicien M. Steichen*
The Evaluation and Management of Pheochromocytomas, *by Steven N. Levine and John C. McDonald*

Volume 18

Preservation of the Anorectum, *by Bruce G. Wolff and Oliver H. Beahrs*
NMR: The New Frontier in Diagnostic Radiology, *by J. Bruce Kneeland, B.C.P. Lee, J.P. Whalen, R.J.R. Knowles, and P.T. Cahill*
New Approaches to Unusual Aneurysms, *by E. Stanley Crawford and Cary L. Stowe*
Selective Variceal Decompression: Current States and Recent Advances, *by J. Michael Henderson and W. Dean Warren*
Horizons in Surgical Oncology, *by John M. Daly and Jerome J. Decosse*
Current Burn Treatment, *by Cleon W. Goodwin*
Implantable Infusion Pumps, *by Henry Buchwald and Thomas D. Rohde*
Complications of Gastric Partitioning for Morbid Obesity, *by Juan Bass and Joel B. Freeman*

Volume 19

Transhiatal Esophagectomy Without Thoracotomy for Carcinoma of the Esophagus, *by Mark B. Orringer*
Treatment of Renovascular Hypertension, *by William J. Fry*
Posterior Sagittal Approach for the Correction of Anorectal Malformations, *by Alberto Peña*
In Utero Surgery, *by Kevin C. Pringle*
Proximal Gastric Vagotomy: The First 25 Years, *by Philip E. Donahue, Hsu-Shan Tsai, Junichi Yoshida, and Lloyd M. Nyhus*
In-Situ Saphenous Vein Arterial Bypass for the Treatment of Limb Ischemia, *by Robert P. Leather and Allastair M. Karmody*

Advances in Surgery®

Editor-in-Chief

Ronald K. Tompkins, M.D.

Chief, Division of General Surgery, Department of Surgery, UCLA Center for the Health Sciences, Los Angeles, California

Associate Editors

Charles M. Balch, M.D., F.A.C.S.

Head, Division of Surgery, Chairman, Department of General Surgery, The University of Texas, M. D. Anderson Cancer Center, Houston, Texas

John L. Cameron, M.D.

Professor and Chairman, Department of Surgery, The Johns Hopkins Hospital, Baltimore, Maryland

Bernard Langer, M.D.

The R. S. McLaughlin Professor and Chairman, Department of Surgery, University of Toronto, Banting Institute, Toronto, Ontario, Canada

John A. Mannick, M.D.

Moseley Professor of Surgery, Harvard Medical School; Surgeon-in-Chief, Brigham and Women's Hospital, Boston, Massachusetts

George F. Sheldon, M.D.

Zack D. Owens Professor and Chairman, Department of Surgery, School of Medicine, The University of North Carolina at Chapel Hill, Chapel Hill, North Carolina

G. Thomas Shires, M.D.

Cornell University Medical College; Professor and Chairman, Department of Surgery, The New York Hospital, New York City, New York

Claude E. Welch, M.D.

Clinical Professor of Surgery, Emeritus, Harvard Medical School; Senior Surgeon, Massachusetts General Hospital, Ambulatory Care Center, Boston, Massachusetts

Volume 22 • 1989

Year Book Medical Publishers, Inc.

Chicago • London • Boca Raton

International Standard Serial Number: 0065-3411
International Standard Book Number: 0-8151-8811-0

Sponsoring Editor: Julie M. Jewell
Assistant Director, Manuscript Services: Frances M. Perveiler
Production Project Manager: Max Perez
Proofroom Manager: Shirley E. Taylor

Vascular Access for Dialysis and Cancer Chemotherapy, *by N.L. Tilney, R.L. Kirkman, A.D. Whittemore, and R.T. Osteen, Jr.*
Developments in the Resuscitation of Critically Ill Surgical Patients, *by Ronald V. Maier and C. James Carrico*
Role of Percutaneous Angioplasty in the Treatment of Peripheral Arterial Disease, *by Brooke Roberts and Gordon K. McLean*

Volume 20

Penetrating Abdominal Trauma: Resuscitation, Diagnostic Evaluation, and Definitive Management, *by Susan E. Briggs, Douglas Hendricks, and Lewis M. Flint, Jr.*
Total Parenteral Nutrition in the Cancer Patient, *by Samuel M. Mahaffey and Edward M. Copeland III*
The Current Management of Acute Pancreatitis, *by David W. Crist and John L. Cameron*
Lasers in General Surgery, *by Stephen N. Joffe and Tom Schröder*
Up-To-Date Treatment of the Patient With Hypergastrinemia, *by Courtney M. Townsend, Jr., and James C. Thompson*
Valid Alternatives in the Management of Early Breast Cancer, *by C. Barber Mueller*
Ambulatory Procedures in Anorectal Surgery, *by Hartley Stern, Robin McLeod, Zane Cohen, and Theodore Ross*
Up-To-Date Management of Small-Bowel Crohn's Disease, *by J. Alexander-Williams and Ian G. Haynes*
Treatment of Motility Abnormalities of the Esophagus, *by Alex G. Little and David B. Skinner*
Modern Management of Biliary Tract Stone Disease, *by Ronald K. Tompkins and Jeffrey E. Doty*
Current Status of Transplantation of the Pancreas, *by David E.R. Sutherland, Frederick C. Goetz, and John S. Najarian*

Volume 21 (out of print)

Contributors

Christos A. Athanasoulis, M.D., M.P.H.

Professor of Radiology, Harvard Medical School; Head, Section of Vascular Radiology, Massachusetts General Hospital, Boston, Massachusetts

Charles M. Balch, M.D., F.A.C.S.

Head, Division of Surgery, Chairman, Department of General Surgery, The University of Texas, M. D. Anderson Cancer Center, Houston, Texas

Larry C. Carey, M.D.

Clinical Professor of Surgery, Department of Surgery, The Ohio State University College of Medicine, Grant Medical Center, Columbus, Ohio

John A. Collins, M.D.

Professor of Surgery, Stanford University School of Medicine, Stanford, California

Michael J. Edwards, M.D.

Senior Surgical Oncology Fellow, Department of General Surgery, The University of Texas, M. D. Anderson Cancer Center, Houston,Texas

E. Christopher Ellison, M.D.

Clinical Assistant Professor of Surgery, Department of Surgery, The Ohio State University College of Medicine, Grant Medical Center, Columbus, Ohio

Lazar J. Greenfield, M.D.

Professor and Chairman, Department of Surgery, University of Michigan Hospital, Ann Arbor, Michigan

Stuart W. Jamieson, M.B., F.R.C.S.

Professor and Head, Division of Cardiovascular and Thoracic Surgery, Director, Minnesota Heart and Lung Institute, Minneapolis, Minnesota

Nancy Kemeny, M.D.

Gastrointestinal Oncology, Memorial Sloan-Kettering Cancer Center, New York City, New York

Jeffrey B. Kramer, M.D.

Resident, Department of Surgery, Washington University School of Medicine, St. Louis, Missouri

Anthony A. Meyer, M.D., Ph.D.

Associate Professor of Surgery, University of North Carolina; Director, Surgical Intensive Care Unit, Medical Director of Critical Care, North Carolina Memorial Hospital; Assistant Director, North Carolina Jaycees Burn Center, Chapel Hill, North Carolina

Ashby C. Moncure, M.D.

Associate Clinical Professor of Surgery, Harvard Medical School; Visiting Surgeon, Massachusetts General Hospital, Boston, Massachusetts

Denis S. Quill, M.Ch., F.R.C.S.I.

Vascular Research Fellow, Department of Surgery, Section of Peripheral Vascular Surgery, Southern Illinois University School of Medicine, Springfield, Illinois

Robert Rutledge, M.D.

Assistant Professor, Department of Surgery, The University of North Carolina at Chapel Hill, Chapel Hill, North Carolina

George F. Sheldon, M.D.

Professor and Chairman, Department of Surgery, The University of North Carolina at Chapel Hill, Chapel Hill, North Carolina

Paul H. Sugarbaker, M.D.

Winship Cancer Center and Department of Surgery, Emory University School of Medicine, Atlanta, Georgia

David S. Sumner, M.D.

Professor of Surgery, Chief, Section of Peripheral Vascular Surgery, Southern Illinois University School of Medicine, Springfield, Illinois

Ronald G. Tompkins, M.D., S.D.

Assistant Professor of Surgery, Harvard Medical School; Assistant in Surgery, Massachusetts General Hospital, Boston, Massachusetts

Ishik C. Tuna, M.D.

Resident, Division of Thoracic and Cardiovascular Surgery, Mayo Clinic, Rochester, Minnesota

Peter A. Vevon, M.D.

Department of Surgery, The Ohio State University College of Medicine, Columbus, Ohio

Thomas W. Wakefield, M.D.

Assistant Professor of Surgery, Section of Vascular Surgery, University of Michigan Hospital, Ann Arbor, Michigan

Claude E. Welch, M.D.

Clinical Professor of Surgery, Emeritus, Harvard Medical School; Senior Surgeon, Massachusetts General Hospital, Ambulatory Care Center, Boston, Massachusetts

Samuel A. Wells, Jr., M.D.

Professor and Chairman, Department of Surgery, Washington University School of Medicine, St. Louis, Missouri

Preface

Volume 22 of the *Advances in Surgery* series is one of the most exciting in recent years. From the up-to-date, definitive statement on the management of metastatic cancer to the liver, to the most recent information on the relationship of the surgeon to the AIDS patient, and the current status of blood therapy, to definitive articles on occult GI bleeding, hepatic trauma, Hodgkin's lymphoma, and the experience with the heart-lung transplantation among others, there is a wealth of surgical and scientific information in this volume.

The articles are current, in-depth, and constitute the state of the art in their particular areas.

The Editorial Board proudly recommends this volume to students, residents, and practicing surgeons.

Ronald K. Tompkins, M.D.

Contents

Management of Metastatic Cancer to the Liver

Paul H. Sugarbaker, M.D.

Winship Cancer Center and Department of Surgery, Emory University School of Medicine, Atlanta, Georgia

Nancy Kemeny, M.D.

Gastrointestinal Oncology, Memorial Sloan-Kettering Cancer Center, New York City, New York

Recent excitement shared by surgeons, medical oncologists, and radiation therapists concerning progress in the treatment of hepatic tumors has resulted from a confluence of advances in biology and technology. The tumor biologist remains in awe as he reviews the data showing 25 to 50% long-term survival of patients who have metastatic colorectal cancer to the liver with simple surgical removal of all clinical evidence of disease. The single institution reports have become so numerous that this phenomenon cannot be denied. Cooperative efforts at obtaining data, as in the hepatic metastases registry, confirm the single institution reports of significant cure of metastatic cancer by surgical removal of the disease. New trends in the use of serial carcinoembryonic antigen (CEA) assays to detect recurrence of cancer following large-bowel resection have led to a greater number of patients whose metastatic disease is at a stage compatible with surgical resection. The number of hepatic resections performed around the United States and Europe has markedly increased in the 1980s. Radiology has made its significant contribution to the clear definition of the surgical problem. Determination of the number of metastases, their location within the liver parenchyma, and their relationship to major vascular structures now provides the surgeon preoperatively with information only available after considerable liver dissection in the past. Liver anatomy has now been appreciated by the surgeon so that its segmental nature is utilized. Resections carried out through the relatively avascular intersegmental planes promise to markedly decrease the blood loss experienced during parenchymal transection. Finally, the surgical techniques themselves have been refined so that suction dissection or ultrasonic dissection is utilized. Clean, bloodless, tumor-free margins of resection equate with low morbidity and mortality and optimal long-term survival. As we move into the 1990s, the oncologist

Adv Surg 22:1–56, 1989

0065-3411/89/22-001–056-$04.00

looks forward to the development of regional and systemic therapies that will augment hepatic resections for metastatic disease. Also, technologies for the local or regional destruction of intrahepatic tumor promise to eliminate liver metastases as a cause of death from metastatic gastrointestinal malignancy.

Surgical Anatomy of the Liver

External Anatomy

The liver is the largest internal organ of the human body, excluding the skin. To perform its manifold metabolic tasks the liver is richly supplied with arterial blood, portal venous blood, and hepatic venous drainage. It also has abundant lymphatic drainage.

Figure 1 shows the external anatomy of the liver. There are two external surfaces of the liver, the diaphragmatic surface and the visceral surface. Unfortunately, the external configuration is of little help interpreting the complex internal anatomy of the liver. Surgically, the left lobe is more easily managed. It is rather flat and very mobile after taking down the triangular ligament, and it is covered by a tough fibrous capsule, Glisson's capsule. It can generally be easily grasped by the surgeon so that traction on intrahepatic structures can be maintained while a dissection proceeds. In contrast, the right lobe of the liver is more spherical in its configuration. It is difficult to maintain traction on portions of the parenchyma that are to be removed, and this makes dissection more treacherous.

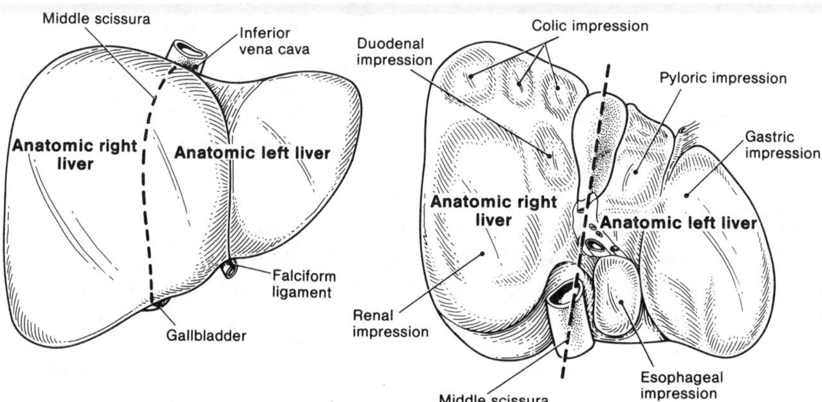

FIG 1.
Diaphragmatic *(left)* and visceral *(right)* surfaces of the liver. *Dashed line* separates anatomic right from anatomic left liver.

External Attachments of the Liver

The liver is suspended within the body from the falciform ligament and triangular ligaments. Both of these structures can be completely dissected off of the liver without any noticeable compromise of its function. The falciform ligament is important in fetal life because it contains the venous drainage from placenta to fetus. What is referred to as the round ligament in adults is the umbilical vein in the fetus. Clinically, the umbilical vein has been used to deliver cytotoxic drugs into the portal system after it has been recannulated. It is seldom open in adult life, but is accomplished by several sizable veins that flow from the liver into the epigastric fat pad and omentum. The falciform ligament marks the course of the left paramedian portal pedicle that separates liver segments 4b and 3. This is a unique anatomic feature of the falciform ligament; all other liver segments are separated by hepatic veins.

Vascular Connections of the Liver

The portal vein receives blood from the small intestine and right colon through the superior mesenteric vein. Blood from the spleen drains through the splenic vein and connects beneath the head of the pancreas with the superior mesenteric vein. Entering the splenic vein at right angles is the inferior mesenteric vein, which drains the left colon and upper rectum (Fig 2). The portal vein receives blood from the colon, superior mesenteric and inferior mesenteric arteries after they go through the intestinal capillary network.

The arterial blood supply to the liver is quite variable.[1] Figure 3 shows the anatomic variations that have been described. There is consistently arterial blood supply to the right and the left lobes of the liver. Generally, there is a single left and a single right artery. It is the origins of these vessels that are so variable. Occasionally, however, three hepatic arteries will exist; in this situation there are usually two arteries to the right lobe. There are three main sources for the right and left hepatic arteries. These are the hepatic artery, the left gastric artery, and the superior mesenteric artery.

The hepatic veins are three in number and are barely visible between liver parenchyma and the vena cava. It is usually poor surgical practice to attempt to dissect these veins free within the suprahepatic space. The veins are completely accessible from within the hepatic parenchyma and this is their proper surgical approach.

There are few or no lymphatic vessels going to the liver but, there is a rich lymphatic drainage from the liver (Fig 4). Minor lymphatic drainage is along the falciform ligament to the para-aortic and paraesophageal lymph nodes. It follows the phrenic lymphatics from the capsular surface of the liver. The majority of the lymphatic drainage from the liver parenchyma is

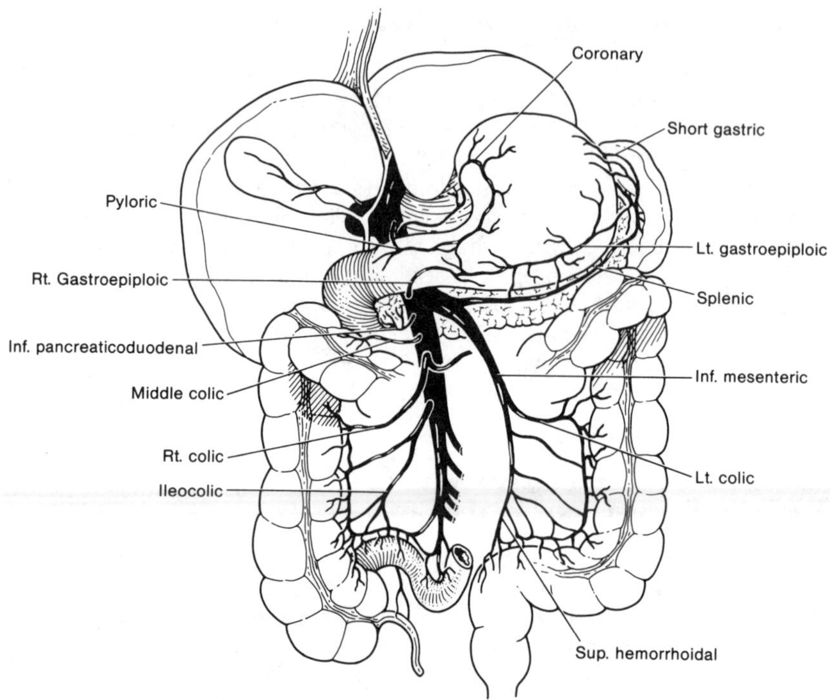

FIG 2.
Splanchnic veins.

retrograde along the porta hepatis into the hepatic celiac and superior mesenteric lymph nodes. From here the drainage is upward into the thoracic duct.[2]

Minor parabiliary veins and arteries exist. The parabiliary veins may become extremely important in providing venous drainage of the viscera if portal vein thrombosis or obstruction occurs. The arterial parabiliary plexus arises from the hepatic and cystic arteries. Other anastomoses are with the superior pancreaticoduodenal arteries. This parabiliary arterial plexus has several important clinical implications. Because of it liver dearterialization is only possible for a very brief time. Also, the plexus accompanies the bile ducts within the liver. The arterial parabiliary arch may cause bothersome bleeding while one is dissecting the structures of the porta hepatis. Disruption may result in necrosis or stenosis of a segment of the biliary tree.

The nerve supply to the liver is poorly understood and the function has not been well described. Apparently there are sensory nerve fibers within Glisson's capsule for pain is experienced upon penetration of the liver by liver biopsy. Also, stretching of Glisson's capsule produces discomfort, as with acute vascular congestion of the liver or an expanding intrahepatic

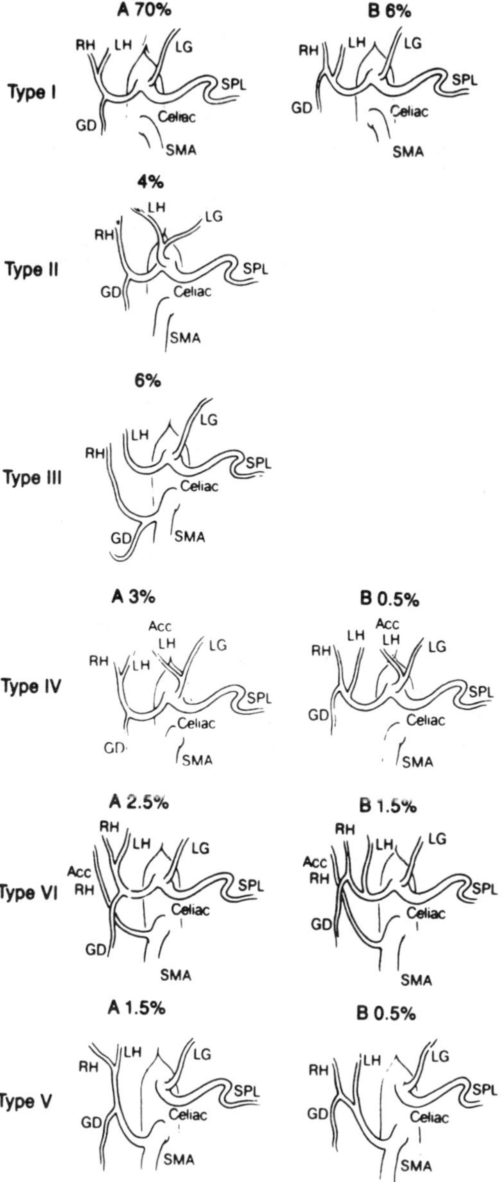

Other 6%

FIG 3.
Arterial blood supply to the liver. (From Daly JM, Kemeny N, Oderman P, et al: Long-term hepatic arterial infusion. *Arch Surg* 1984; 119:936–941. Used by permission.)

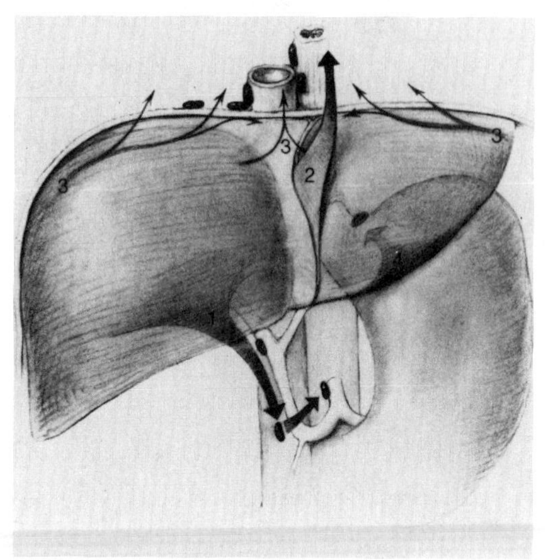

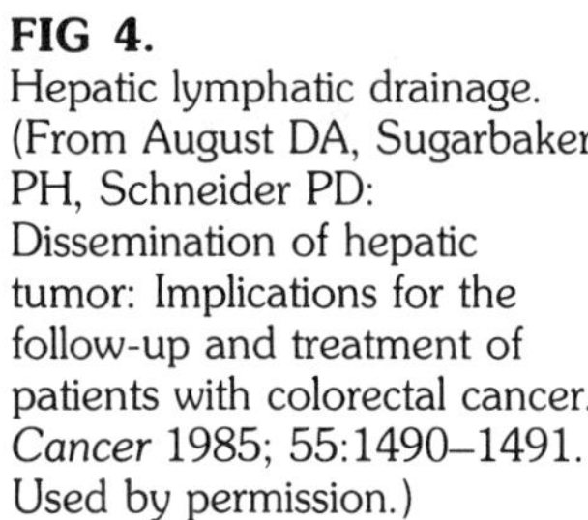

FIG 4.
Hepatic lymphatic drainage. (From August DA, Sugarbaker PH, Schneider PD: Dissemination of hepatic tumor: Implications for the follow-up and treatment of patients with colorectal cancer. *Cancer* 1985; 55:1490–1491. Used by permission.)

tumor mass. Large tumor masses or an abscess within the liver parenchyma will usually not cause any local symptoms. For the most part liver pain is recognized as irritation of adjacent sensory nerve supply to the parietal peritoneum or undersurface of the hemidiaphragm. Irritation of the diaphragm at its periphery is detected at that particular site, whereas irritation of nerve fibers over the major portion of the undersurface of the diaphragm is referred to the shoulder.

The spatial relationships of structures in the porta hepatis are quite consistent. Figure 5 shows the most common anatomic configuration. The common bile duct is the most superficial of the structures within the portal triad and is the first one to be damaged if surgical misadventures occur in the dissection of this area. This anterior location of the hepatic ducts above the artery and portal veins persists within the liver.

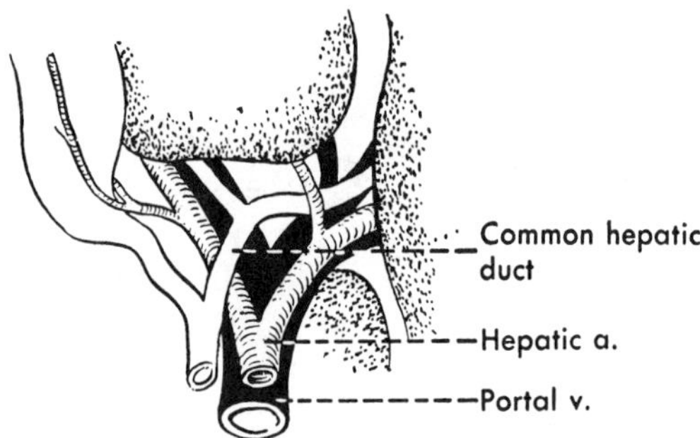

FIG 5.
Relationships of ducts, arteries, and veins within the parahepatis. (From Hollinshead WH: Anatomy for surgeons, in *The Thorax, Abdomen and Pelvis*. New York, Harper & Row, 1971, vol 2, p 319. Used by permission.)

Internal Anatomy of the Liver

The anatomy of the liver within its parenchyma is considerably more complex than in most other organs. There is an extensive and complex vascular and duct system that is obscured by the large amount of hepatic parenchyma. Understanding intrahepatic anatomy is further complicated because there is a dual segmentation. This dual division of intrahepatic structures is comprised of two different vascular trees. There is a division of the liver parenchyma by portal venous segmentation and another division of the parenchyma by the hepatic venous segmentation. Taken together these two systems define the segmental anatomy of the liver.

Division of the Liver Through Portal Venous Segmentation

The hepatic ducts, hepatic arteries, and portal veins all run closely together within the liver parenchyma as part of the liver triad. Additional structures that should be mentioned as a consistent part of the triad are the numerous and large lymphatic vessels. Figure 6 shows the branches of the portal vein, hepatic artery, and intrahepatic bile ducts.[4]

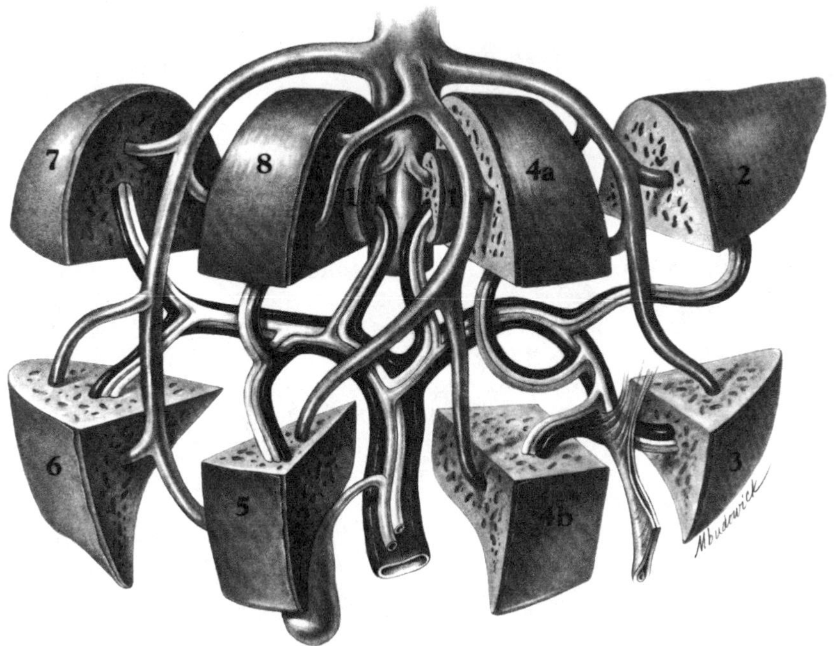

FIG 6.
Segmental hepatic anatomy. (Modified from Bismuth H: Surgical anatomy and anatomical surgery of the liver. *World J Surg* 1982; 6:3–9.)

The portal segmentation is vertically defined by scissurae, which exist between the major branches of the portal vein. The main portal scissura (Cantlie's line) is defined by an imaginary line that runs from the middle of the vena cava to the middle of the gall bladder forsa. The middle hepatic vein exists within the plane beneath this line. The line is 20° right of a sagittal plane through the middle of the vena cava.[5]

A second scissura important to an understanding liver anatomy is the right portal scissura. It is parallel to the main scissura and courses between the two major branches of the right portal vein. The right portal scissura separates segments 5 and 8 from 6 and 7. This scissura is not evident on the surface of the human liver but is clearly evident on the surface of dog and pig livers. The right hepatic vein lies within the liver below the right portal scissura.

The left portal scissura lies beneath the falciform ligament extending from the origin of the left hepatic vein midway across the dome of the left lobe of the liver. The left hepatic vein lies within the liver beneath this line. The left hepatic vein courses at an angle of 90° toward the left. The scissura continues as the falciform ligament, which contains the left paramedian portal triad. This is the only place in the liver where the portal triad vertically separates liver segments.

Portal Segmentation of the Anatomic Left Liver

As the portal vein divides just external to the liver parenchyma it divides into two branches. The division between the right and left portal vein can usually just be visualized at the visceral surface of the hepatic parenchyma. The left portal pedicle is long, measuring approximately 3 cm in length. This makes an anatomic left liver resection easier because one has a distance of approximately 3 cm, any point at which the portal vein can be divided from within the liver. The left portal pedicle divides into two branches. The left lateral portal pedicle is the branch to segment 2 (see Fig 6). The left paramedian pedicle provides the blood supply to segments 3 and 4. Medial branches off this vein supply segment 4. Usually there are two prominent branches so that segment 4 is surgically divided into 4 posteriorly (4a) and 4 anteriorly (4b). This left paramedian vein is in fetal life the main constituent of the umbilical vein and it is located just deep to the falciform ligament within the umbilical sulcus.

The quadrate lobe is that portion of the liver to the left side of the gallbladder up to the falciform ligament. The width of the quadrate lobe measures the length of the left portal pedicle. When the lobe is rectangular the pedicle is long; when the quadrate lobe is diminished the left pedicle is short.

The Anatomic Right Liver

The right portal pedicle is generally much shorter than the left portal pedicle. The right portal pedicle divides almost immediately off the main portal vein into a right paramedian pedicle and a right lateral pedicle (see Fig 6). The right paramedian pedicle courses anteriorly and then arches posteriorly. Anteriorly it gives rise to the portal branches to segment 5 and posteriorly gives rise to branches to segment 8.

The right lateral pedicle continues in the direction of the right portal pedicle and in a plane parallel the under surface of the liver. It has two branches: one anteriorly to supply segment 6 and another posteriorly to supply segment 7.

The Caudate Lobe

The caudate lobe is supplied with portal blood by several small veins originating from the posterior surface of the right or left portal pedicles. The position of the caudad lobe is variable as to whether its blood supply is primarily from the left portal pedicle, the right portal pedicle, or both (Fig 7). This variation in location of the caudate lobe can cause a major resection to be relatively simple or more difficult. If it overloads to the right side and one is performing a right lobectomy, one must transect the caudate lobe and of course the same on the left. The caudate lobe is separated from the anatomic right and left liver by the right and left dorsa portal fissures.

Segmentation of the Liver by the Hepatic Veins

The hepatic venous anatomy is considerably simpler than the portal segmentation. There are three hepatic veins. They lie above the portal structures within liver parenchyma. In dissecting through the liver, the major veins are equidistant between the diaphragmatic surface and the major portal structures. The left vein drains the smaller anatomic left liver and the large right hepatic vein drains the anatomic right liver. The middle hepatic vein lies directly beneath the main portal scissura and drains both anatomic right and left livers. In an anatomic right liver resection one stays just to the right of the middle hepatic vein. In an extended right liver resection one stays to the left of the middle hepatic vein.

The left hepatic vein may join the middle hepatic vein to form a single

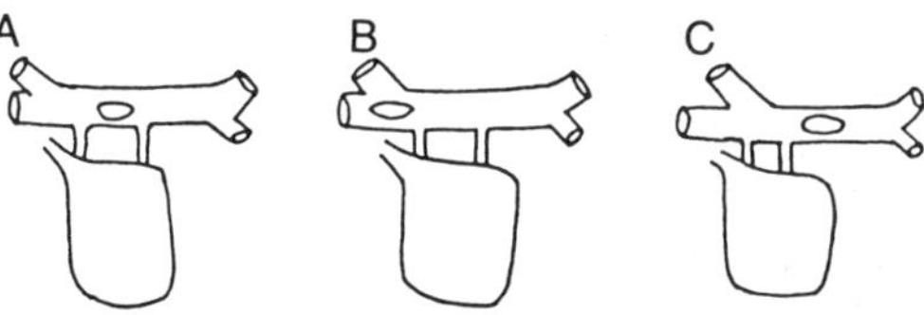

FIG 7.
Variable blood supply of the caudate lobe. **A,** belongs to anatomic right and left livers; **B,** only to the left liver; **C,** only to the right liver, controlled hepatectomies, and exposure of the intrahepatic bile ducts. (Modified from Couinaud: *Anatomical and Technical Study*. Paris, France, 1981. Used by permission.)

vessel that enters immediately the inferior vena cava. It may receive the left inferior phrenic vein. A frequent bothersome bleeding problem during dissection around the left hepatic veins is bleeding from inadvertent injury to the left phrenic vein as it enters the left hepatic vein.

The right hepatic vein is the largest vessel of the three. It has three branches: the superior, middle, and inferior branches. The right hepatic vein follows the right portal scissura over most of its course. It gives off the right inferior veins to the lower portion of the right lobe of the liver.

The caudate veins drain directly from the caudate lobe into the anterior face of the retrohepatic vena cava. They number between one and five major veins. They present a particular hazard in performing a major liver resection unless they are ligated and then divided in continuity, prior to any attempt at a parenchymal resection. If these veins are pulled out of the vena cava, severe hemorrhage can result.

Diagnosis of Hepatic Tumors

Liver as a Common Site for Cancer Spread

Because of its large size and its protected position beneath the right side of the rib cage, the liver is not readily examined by routine methods for physical diagnosis. Yet because of its rich blood supply and direct access of hematogenously disseminated tumor cells from the GI tract, the liver is a common site for the spread of cancer. According to Pickren et al., approximately 50% of patients with large-bowel cancer will eventually develop liver metastases.[6] The same is true for gastric cancer. Patients with pancreas cancer will show liver metastases at some time in their course in approximately 75% of patients. Also, endocrine tumors such as gastrinoma, insulinoma, or carcinoid frequently metastasize to the liver.

Diagnosis From Medical History

Even large tumors within the liver parenchyma often cause no symptoms.[7] The liver itself, including the intrahepatic bile ducts, does not contain a well-developed sensory nerve supply. Glisson's capsule does contain somatic sensory fibers, and penetration of the capsule by a needle or its acute distention caused by liver swelling will result in pain or discomfort. Often, a mass lesion in the liver causes pain by irritation of the undersurface of the hemidiaphragm. Tumors that rub against the central portion of the diaphragm will cause pain in the shoulders. This is referred pain caused by irritation of phrenic nerve fibers. Irritation of the periphery of the diaphragm causes stimulation of the intercostal nerve and that pain is detected at the site of irritation (Fig 8).

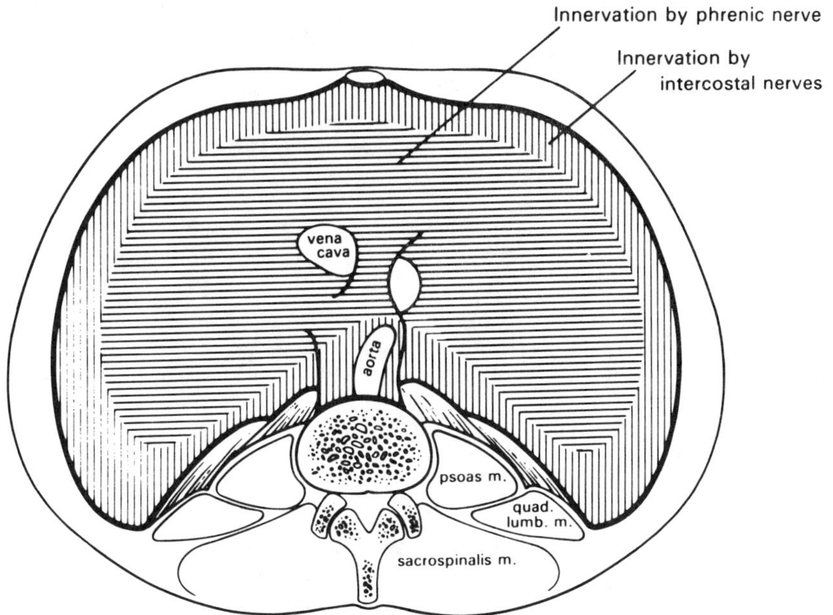

FIG 8.
Sites of pain reported from metastases on the diaphragmatic surface of the liver. Irritation of the periphery is detected by somatic sensory fibers and is felt at the tumor site. Irritation of the large central portion of the right or left hemidiaphragm is felt in the shoulders. (From Sugarbaker PH, Reinig JW, Hughes KS: Diagnosis of hepatic metastases, in Rosenberg SA (ed): *Surgical Treatment of Metastatic Disease*. Philadelphia, JB Lippincott Co., 1987. Used by permission.)

Physical Examination

Physical examination of the liver is difficult, often impossible. Only in asthenic individuals can a small portion of the left lobe of the liver be directly palpated in the normal individual. For liver nodules to be detected by physical examination they generally must be very large. Often, a large tumor mass may displace the liver caudally and result in an unusually large but normally textured organ.

Laboratory Test

The liver function tests frequently used to detect metabolic liver dysfunction are usually not helpful in the diagnosis of hepatic metastases. An exception to this is the CEA assay. Approximately 90% of the patients who have hepatic metastases from colorectal cancer will have an elevated carcinoembryonic antigen assay.[8] Other tests such as the lactic dehydrogenase (LDH) and alkaline phosphatase may be used to screen patients preoperatively for liver abnormalities.[9] However, the truism, "negative means nothing," must be used in interpreting these tests. Often times, before the liver function test results become abnormal, metastases are evident by physical examination and the clinical value of the laboratory test is minimal.

Radiological Examination of the Liver

Determination of the presence or absence of hepatic metastases in patients with cancer is of great importance in making decisions about the disease. For this reason many different radiologic tests have been developed and their utility tested in clinical studies. Smith and colleagues determined that the liver spleen scan, the liver ultrasound, and the liver computed tomographic (CT) scan (scans performed without the use of contrast materials) were equally accurate in detecting hepatic mass lesions.[10] The size threshold for tumor identification was approximately 3 cm for all three tests. All three of these routine radiologic studies were considered equivalent for the radiologic study of hepatic metastases.

For resection of hepatic metastases, accurate descriptions of the number and location of the lesions are of great importance in selecting patients for resection. The CT scan has been utilized with several contrast agents to provide a large amount of additional information. In CT portography, a bolus of soluble contrast is rapidly injected into the superior mesenteric artery while the CT is being performed.[11] Because the liver parenchyma is more richly vascularized by portal blood than are tumor nodules, the parenchyma is highlighted and the tumor nodules appear as filling defects. Tumor nodules as small as 1-cm diameter are routinely detected. Also, the portal vein and its branches are distinctly seen and the relationship of tumor masses to the portal structures can be readily determined. An example of CT portography in a patient with hepatic metastases is shown in Figure 9.

Bernardino and colleagues have explored the use of the delayed CT scan in patients with hepatic metastases. If one waits four to six hours after the intravascular administration of soluble contrast material, approximately 10% of the dye is excreted in the bile.[12] This makes the liver parenchyma more dense than tumor tissue and more dense than the portal veins and hepatic veins. An example of a delayed CT scan is shown in Figure 10. This simple examination is extremely accurate in detecting small lesions not seen by other radiologic tests within the liver. It shows the relationship of tumor masses to the hepatic vessels and provides a general assessment of hepatocyte function. Cirrhotic livers will not image by delayed CT.

Magnetic resonance imaging (MRI) is emerging as a prominent new radiologic test by which to study the liver. Both the T1 and T2 effects have been studied. The experience of Reinig and colleagues suggests that MRI

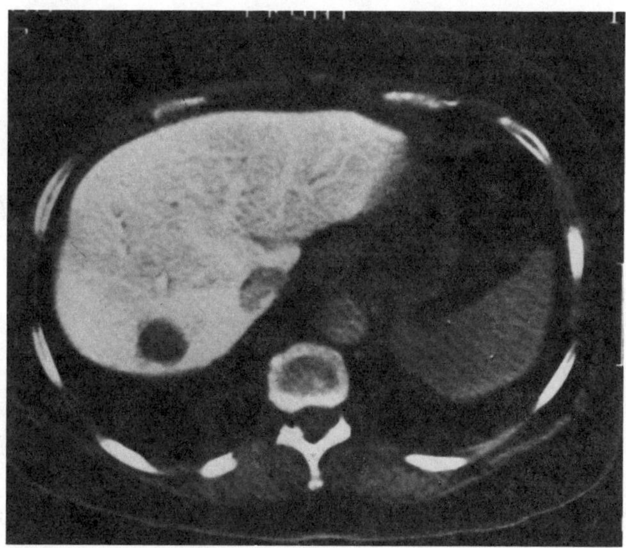

FIG 9.
Computed tomography (CT) for the precise definition of liver metastases. A bolus of soluble contrast is infused through the superior mesenteric artery while the liver CT is performed. The portal structures and liver parenchyma are highlighted. Metastases that obtain their major blood supply from the hepatic artery show clearly as filling defects. The relationships of the tumor to portal vein and its branches are revealed.

is as accurate as CT or delayed CT in the detection of hepatic lesions.[13] Unfortunately, MRI does not give as much information about the remainder of the abdominal cavity as does the CT scan. It does enable accurate detection of small lesions within the liver down to 1 cm in diameter. These are lesions that may be missed by surgical palpations of the liver. As MRI increases in its availability and as the radiologist learns more about its proper use, it may emerge as an important tool for the preoperative assessment of metastatic cancer in the liver.

Hypervascular liver metastases from endocrine tumors, hepatocellular carcinoma, and some metastases from GI cancer can be visualized well with arteriography. A majority of metastatic lesions, however, are not well shown. Arteriography is often valuable in differentiating benign lesions such as hemangioma from metastases. Computed tomographic scans following contrast infusion or the T2-weighted spin-echo MRI can also help in this differentiation. The major role of arteriography in hepatic tumors is not in diagnosis but in therapy planning. Preoperative delineation of the hepatic arterial anatomy is helpful in defining the structures to be ligated within the portahepatis prior to performing a major liver resection.

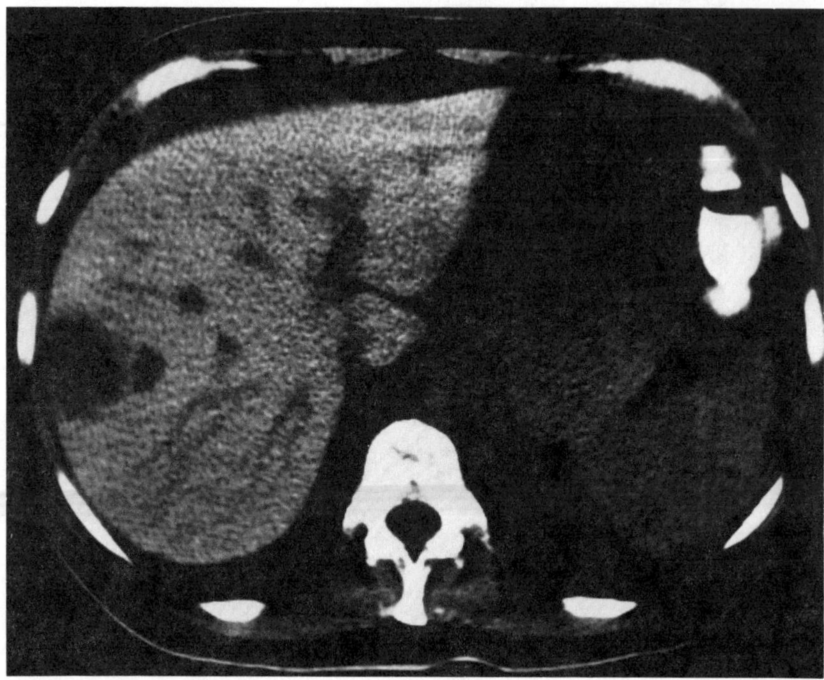

FIG 10.
Delayed computed tomogram for precise definition of liver metastases. If 50 gm of iodine are infused intravascularly, sufficient contrast material will accumulate in the bile to increase the density of liver parenchyma four to six hours later. The iodine will then function as a liver contrast agent.

Intrahepatic Examination of the Liver

Surgical palpation of the liver is still the most accurate way to detect hepatic lesions. Minute surface lesions not currently detectable by any radiologic test are readily found and their benign or malignant nature determined by biopsy. Lesions of 1 to 2 cm within the liver parenchyma can be detected accurately in the left liver. However, the thick right liver can hide lesions that cannot be palpable but that may be up to 2 cm in diameter. The sensitivity (true positive percentage) of direct surgical examination is approximately 95%.[6, 14–17] For this reason accurate hepatic imaging prior to surgical removal of hepatic metastases is essential.

Recently, intraoperative ultrasonography has become available for endocrine tumors and hepatomas. The utility of this examination has been demonstrated for bile duct stones, for primary hepatic malignancy, and for endocrine metastases to the liver.[18, 19] Currently, studies are underway to determine the accuracy of intraoperative ultrasonography for hepatic metastases from colorectal or other gastrointestinal primary tumors.

At present, the major role of intraoperative ultrasonography comes from the ability to define the segmental anatomy of the liver. With this tool the precise anatomic location of a metastases within one or more of the eight anatomic liver segments can be determined and the entire segment removed with more precision.[20]

Selection of Patients for Hepatic Resection

Studies from the Mayo Clinic by Wagner and colleagues show that the only currently available curative treatment for metastatic solid tumors to the liver is hepatic resection (Fig 11).[21] Surgical removal of hepatic metastases has produced a 20 to 40% five-year survival following removal of large-bowel cancer metastases and should be accepted as a standard therapy for selected patients (Fig 12).[30] Occasionally, long-term survivors have

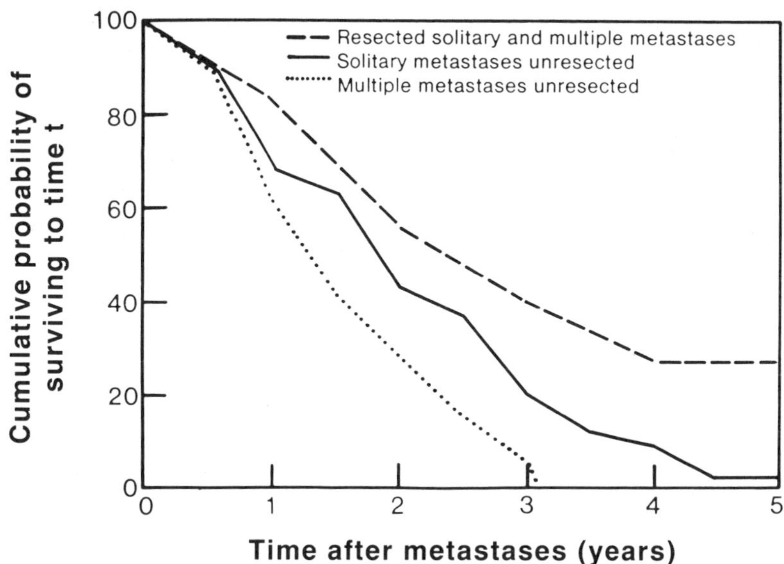

FIG 11.
Comparison of survival of resected and unresected hepatic metastases from colon cancer. *Top survival curve* shows the results over five years for 116 patients with solitary and multiple hepatic metastases that underwent potentially curative hepatic resections. *Lower curves* show solitary and multiple hepatic metastases without extrahepatic disease that were not resected. (Modified from Wagner JS, Adson MA, Van Heerden JA, et al: The natural history of hepatic metastases from colorectal cancer. *Ann Surg* 1984; 147:502–508.)

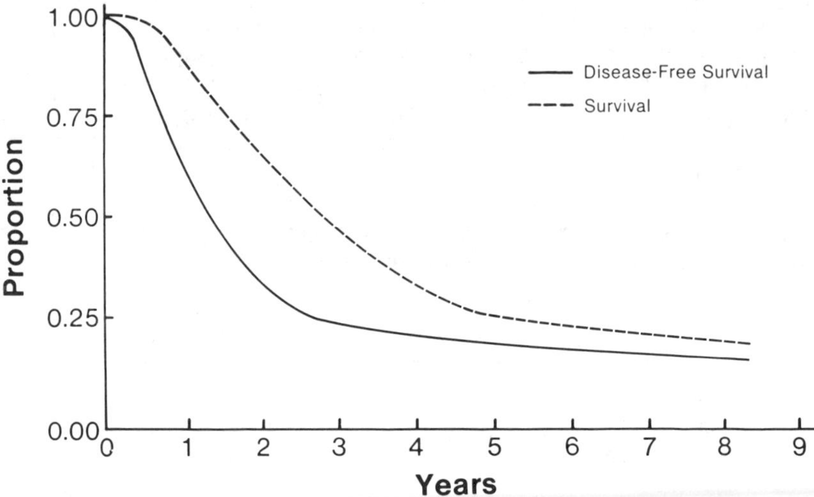

FIG 12.
Disease-free survival and survival of patients who had a liver resection for colorectal metastases. Approximately one fourth of patients are cured of their metastatic disease by surgery (Hepatic Metastases Registry data).

been reported following hepatic resection for metastatic Wilm's tumor, melanoma, leiomyosarcoma, pancreatic cancer, gastric cancer, renal cell cancer, and adrenal carcinoma. In addition, resection of metastatic endocrine tumors from the liver occasionally leads to a marked palliation and, occasionally, cure. This is particularly true with carcinoid tumors. Although the morbidity and mortality for hepatic resection are low, an operation of this magnitude should not be undertaken lightly. The clinical features by which the surgeon selects patients for resection have been studied by many groups.[1, 21–47] Our discussion will focus on the data provided by the Hepatic Metastases Registry.[21]

Numbers of Hepatic Metastases

In the past, most surgeons recommended that resection be performed only in patients with solitary metastases. Others suggested that more than one lesion might be removed in a good-risk patient if lesions were confined to a single lobe of the liver. The data from the Hepatic Metastases Registry do not support this concept. Patients with one metastasis removed have essentially the same prognosis statistically as patients with two or three metastases. Those with over three metastases have only a slightly worse progress. From this data it is impossible to exclude patients from a curative resection based on number of metastases (Fig 13). The author has one patient with six metastases removed on two occasions who is a seven-year

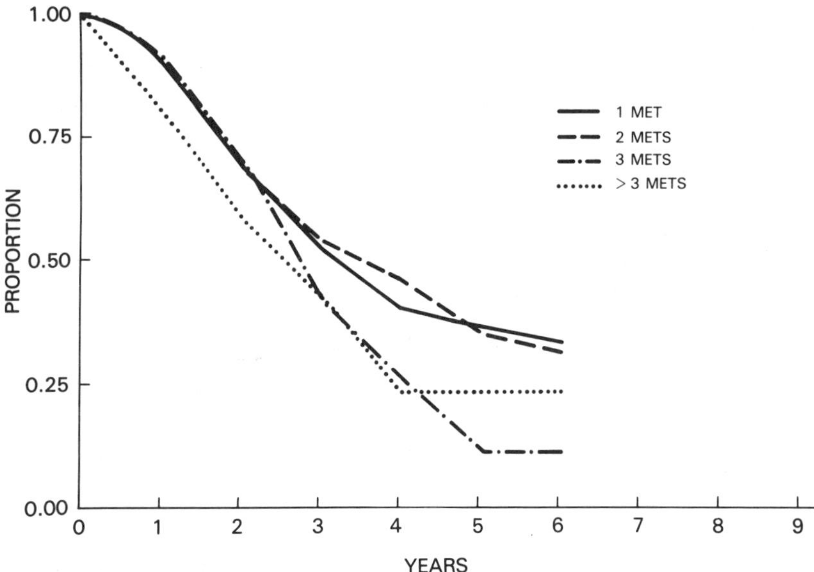

FIG 13.
Prognosis as determined by number of hepatic metastases resected. (From Hughes KS, Sugarbaker PH: Treatment of hepatic metastases, in Rosenberg SA (ed): *Surgical Treatment of Metastatic Disease.* Philadelphia, JB Lippincott Co, 1987. Used by permission.)

survivor. Current practice may be to recommend resection of four or fewer metastases in patients with metastatic colorectal cancer.

Location of Tumor Nodules as a Prognostic Variable

In the registry data, when only patients with more than one metastasis were examined, those with metastases on one side of the liver had the same five-year survival and disease-free survival rates as patients with metastases in both the right and left livers. The distribution of metastases within the liver may have profound implications for the surgical techniques involved in liver resection but does not in itself have an effect on the prognosis (Fig 14).

Stage of the Primary Tumor

The strongest prognostic variable in patients with gastointestinal malignancy is the status of the lymph nodes. Patients with positive lymph nodes have approximately a 30% five-year survival, whereas those with negative lymph nodes have a 60% five-year survival. A similar phenomenon occurs in patients with hepatic metastases. As shown in Figure 15, Dukes' stage

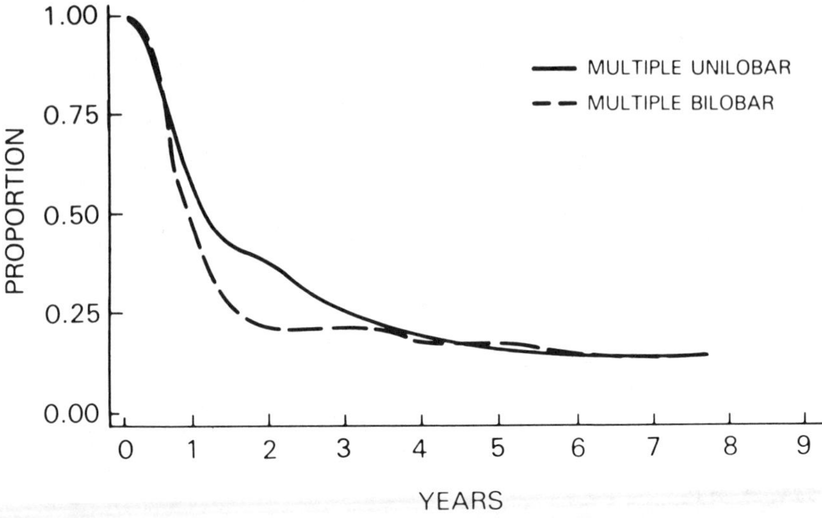

FIG 14.
Prognosis as determined by distribution of metastases within the liver, multiple metastases on one side of the liver as compared to lesions on both right and left sides of the liver. (From Hughes KS, Sugarbaker PH: Treatment of hepatic metastases, in Rosenberg SA (ed): *Surgical Treatment of Metastatic Disease.* Philadelphia, JB Lippincott Co, 1987. Used by permission.)

B patients with potentially curative colon resections and hepatic metastases have a 40% five-year survival, whereas those who had a Dukes' stage C primary tumor have a 20% five-year survival. Apparently, in patients with hepatic metastases, the status of the lymph nodes makes a strong statement about the biologic character of the malignant process. If hepatic metastases can be surgically removed, recurrence in the liver is not frequent and the likelihood of disease recurrence elsewhere (estimated by Dukes' stage) determines the prognosis. Lymph node invasion signifies a tumor biology likely to result in distant disease spread by that tumor.

It should be noted, however, that patients with Dukes' C adenocarcinoma of the large bowel with hepatic metastases have approximately 20% five-year survival. Therefore, because a patient had Dukes' C primary lesion does not in any way mean that hepatic resection should not be performed.

Pathologic Margin of the Resected Specimen

In the hepatic metastases registry data, the patient who had a margin greater than 1 cm had an improved survival (Fig 16). If patients had a margin less than 1 cm in diameter or a positive margin on resection, there

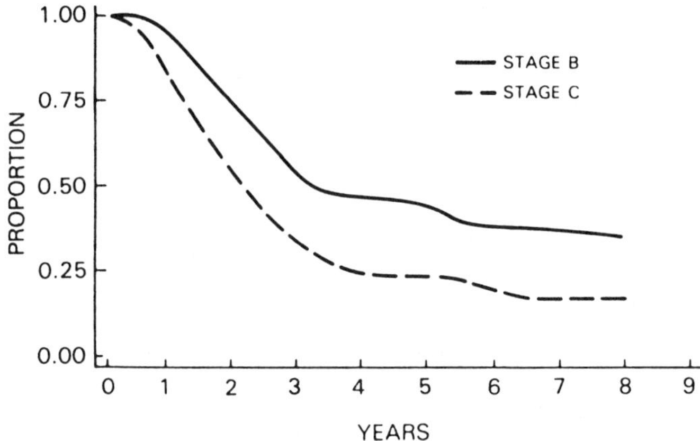

FIG 15.
Prognosis as determined by Dukes' classification. (From Hughes KS, Sugarbaker PH: Treatment of hepatic metastases, in Rosenberg SA (ed): *Surgical Treatment of Metastatic Disease*. Philadelphia, JB Lippincott Co, 1987. Used by permission.)

was a reduced five-year survival. However, even in those patients with narrow or positive margins long-term survival is seen.

Preoperative CEA Level

Patients with a preresection CEA level of less than 5 mg/ml do better than patients with an elevated CEA (40% survival vs. 25%). Patients should not be denied a resection because the CEA is high but an elevated CEA is a poor prognostic indicator.

Disease-Free Interval

The length of time between colon resection and hepatic resection does have an impact on prognosis. If patients had a disease-free interval of less than one month there was a 17% five-year survival, a disease-free interval of one month to a year gave 22% five-year survival, and if that interval was greater than a year there was a 26% disease-free survival. This statistic probably reflects the rate of progression of the primary tumor but also may indicate that tumors that grow faster are more likely to disseminate widely from liver to systemic sites.

Presence of Extrahepatic Metastases

Patients with extrahepatic metastases that were removed along with the disease in the liver had no significant difference in survival from patients with only hepatic metastasis, but there was a trend toward reduced sur-

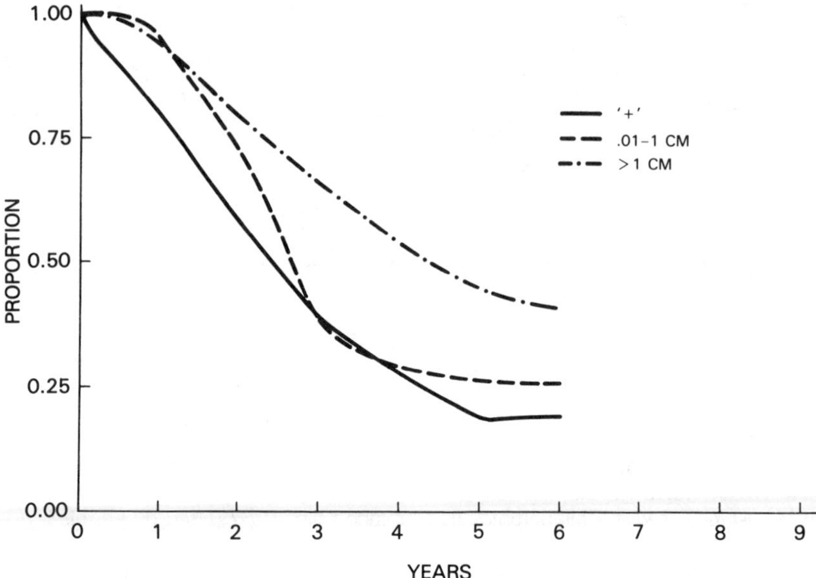

FIG 16.
Prognosis as determined by pathologic margin of resected specimen. (From Hughes KS, Sugarbaker PH: *Treatment of Hepatic Metastases,* in Rosenberg SA (ed): *Surgical Treatment of Metastatic Disease,* Philadelphia, JB Lippincott Co, 1987. Used by permission.)

vival. Data reviewed by Wagner at the Mayo Clinic showed reduced survival when extrahepatic disease was resected.[22] This group included patients with lung metastases resected simultaneously, patients with anastomotic recurrence resected simultaneously, and patients with peritoneal implants resected simultaneously. It does not include patients who had contiguous involvement of adjacent structures such as invasion into the diaphragm. From these data it seems reasonable to suggest that some good-risk patients who can be made clinically disease-free by hepatic surgery plus a resection of tumor at another site should undergo this potentially curative surgery.

In the registry data, one site of spread that did seem to abrogate the beneficial effects of hepatic resection was disease in the hepatic lymph nodes. August and co-workers identified the hepatic lymph nodes as a site for metastatic spread of liver secondaries. If the tumor biology is such that metastases from the liver to the local lymph nodes occur, the chances for gaining control through liver resection must be extremely small. We have adopted this clinical factor as an absolute contraindication to hepatic resection.

Clinical Features That Lack Prognostic Significance

Age, size of solitary lesions, type of resection (metastasectomy vs. major resection), and distribution of metastases are of little or no prognostic value. One prognostic feature related to size may be of some interest to surgeons. In an analysis of the Registry data the patients with large hepatic metastases greater than 4 cm in diameter survived less frequently with a metastasectomy than with an anatomic right or left resection. It may be that incomplete removal of a liver segment containing metastatic disease leaves that portion of the liver at greater risk for local recurrence. Alternatively, removal of large lesions with minimal margins may predispose to traumatic dissemination of cancer at the time of surgery. Also, large lesions resected by metastasectomy may, of necessity, have a less adequate free margin.

Contraindications to Hepatic Resection

Certainly, clinical criteria for selection of patients for hepatic resection have been greatly expanded (Table 1). Few people who can be made clinically disease-free should be denied the potential benefits of this surgical procedure. Only if one sees the mortality of the resection as 20% or more should the physical status of the patient be considered a contraindication. Another absolute contraindication to surgery is the presence of disease either within the liver or at another site that cannot be removed with curative intent. Multiple pulmonary metastases, peritoneal seeding, or retroperitoneal lymph node involvement should be considered absolute contraindications. However, a few foci of resectable disease in the lungs, or isolated recurrence within the abdomen, especially at the anastomotic site, should not be considered contraindications to hepatic resection of metastatic disease. Metastatic disease within the hepatic lymph nodes should be considered an absolute contraindication to hepatic resection, even though these nodes could be removed to make the patient clinically disease-free (Table 2).

Reresection of Hepatic Metastases

Approximately one third of the patients who fail hepatic resection will be found to have the cancer recurrence only in the liver.[49] In these patients careful diagnostic studies for metastatic disease should be undertaken. If no other sites of disease recurrence are found and if the liver tumor can be removed, this should be done. The experience with reresection of hepatic metastases has been summarized by Sugarbaker and colleagues.[50] He collected data on 10 patients who had undergone a second hepatic resection with curative intent. Those patients seem to represent a select group who did very well with a second liver resection. Nine of these 10 patients are free of disease with a minimum of 2-year followup.

TABLE 1.
Prognostic Features as Defined by the Hepatic Metastases Registry for Patients Undergoing Resection of Hepatic Metastases in the Absence of Extrahepatic Disease*

Prognostic Factor	Survival†	Disease-Free Survival‡
No. of metastases		
1	37%	25%
2	37%	25%
3	7%	0%
≥4	23%	7%
Multiple (not specified)	18%	15%
Pathologic margin on liver specimen:		
0	19%	13%
>0 but <1 cm	25%	15%
>1 cm	47%	33%
Distribution of multiple metastases		
Unilobar	30%	16%
Bilobar	20%	13%
Stage of the primary tumor		
Dukes' B (neg, mesenteric nodes)	47%	28%
Dukes' C (pos, mesenteric nodes)	23%	18%
Disease-free interval		
<1 mo	27%	17%
1 mo to 1 yr	31%	22%
>1 yr	42%	26%
Age		
<40 yr	37%	27%
40–70 yr	33%	21%
>70 yr	31%	18%
CEA level prior to liver resection		
0–5 ng/ml	47%	42%
>5 and <30	30%	19%
>30	28%	14%
Size of solitary lesions		
<8 cm	38%	27%
>8 cm	27%	21%
Size of largest lesion in multiple metastases		
<2 cm	27%	18%
2–4 cm	17%	10%
4–8 cm	27%	18%
>8 cm	37%	18%

Type of resection of solitary lesion		
Wedge	35%	21%
Anatomic	41%	29%
Type of resection and size of solitary lesions		
Anatomic, met <4 cm	45%	28%
Wedge, met <4 cm	37%	25%
Anatomic, met >4 cm	35%	25%
Wedge, met >4 cm	20%	12.5%

*From Hughes KS, Sugarbaker PH: Treatment of hepatic metastases, in Rosenberg SA (ed): *Surgical Treatment of Metastatic Disease*. Philadelphia, JB Lippincott Co, 1987. Used by permission.
†Five-year actuarial survival.
‡Five-year actuarial disease-free survival.

Patterns of Recurrence

Steele and co-workers suggested that patients who fail the surgical treatment of hepatic metastases usually do so because of disease at other anatomic sites.[51] More often than not, the liver remains free of metastatic disease through simple surgical removal of cancer.[52] Figure 17 shows the data from the Hepatic Metastases Registry regarding patterns of failure.[49] When one considers only the first site of recurrence, roughly one third of the patients recurred in the liver only, one third recurred at other distant sites including the lungs, and one third remained disease-free. Figure 18 shows not only the sites of recurrence seen initially but also those with prolonged follow-up. Note that the number of combined recurrences is markedly increased. Recurrences isolated to the liver only are infrequently

TABLE 2.
Contraindications to Hepatic Resection of Colorectal Metastases to the Liver

Operative mortality of 20% or greater
Moderate to severe cirrhosis
More than four hepatic metastases
Unresectable disease at another site
Involvement of hepatic lymph nodes

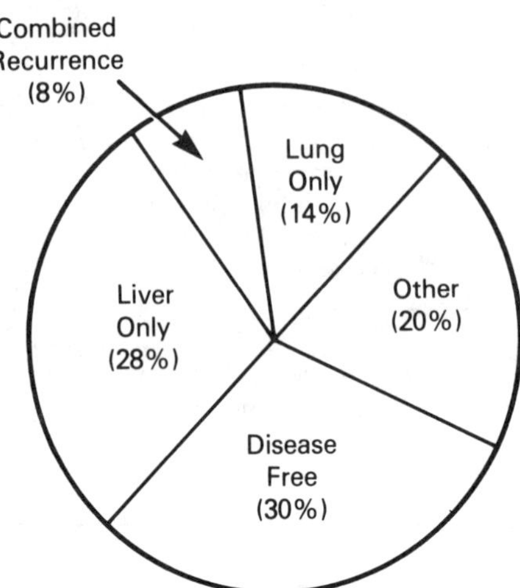

FIG 17.
Initial sites of surgical treatment failure after surgical resection of hepatic metastases. (From Hughes KS, Sugarbaker PH: Treatment of hepatic metastases, in Rosenberg SA (ed): *Surgical Treatment of Metastatic Disease.* Philadelphia, JB Lippincott Co, 1987. Used by permission.)

observed. As suggested by Steele and co-workers, there is a need for effective systemic adjuvant therapy.[51]

Hepatic Resection for Endocrine Tumors

Palliative resection of the liver for symptomatic metastases from endocrine tumors is not uncommon. Hughes selected 54 patients from the literature. He found that alleviation of symptoms was reported in 33 of 36 patients to whom follow-up was available. Palliation lasted up to 78 months in these patients.[48] Foster et al. and Martin et al. suggested that hepatic re-

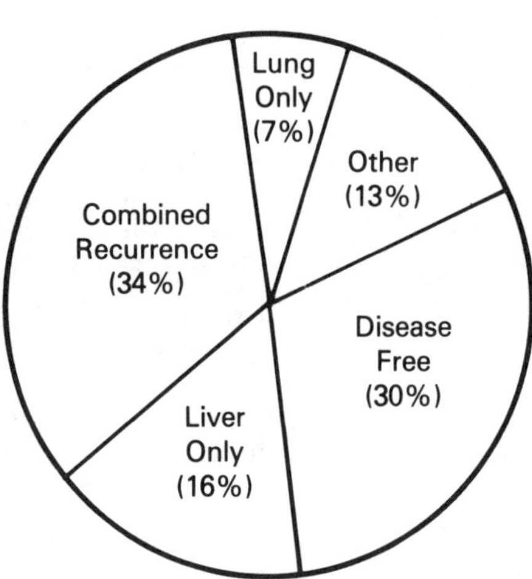

FIG 18.
Initial plus late sites of surgical treatment failure after surgical resection of hepatic metastases. (From Hughes KS, Sugarbaker PH: Treatment of hepatic metastases, in Rosenberg SA (ed): *Surgical Treatment of Metastatic Disease.* Philadelphia, JB Lippincott Co, 1987. Used by permission.)

section to palliate the disabling symptoms of the carcinoid syndrome should be considered if 90% of the functioning tumor can be removed.[32, 53]

Norton and co-workers from the National Cancer Institute have reported a curative approach to the treatment of metastatic gastrinoma.[54] Resection of the primary tumor in the pancreas along with the hepatic spread of the disease may be considered a curative approach in some patients. In others, palliative efforts may be well worth the risks of surgery. The goal of surgery should be to remove all disease possible if a curative approach is not technically feasible.[55]

Noncolorectal, Nonendocrine Metastases

Table 3 presents the literature concerning liver resection for metastatic cancer from noncolorectal, nonendocrine primary sites.[48] Long-term survivors

TABLE 3.
Liver Resection for Metastatic Cancer from Noncolorectal, Nonendocrine Sites*

Cancer Type	Postoperative Survivors	5-Year Survivors	Died of Recurrence After 5 Years
Wilms' tumor	20	6 (14 yr and 17 yr)	?
Renal cell cancer	11	3 (5 yr, 7 yr, and 12 yr)	0
Adrenal carcinoma	4	2 (6 yr and 7 yr)	0
Leiomyosarcoma	16	2 (12 yr)	1
Melanoma	13	1	1
Pancreatic cancer	8	1	1
Stomach cancer	23	0	. . .
Other adult sarcomas	9	0	. . .
Breast cancer	7	0	. . .
Ovarian cancer	5	0	. . .
Uterine and cervical cancer	7	0	. . .
Lung cancer	2	0	. . .
Esophageal cancer	3	1 (13 yr)	. . .
Rhabdomyosarcoma	1	0	. . .
Neuroblastoma	1	0	. . .
Thyroid cancer	1	0	. . .
Choriocarcinoma	1	0	. . .
Periampullary cancer	1	0	. . .

*From Hughes KS, Sugarbaker PH: Treatment of hepatic metastases, in Rosenberg SA (ed): *Surgical Treatment of Metastatic Disease.* Philadelphia, JB Lippincott Co, 1987. Used by permission.

with Wilms' tumor, renal cell cancer, adrenal cancer, leiomyosarcoma, melanoma, and pancreas cancer have been reported. Sheele and co-workers from Erlanger, West Germany, have recently reported long-term survival with hepatic resection in patients with metastatic gastric cancer (personal communication, 1987). Undoubtedly, the more aggressive biologic character of the noncolorectal and nonendocrine tumors will require a more highly selected group of patients for liver resection. The lower biologic grade of the tumor that arises from colonic epithelium and the anatomic nature of the large bowel that provides local disease control as compared with pancreatic or gastric cancer may account for favorable results with surgery for metastatic disease from colorectal cancer.

Surgical Treatment of Hepatic Metastases

The year 1988 will make the 100th year since Garre was reported to have performed the removal of a liver tumor (Table 4). Certainly the modern era of liver surgery has begun. More and more surgeons will be methodi-

TABLE 4.
100 Year Evolution of Techniques for Hepatic Surgery for Metastatic Colorectal Cancer

Date	Author	Country	Comment
1888	Garre[56]	Germany	Metastasectomy
1889	Keen[57]	USA	Left lateral segmentectomy
1908	Pringle[58]	Great Britain	Inflow occlusion
1910	Wendel[59]	Germany	Right lobectomy; partial hilar dissection
1952	Lortat-Jacob & Robert[60]	France	Preliminary hilar ligation for anatomic lobectomy
1953	Healey[61]	USA	Segmental anatomy
1958	Lin[62]	Taiwan	Finger fracture technique
1960	Couinaud[63]	France	Segmental nomenclature and resections
1971	Storm & Longmire[64]	USA	Liver clamp
1975	Starzl[65]	USA	Right trisegmentectomy
1976	Wilson & Adson[31]	USA	Successful resection CRC metastases
1977	Foster & Berman[32]	USA	Liver tumor survey
1979	Hodgson[66]	USA	Ultrasonic dissection
1981	Fortner[67]	USA	Electrocautery
1982	Starzl[68]	USA	Left trisegmentectomy
1986	Hughes[21]	USA	Hepatic metastases registry

cally utilizing the new technology, oncology, and anatomy developed by so many.[1, 21, 31, 32, 56–68]

Pre- and Postoperative Care

Preoperatively, the patient should be carefully evaluated for systemic spread of tumor. This involves CT of the chest, abdomen, and pelvis. Patients with a primary large-bowel cancer should have a barium enema or a colonoscopy to rule out locally recurrent cancer or a second primary large-bowel cancer. Other more complex radiologic studies are done only as suggested by clinical evaluation. The day before surgery the patient should have a mechanical bowel preparation. Vitamin K is given by intramuscular injection. A thorough preoperative scrub of the skin is indicated. Postoperatively fresh frozen plasma is frequently needed to maintain an adequate prothrombin level. Albumin may be needed if edema from hypoproteinemia occurs.

Incisions

The incision is carefully planned to suit the expected procedure. For large tumors, a thorocoabdominal incision may be needed to keep blood loss at a minimum, deal with surgical misadventures should they occur, and keep traumatic tumor manipulation to a minimum. Not infrequently, tumors on the diaphragmatic surface of the right lobe of the liver are adherent to the undersurface of the right hemidiaphragm. If this is so, excision of that portion of the diaphragm must be performed to prevent spillage of tumor cells. For very large, especially left-sided tumors, a midline abdominal incision with a sternal split is occasionally the optimal incision. For most hepatic resections a large right subcostal abdominal incision is adequate. Alternatively, a generous bilateral subcostal incision may be preferable.

Abdominal Exploration

Initially, a small incision is made to explore the abdominal cavity. A complete examination should include a biopsy sampling of hepatic lymph nodes if these nodes are suspicious for malignant disease. The studies of Lefor and colleagues show that approximately one third of the patients who are explored for removal of hepatic metastases, but in whom disseminated disease is uncovered at the time of exploration, have positive hepatic lymph nodes.[69] Another important site of disseminated disease is the peritoneal surfaces. Small nodules of tumor on the serosal surface of the pelvic viscera, beneath the right hemidiaphragm, or within the greater omentum are all that may be found. Approximately one third of the patients denied hepatic resection because of disseminated disease were found to have tumor on peritoneal surfaces. A third common site of disease spread is the large-bowel cancer resection site and this should be carefully palpated. Finally, the liver itself should be carefully inspected. Usually patients with four or fewer metastases that can be completely resected go on to hepatic resection. If all these common sites of extrahepatic disease are negative for tumor spread and if the liver cancer is potentially resectable, then the incision should be enlarged and the resection of liver tissue carefully planned out.

Mobilization of Hepatic Tissue

The first step in the hepatic resection is complete mobilization of the portion of the liver to be removed. This is necessary so that tissue to be dissected can be placed on stretch during parenchymal dissection. Also, this allows the margins of resection to be marked out using electrocautery both above and below the portion of the liver to be removed. One is then able to dissect straight through the liver parenchyma. Finally, if the tumor mass is dissected free of all fascial attachments, it then becomes easier to determine adequate margins of resection. Adequate mobilization for an anatomic right or left resection means complete division of the triangular ligament and the fascial attachments of the liver over the vena cava. In an anatomic right liver resection, care is taken not to traumatize the right adrenal gland. Also, from one to four veins passing from the caudate lobe directly into the liver should be ligated in continuity and then divided. Division of these caudate veins adds a great deal to the mobility of the anatomic right or left liver and facilitates their removal. Moreover, when traction is placed on the portion of the liver to be excised, this traction may tear the vena cava if these caudate veins are not divided prior to parenchyma dissection.

Preliminary Ligation of Hilar Vessels

One must determine if a cholecystectomy should be performed. It is always indicated for an anatomic right or left liver resection and is required for resection of segment 4 or 5. Dissection of the gallbladder should be the first step toward defining the anatomy of the porta hepatis. Preliminary occlusion of the right portal vein and right hepatic artery in an anatomic right liver resection lobe will facilitate the accurate placement of the parenchymal incision. A vessel loop is placed around the hepatic artery and then passed around it again. A Romel tourniquet is used to occlude the hepatic artery. The duct is usually avoided, as its dissection is unnecessary at this point. The branches of the duct will be secured as the liver parenchyma is transected. A vessel loop is passed around the right branch of the portal vein and the Romel tourniquet is used to occlude the right portal vein.

The line of demarcation produced by preliminary occlusion of the hilar vessels clearly indicates the portion of the liver supplied by these vessels. In patients with small tumors, preliminary ligation of the hilar vessels may not always be necessary. However, in patients with large tumor masses that distort normal liver configuration, demarcation of the division between anatomic right and anatomic left liver may be of great help. Also, in patients who have had considerable liver hypertrophy, the same is true. The line of demarcation is heavily scored, approximately one-half cm into the liver parenchyma, using a YAG laser scalpel or the electrocautery. This is done circumferentially around the liver so that the line of transection on the diaphragmatic and visceral surfaces is readily recognized at any point in time during the parenchymal dissection.

Inflow Occlusion

The entire portal pedicle is encircled by a Penrose drain. Vascular flow is interrupted (Pringle maneuver). This continues for 20 minutes and then blood flow is reestablished.[70] Inflow occlusion keeps blood loss during parenchymal dissection at an absolute minimum.

Parenchymal Dissection

Using the ultrasonic dissector, a suction dissector, or a fracture technique, the parenchyma is divided, taking care not to traumatize major vascular or ductal structures prior to their ligation. Minor bleeding points on the parenchyma that exists between the major vessels are electrocoagulated or laser coagulated using the YAG laser. Smaller ducts and vessels up to 1 mm are coagulated and divided using the electrocautery on coagulation current. Vessels above 1 mm in diameter are secured with silk ties. Metal clips on the patient side of the dissection should be discouraged. These clips, especially when they are used early in the parenchymal dissection, are liable to cut through or be wiped off and result in a bile fistula. If used in great number they interfere with follow-up CTs of the liver. Mark the major vascular structures with a single metal clip so that in follow-up radiologic studies the relationship of new metastases to these major vascular structures is readily apparent. Clips are avoided even on the specimen side of the dissection because with strong traction on the specimen these clips are often dislodged, resulting in unnecessary blood loss.

Complete control of the parenchyma dissection needs to be maintained at all times. Oftentimes toward the end of the dissection with a major liver resection the surgeon becomes so concerned with the complex anatomy and the progressive blood loss that the tumor margin is insufficiently monitored. Of great importance is a full 2 cm of normal tissue between the tumor mass and the margin of resection. According to the studies of the Hepatic Metastases Registry the presence of an adequate margin of resection is one of the most important prognostic variables.

Closed Suction Drainage

The closure is performed after copious irrigation. Sometimes the small bleeding points on the surface of the liver must be electrocoagulated or YAG laser coagulated. A closed suction drain is placed in the bed of the excised liver; usually the end of the drain is placed through the foramen of Winslow. If the chest was opened, a large-bore chest tube is secured.

Techniques for Parenchymal Dissection

As the indications for hepatic resection have expanded and more liver surgery has been performed, surgeons have worked to improve their techniques for dissecting through hepatic parenchyma. Several studies in experimental animals and one in humans were initiated. The ideal instrument for hepatic resection will allow skeletization of vascular and ductal structures, achieve small vessel hemostasis, and leave minimal devitalized tissue behind. Currently, combinations of suction dissection, ultrasonic dissection, microwave, electrocautery YAG laser, and fracture techniques are being employed.[71–76] Continued research in this field promises to maintain a steady flow of valuable information about an important surgical technology.

Resection Anatomic Right or Left Liver

Adequate exposure is achieved and the portion of liver to be resected is mobilized including ligation of the caudate lobe veins. The gallbladder is removed. This structure then guides the surgeon to an accurate dissection of the porta hepatis.

Romel tourniquets are placed around the right or left branch of the hepatic artery and the right or left branch of the portal vein in the hilum. These tourniquets are secured around the vessels so that the line of demarcation across the liver is easily visualized. There is no reason to ligate the vessels at the hilum because they will be ligated again within the hepatic parenchyma as the liver is removed as a specimen. The liver capsule is scored to mark the line of liver transection. The surgeon's nondominant hand is placed beneath the liver and upward traction applied. This places traction on liver parenchyma at its line of transection and minimizes back bleeding through hepatic veins. Small vessels and ducts are divided by electrocoagulation or YAG laser. Larger structures are skeletonized, tied in continuity, and divided. Metal clips are not used because they are associated with bile leaks from transected parenchyma. As the main hepatic veins are encountered, they are clamped and oversewn at their entrance into the vena cava (Fig 19).

Extended Resections of Anatomic Right or Left Liver (Formerly Called Trisegmentectomy Technique)

In performing an extended liver resection the complete caudate lobe is removed. It is of importance that all caudate veins on both the right and left anterior surface of the vena cava be ligated and then divided prior to starting the parenchymal dissection.

Preliminary ligation and division of the hilar structures is absolutely essential in performing an extended resection of the anatomic right or left

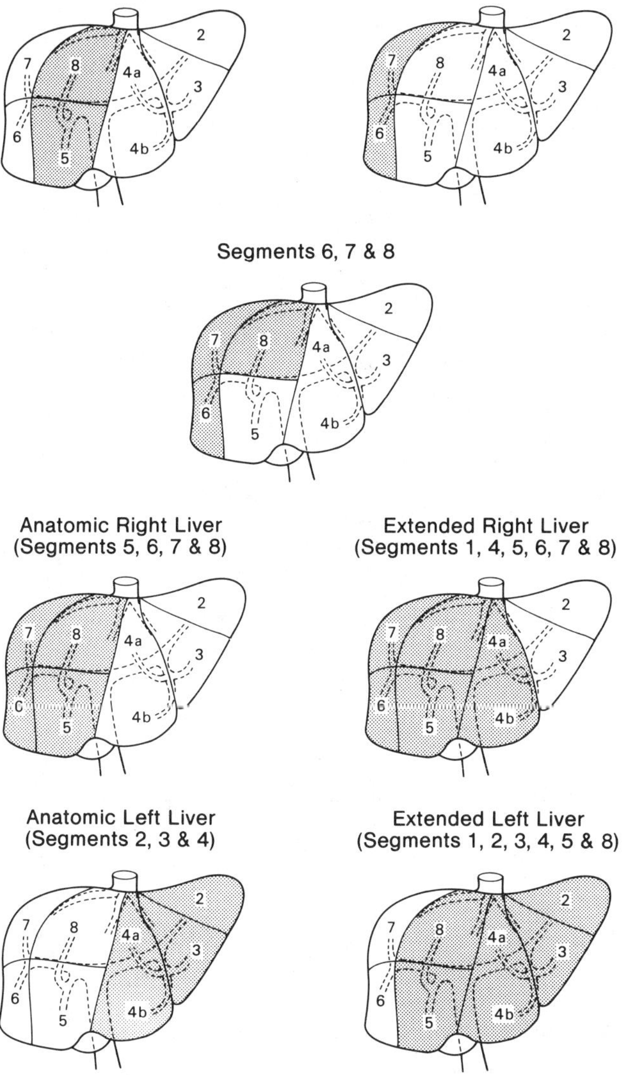

FIG 19.
Hepatic resections for metastatic disease.

liver. In the right extended resection one ligates and divides the right hepatic artery and the right hepatic duct. Then the right portal vein is isolated and divided between vascular clamps and oversewn to give a smooth proximal stump. The ties on the distal artery, duct, and portal vein are left long so that these structures can be placed on traction in performing subsequent dissection. After performing the preliminary hilar ligation one follows the left hepatic duct, left hepatic artery, and left portal vein out into the liver parenchyma until the vascular and ductal structures to segment 4 are divided and an adequate margin is achieved around the tumor mass. Then one dissects along the umbilical fissure back toward the hepatic veins. The left hepatic vein is carefully avoided. The right and middle veins are clamped with vascular clamps and oversewn as they enter the vena cava.

In performing the extended resection of the anatomic left liver one divides the left hepatic artery and left hepatic duct, and oversews the left portal vein. Then the right artery, duct, and vein are followed into the liver until the vessels and ducts to segments 5 and 8 are ligated and divided. Only after one achieves an adequate margin around the tumor does one come up through the parenchyma and move toward the origin of the right hepatic vein.

Hepatic Metastasectomies (Formerly Called Wedge Resections)

In performing a metastasectomy, inflow occlusion (Pringle maneuver) is performed by passing a Penrose drain around all of the portal structures. Alternatively, one may wish only to encircle the portal vein and the hepatic artery, excluding the common bile duct. In performing the Pringle maneuver approximately 20 minutes of ischemia time should be used before releasing the clamp and allowing liver blood flow to resume. A large suture is placed around the tumor mass so that strong traction on the metastasectomy specimen can be maintained during the parenchyma dissection. Under inflow occlusion a 2-cm rim of normal liver is left intact on the tumor nodule. In moving through parenchyma, large vessels and ducts are tied and small structures are divided with electrocautery. Following removal of the specimen the inflow occlusion is released and bleeding points that were not controlled during the dissection are secured with electrocautery or with a purse string suture around the bleeding point.

Segmentectomy Techniques

Resection of Segment 1: The Caudate Lobe

Wide exposure with complete dissection of the caudate lobe off of the vena cava is required. An approach from the right, left, or both sides of the portal triad is determined by the anatomy (see Fig 7). Removal of tumor from the caudate lobe is usually not difficult and does not usually involve transection of a major branch of the portal segmentation.

Resection of Segments 2 and 3 (Formerly Called Left Lateral Segmentectomy)

Because the left lobe of the liver is flat, covered by a well-developed Glisson's capsule, and easily exposed, resection of segments 2 and 3 is generally not difficult (Fig 20). One stays just to the left of the umbilical fissure so that vessels to segment 4 are not compromised. Vessels and ducts to segments 2 and 3 are secured as they exit from the left portal pedicle. The left hepatic vein is secured from within the liver parenchyma.

Resection of Segment 4

Segment 4 dissections are relatively simple because the deep margin of the dissection, the left portal pedicle, is usually long and devoid of branches. As a first step of the procedure, the gallbladder is removed. The right lateral margin is the middle hepatic vein. The middle hepatic vein is secured early in the dissection. This is done from within liver parenchyma by dissecting along the course of the middle vein for approximately 1 cm before it is secured with a vascular clamp and oversewn proximally. The left lateral margin is the umbilical fissure. One dissects along the right side of the umbilical sulcus, dissecting full thickness through the liver until the left portal pedicle is encountered. This is carefully preserved. One further dissects along the left paramedial portal pedicle, ligating several large branches that course medially off this vein to segment 4. One completes the dissection by transecting parenchyma along the main portal scissura to release the specimen.

Collateral Venous Circulation Between Right, Middle, and Left Hepatic Vein

Anastomosis between the main vessels or between tributaries of the hepatic veins is consistent. These abundant interconnections allow one to surgically ligate one of the three hepatic veins with no hepatic dysfunction. For this reason in performing segmental resections one is guided by the portal segmentation rather than the hepatic venous segmentation. This concept was not well understood by surgeons in the past. It has helped revise the modern surgical approach to liver resection. For example, in performing segmentectomies on the right liver the large right hepatic vein will be removed when excising segments 7 and 8 together. Venous drainage from segments 5 and 6 will not be impaired because of the venous collateral through the middle and right hepatic veins.

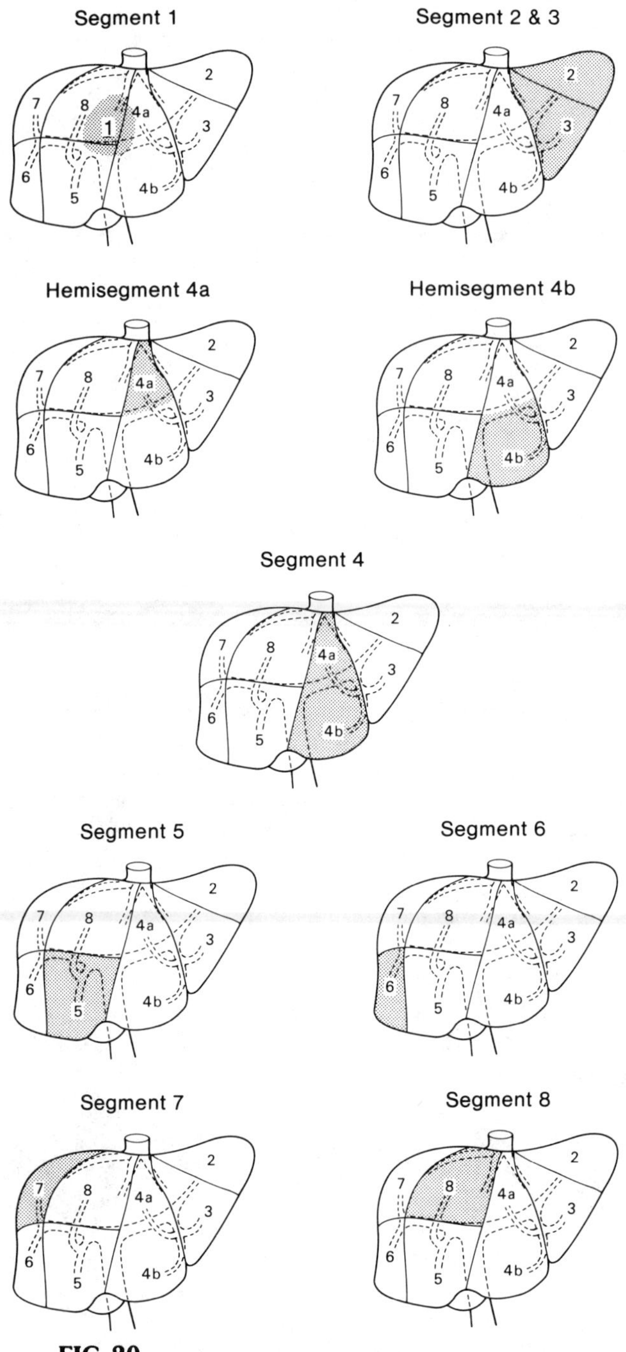

FIG 20.
Segmental hepatic resections for metastatic disease.

Resection of Segments 5 and 6

Segment 5 extends horizontally from the middle of the gallbladder fossa to half way to the right edge of the liver. To remove this segment the anterior branches of the right paramedian vein are skeletonized as they come off the right portal pedicle and then ligated and divided. One must remove the gallbladder to excise segment 5. Care must be taken not to damage vessels and ducts to segment 8.

Removal of segment 6 is generally not difficult because it involves removal of a terminal portion of portal segmentation. Removal of segment 6 involves ligation of the anterior branch of the right lateral portal vein.

Resection of Segment 7

Removal of segment 7 is also not a difficult procedure. One finds that the majority of the vessels are terminal portal veins or hepatic veins. Good mobility of the right lateral portion of the liver is secured by ligation of the caudate veins. Traction on segment 7 allows one to dissect through parenchyma just to the right of the right hepatic vein. Completion of the dissection involves removal of the cranial half of the tissue lateral to the right portal scissura.

Resection of Segment 8

Segment 8 lies between the right and main portal scissura. Removal involves dissecting along these veins down to the right portal pedicle. The posterior branch of right paramedian portal vein, artery, and biliary duct are ligated.

Systemic Chemotherapy

The effect of systemic chemotherapy on hepatic metastases depends on the primary site of metastatic disease and the doses of agents used. Since certain tumors are responsive to chemotherapy, even when liver metastases develop, systemic chemotherapy may be the appropriate treatment.[77–87] Colorectal carcinoma metastasizes to the liver in approximately 50% of the patients with advanced disease.[88, 89] The standard chemotherapeutic agent for advanced colorectal carcinoma has been 5-fluorouracil (5-FU) with an average response rate of 20% and a median response duration of six months.[90] In a series where response was clearly defined and where response in liver metastases was indicated, the average response rate for all sites was 17%, and for patients with liver metastases the response was 22%.[116] Some of the newer combinations and the responses obtained in liver metastases are listed in Table 5. Generally it is rare to obtain response rates higher than 30% and in most cases this is only possible with considerable systemic toxicity.

TABLE 5.
Response of Liver Metastases From Colorectal Carcinoma to Systemic Chemotherapy*†

Investigator	No. of Patients	% Response	Metastases	% Response
FU				
Moertel[91]	144	15	118	23
Baker[92]	42	10	11	0
Siefert[93]	36	17	5	20
Grage[94]	31	31	31	23
FU + MECCNU ± VCR				
MacDonald[96]	25	40	14	14
Baker[92]	12	32	41	31
Buroker[97]	133	16	93	18
Kemeny[98]	69	11	41	11
FU + MECCNU VCR + Strep				
Kemeny[98]	35	34	29	30
Kemeny[99, 100]	75	32	60	37
CF + FU				
Machover[101]	86	39	73	30
Meth + FU				
Kemeny[102]	43	32	33	31
Mit C + DDP VCR + FU				
Pandya[103]	23	48	15	30
DDP + FU				
Loehrer[104]	38	29	22	16
Kemeny[105]	105	28	77	20

*From Sugarbaker PH, Kemeny N: Metastatic cancer to the liver, in DeVita V, Hellman S, Rosenberg SA (eds): *Principles and Practice of Oncology*. Philadelphia, JB Lippincott Co, 1988. Used by permission.

†FU = 5-fluorouracil; CF = leucovorin; DDP = cisplatin; MitC = mitomycin C; Strep = streptozotocin; Meth = methotrexate.

Other common gastrointestinal malignancies in which patients develop hepatic metastases are gastric and pancreatic carcinoma. In a series of 307 patients at the Mayo Clinic, 22% eventually developed liver metastases.[106] Systemic treatment for gastric carcinoma produces an average response rate of 31%. For hepatic metastases the response rate is 28%.[107–115] In the few studies documenting response in liver metastases from pancreatic carcinoma, the mean response rate is 22% and the mean survival is 3.1 months.[116]

In conclusion, for most malignancies the responses obtained in patients with liver metastases mirror the overall response rate. For gastrointestinal malignancies, especially colorectal and pancreatic, this usually means a low response rate.

Regional Chemotherapy

The reason for using hepatic arterial infusion is to achieve higher drug levels in tumorous areas of the liver and lower systemic drug levels. This is possible because malignant lesions in the liver establish neovascular connections with the arterial circulation, and therefore, most of their blood supply comes from the hepatic artery, while the normal hepatocytes derive a majority of their blood supply from the portal circulation. This observation was made on pathological data from animal tumors,[117] and in a human study[118] using labeled 5-fluoro-z-deoxyuridine (FUDR).

Chemotherapeutic drugs that are most attractive for regional infusion are metabolized by the liver during a single pass, thus ensuring lower systemic drug levels and reduced systemic toxicity.[119] Ensminger and colleagues[120] assayed drug levels from hepatic venous catheters and showed that the hepatic extraction of FUDR was fourfold higher after hepatic arterial injection compared with systemic injection. With hepatic arterial infusion, 94 to 99% of FUDR was extracted in a single pass through the liver. The ability to administer a higher dose to the liver alone exposes tumors to a higher drug concentration than can be achieved with systemic therapy. Since most drugs have a steep dose-response curve, their antitumor effects are increased by hepatic arterial infusion. Based on extraction data, the value of certain drugs for hepatic arterial infusion are listed in Table 6.

Collins reviewed the pharmacologic principles of regional delivery.[122, 123] He emphasized the need for drugs with a high total-body clearance and infusional sites with a low regional exchange. Since intraarterial therapy has a high regional exchange rate (100 to 1,500 ml/minute), drugs with a high clearance rate are needed. Drugs such as FUDR, 5-FU, and cytarabine (ARA-C) have high total-body clearance.[123]

In summary, intraarterial infusion into the hepatic artery is effective because (1) a high concentration of the chemotherapeutic agent can be delivered to a localized area, (2) a significant amount of drug is extracted after the first pass, and (3) the blood flow of the artery receiving the infusion is small.

Early treatment plans with intraarterial infusion of chemotherapy required the use of an external pump. It was cumbersome for doctor and patient alike. Both responses and toxicities were noted.[124–139]

The development of a totally implantable infusion device provided a new stimulus for the infusion advocates.[135] Use of an implantable pump

TABLE 6.
Drugs for Hepatic Arterial Infusion*

Drug	Half-Life (min)	Estimated Increased Exposure by Hepatic Arterial Infusion
Fluorouracil (5-FU)	10	5–10-fold
5-Fluoro-2-deoxyuridine (5-FUDR)	<10	100–400-fold
Bischlorethylnitrosourea (BCNU)	<5	6–7-fold
Mitomycin C	<10	6–8-fold
Cisplatin	20–30	4–7-fold
Adriamycin (doxorubicin hydrochloride)	60	2–fold
Dichloromethotrexate (DCMTX)	. . .	6–8-fold

*From Sugarbaker PH, Kemeny N: Metastatic cancer to the liver, in DeVita V, Hellman S, Rosenberg SA (eds): *Principles and Practice of Oncology*. Philadelphia, JB Lippincott Co, 1988. Used by permission.

delivery system gave several potential advantages: (1) reduction in catheter-related sepsis; (2) ease of drug administration, and (3) greater patient acceptance because there are no bulky external devices. Placement of the catheter at laparotomy eliminates the problem of catheter displacement and allows better determination of the presence of intraabdominal extrahepatic disease.

Surgical Technique of Hepatic Artery Catheterization

The surgical technique has been described by several groups.[138, 140] In most patients, catheterization of the gastroduodenal artery is performed after ligation of the right gastric artery and dissection of the common hepatic, proper hepatic, and gastroduodenal arteries. The beaded Silastic catheter is inserted retrograde so that its tip lies at the junction of the common hepatic and gastroduodenal arteries (Fig 21). It is important to ligate all branches of the hepatic artery above the catheter such as the supraduodenal artery which arises from the common hepatic artery.

In some patients, retrograde catheterization of the splenic artery is required and is performed after proximal ligation of the right gastric and gastroduodenal arteries (distal to the take-off of the left hepatic artery) and ligation of the left gastric artery. The Silastic catheter is inserted so that its

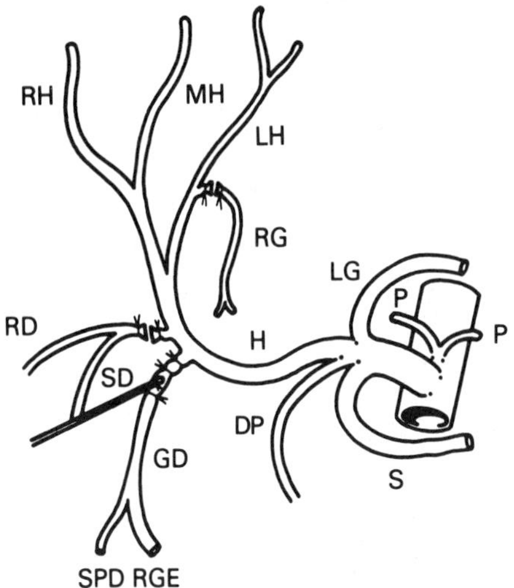

FIG 21.
Techniques for arterial catheterization for long-term infusion of chemotherapy.

tip lies within the celiac artery. In patients with the right hepatic arising off the superior mesenteric artery the gastroduodenal artery is catheterized to allow infusion of the left hepatic artery. The replaced right artery is cannulated directly using a tapered Holter arterial catheter to allow continued blood flow through the nonoccluded right hepatic artery.

Following placement of the arterial catheter, 2.0 ml of a fluorescein solution is injected into the pump's side port. The abdominal contents are exposed to a Wood's ultraviolet light to establish a homogenous uptake in the liver and absence of infusion of the stomach and duodenum. The implantable pumps are then placed into a subcutaneous pocket in the left or right lower quadrant below the belt line.

The first report with the implantable pump and continuous FUDR therapy suggested an 83% response rate.[139] Other investigators using this method could not equal these results (Table 7). The mean response rate of 44% in ten trials is higher than the mean response rate obtained with systemic chemotherapy. In these studies 42% of patients had prior chemotherapy treatment.

Toxicity of Continuous Infusion Intrahepatic Therapy Via Implantable Pump

Gastrointestinal Toxicity

Although the operative and technical complications with the implantable pump have been minimal, there have been chemotherapy complications.[137] Endoscopically documented GI ulcerations were reported in 30% of patients. The most likely mechanism for GI tract toxicity from hepatic arterial infusion is inadvertent perfusion of the stomach and duodenum

TABLE 7.
Hepatic Artery FUDR Infusion With Internal Pump: Responses*

Investigator	No. of Patients	% Prior Chemotherapy	PR†	% ↓ CEA	Median Survival (mo)	% >50 Liver Involvement
Niederhuber[140]	70	45	83	91	25	. . .
Balch[141]	50	40		83	26	. . .
Kemeny[137]	41	43	42	51	12	53
Shepard[142]	53	42	32	. . .	17	. . .
Cohen[143]	50	36	51	. . .	. . .	18
Weiss[144]	17	85	29	57	13	. . .
Schwartz[145]	23	. . .	15	75	18	. . .
Johnson[146]	40	. . .	47	. . .	12	34
Kemeny[147]	31	50	52	. . .	22	. . .
Ramming[148]	55	. . .	8	88	11	. . .

*From Sugarbaker PH, Kemeny N: Metastatic cancer to the liver, in DeVita V, Hellman S, Rosenberg SA (eds): *Principles and Practice of Oncology*. Philadelphia, JB Lippincott Co, 1988. Used by permission.
†PR = partial response.

with drug through small vessels from the hepatic artery. Hohn and colleagues found no ulcer disease in their patients and believed this was related to their surgical techniques, which involve very careful denuding of the vessels arising from the hepatic artery distal to the arterial cannulation.[138]

Hepatic Toxicity

Another frequent side effect of hepatic arterial infusion is hepatic toxicity. Kemeny and co-workers found bilirubin elevations above 3 mg/ml in 20% of the patients and transaminase elevations in 71%.[137] In several studies the incidence of hepatic toxicity was quite similar.[137, 138, 140–148] Approximately 25% of the patients developed bilirubin elevation.[149]

There may be two different types of hepatic toxicity. In some patients it is like hepatitis with documented hepatocyte necrosis and cholestasis on liver biopsy.[150] Other patients have a clinical picture compatible with pericholangitis and fibrosis of biliary radicals. In early stages of hepatic toxicity liver enzyme elevations will usually return to normal when the drug is withdrawn and the patient is given a rest period. In some patients jaundice does not improve. These patients may develop biliary strictures, most commonly at the bifurcation of right and left hepatic ducts, but also in the common bile duct or intrahepatic radicals. Percutaneous cholangiography or endoscopic retrograde cholangiopancreatography show these lesions are similar to idiopathic sclerosing cholangitis. Since the ducts are sclerotic, sonograms are usually normal. Computed tomography of the liver and should be done to exclude progressive malignancy as a cause of strictures. In some patients drainage procedures by transhepatic cholangiogram may be helpful.

Close follow-up will greatly help to avoid biliary sclerosis. If bilirubin elevation is observed, no further treatment should be given until it returns to normal. In some patients who cannot tolerate a low dose for two weeks, it may be possible to continue treatment by giving the FUDR infusion for one week rather than the usual two weeks. The reports that describe more extensive surgery[147, 149] had a lower rate of gastroduodenal ulceration, but a higher rate of biliary sclerosis. Efficient gastric devascularization may allow more direct hepatic arterial infusion, thereby increasing the rate of biliary sclerosis.

Cholecystitis as a Toxicity

Another side effect of hepatic arterial infusional chemotherapy is the development of cholecystitis, which has been reported to occur in as many as 33% of patients.[151] In most recent series the gallbladder has been removed at the same time of catheter placement to prevent this complication and to avoid the confusion of these symptoms with other hepatic side effects from pump treatment.

Systemic Toxicity

Systemic side effects of chemotherapy are almost never seen with continuous infusion intrahepatic therapy. Myelosuppression does not occur with FUDR. While intrahepatic mitomycin or BCNU may depress platelet counts, this occurs to a lesser degree than with systemic administration. Nausea and vomiting is not usually seen from FUDR infusion, but if present, one should suspect that ulcer disease or gastritis has developed. Diarrhea, which is frequently a problem with systemic FUDR infusion, is rarely seen with intrahepatic infusion. If it occurs, one should suspect high systemic drug levels caused by catheter disruption or shunting through the liver to lung or bowel to systemic circulation.

Randomized Studies to Demonstrate Efficacy of Arterial Infusion

To understand the impact of hepatic infusional therapy on survival of patients with hepatic metastases, randomized studies were initiated where patients were stratified for parameters known to affect response and survival. The strong influence of the percent of liver involvement on survival has been shown by many investigators.[152–155]

The high response rates with long-term continuous infusion of FUDR into the hepatic artery caused widespread use of this treatment throughout the United States in 1980 to 1985. To critically evaluate the effects of

TABLE 8.
Randomized Studies of Intrahepatic vs. Systemic Chemotherapy for Hepatic Metastases

Group	No. of Patients	Intrahepatic		Systemic		
		Drug	% Response	Drug	% Response	
MSKCC[156]	163	FUDR	50	FUDR	20	$P = .001$
NCOG[157]	143	FUDR	37	FUDR	10	$P = .002$
NCI[154]	64	FUDR	62	FUDR	17	. . .
Consortium[155]	43	FUDR	56	5-FU	38	. . .
City of Hope[147]	41	FUDR	56	5-FU	0	. . .

continuous arterial infusion several randomized trials were established (Table 8). An early study to compare FUDR intrahepatic infusion to systemic FUDR infusion was initiated at the National Institutes of Health. This group showed a significant increase in response rate, 62% vs. 17%, respectively.[156] If patients with positive nodes are excluded, the two-year survival was 47% vs. 13%, respectively ($P = .03$). This study showed that patients whose hepatic cancer had less tendency to metastasize outside of the liver could be benefited. However, in the group of patients as a whole there were no survival advantages. Another randomized study begun by a consortium of four institutions was unable to enter enough patients and closed after 43 patients had entered.[157] The response rates were 38%, 58%, and 56% for systemic 5-FU, intrahepatic FUDR, and combined systemic and intrahepatic groups, respectively (see Table 8).

The study from Memorial Sloan-Kettering Cancer Center compared intrahepatic infusion with systemic infusion.[158] The dose of FUDR in the intrahepatic arm was 0.3 mg/kg a day for 14 days, and in the systemic arm the dose was 0.125 mg/kg a day for 14 days. All patients underwent exploratory laparotomy to assess the percent of liver involvement and to determine that there was no extrahepatic disease. At surgery, 33 of 162 patients were found to have disease outside of the liver not detected on CT and were thus excluded from analysis.

This study demonstrated a significantly higher response rate (>50% reduction in measurable disease) with hepatic therapy, 50% vs. 20% for systemic infusion ($P = .001$). Thirty-one of the systemic patients crossed over to intrahepatic therapy after tumor progression. Twenty-five percent had a partial response, and 22% showed stabilization of disease. The median survival for the intrahepatic and systemic groups was 17 and 12 months, respectively ($P = 0.424$). Survival information is difficult to interpret because 60% of the patients in the systemic group crossed over and received intrahepatic therapy.

A similar randomized study by the Northern California Cooperative Cancer Group also used FUDR infusion in both the intrahepatic and systemic arms of the study and had similar response rates. They reported a 37% partial response rate in the intrahepatic infusion group and 12% in the systemic FUDR infusion group.[159]

A major problem with direct hepatic therapy is the development of extrahepatic disease. Even though beneficial effects occur in the liver, patient survival may not be prolonged in only a minority of patients.

It is still too early to make definite conclusions about the use of intrahepatic infusional therapy, but certain points appear valid. First, there are five randomized trials demonstrating a significantly higher response rate with intrahepatic infusion versus systemic infusion in the treatment of hepatic metastases from colorectal carcinoma. Second, some studies demonstrate a survival advantage between groups who never received intrahepatic treatment and those who did. Should this treatment be offered to all patients in the community? There is a definite "learning curve," so that in the hands of surgeons and physicians who are not familiar with this type of treatment there may be more toxicity and lower response rate. Before hepatic infusional therapy via the hepatic pump becomes a standard treatment, more work needs to be done on (1) clearly defining whether there is a survival advantage, (2) working on ways to decrease biliary sclerosis, and (3) perhaps developing ways to increase response rate, particularly complete responses.

Radiation Therapy

The tolerance of the normal liver to radiation limits the total radiation dose and the use of this modality to treat hepatic metastases.

The role of radiation in palliation of symptoms from liver metastases has been demonstrated.[158–163] With an average dose of 2,500 rad in 3 to 3.5 weeks, Prasad and colleagues treated 27 patients (41% had failed to respond to chemotherapy) and reported symptomatic pain relief in 70%, with an average survival of four months.[160] Jaundice and ascites improved in 28% and 50% of patients, respectively; however, no follow-up radiologic studies were available. The average response rate obtained with the combined treatment is not higher than that obtained with FUDR intrahepatic infusion alone.[164–173]

Another means by which to deliver radiotherapy to the liver is interstitial radiation. This offers an opportunity for a higher dose to a smaller area and sparing of the normal liver. With a high-intensity iridium 192 source, doses of 5,000 rad can be delivered in a single treatment. In a pilot study Dritschillo and colleagues positioned afterloading catheters by sonography in six patients with tumors ranging from 2.5 to 9.5 cm.[174] One patient had a 25% regression, while the others remained stable, with little toxicity.

Other Therapeutic Modalities

Hepatic Arterial Occlusion

The rationale for treating liver cancer by occlusion of the hepatic artery has been present since 1952.[175] It is based on the fact that liver metastases have a single blood supply from the hepatic artery. The normal liver has a dual blood supply by both the portal vein and hepatic artery. Few studies use arterial occlusion alone; therefore, it is difficult to interpret the effect of ligation itself on survival.[176–187] No randomized controlled studies have been performed.

Arterial Embolization

Although gross regression with tumor necrosis has been reported after ligation, there is usually a rapid reestablishment of arterial blood flow through the development of arterial collaterals and consequently a regrowth of tumor. The rationale for arterial embolization is that repeated treatments will cause repeated episodes of tumor ischemia but diminish the development of collateral circulation. Beneficial effects with hepatic arterial embolization have been seen in patients with endocrine tumors. Since these tumors are slow growing and rarely metastasize outside the liver, a reduction in the mass of the tumor often gives significant palliation. In a series of patients with apudoma treated at the M.D. Anderson Hospital, eight of 14 patients responded who underwent embolization after failure of systemic or hepatic chemotherapy.[188] Five of six patients experienced a dramatic improvement in the symptoms of the carcinoid syndrome and reduction in 5-hydroxyindole acetic acid (5-HIAA) levels. Nine of 13 patients with carcinoid syndrome treated by Maton noted improvement in symptoms. He emphasized the requirement for blocking pharmacologically active substances produced by the tumor prior to embolization. Patency of the portal vein must be present to avoid hepatic necrosis as a complication of embolization. Almost all patients have fever, leukocytosis, and hepatic pain, and some develop hepatic abscesses, gas formation, or urate nephropathy.[190, 191] Using both hepatic artery occlusion and chemotherapy, Moertel noted systemic relief in nine of ten patients with carcinoid tumor.[190]

It is clear from these studies that embolization will decrease symptoms in patients with endocrine tumors and actually cause reduction in tumor size, but it is not clear whether these measures prolong survival, but they clearly improve quality of life.

Microspheres

Another way to avoid revascularization after hepatic arterial ligation and to achieve temporary occlusion of the hepatic artery is by the use of microspheres.[192–198] Starch microspheres or collagen particles are approximately 40 μm in diameter and are degraded by naturally occurring enzymes. When injected into the hepatic artery, they lodge in the arteriolar capillary bed and partially stop flow until they undergo degradation (approximately 30 minutes). If the tumor has a single blood supply (the hepatic artery) and the normal liver has a dual blood supply (hepatic artery and portal vein), then the blood flow through tumor will be markedly slowed. This increases the time over which tumor is exposed to the chemotherapeutic agent.[193] Drugs with a short half-life and/or low extraction efficiency are the best to use with microspheres.[194] Intrahepatic injection of labeled 5-FU and microspheres resulted in increased tumor labeling in the livers injected with the microspheres and a reduced peripheral blood ^{14}C FU level compared with 5-FU alone.[195] Using intrahepatic injections of adriamycin or mitomycin C plus microspheres, there was a reduction in systemic levels of drugs.[196, 198]

Yttrium 90 Microspheres

Another type of microsphere is a resin particle in which yttrium 90 has been entrapped, providing the opportunity for "internal radiotherapy." Grady and colleagues reported six responses in 16 patients treated with intraarterial yttrium 90 microspheres and hyperthermia. Toxicity included radiation hepatitis and peptic ulceration.[199] Ariel and co-workers treated 65 patients with hepatic metastases from colorectal carcinoma using infusion of 5-FU (1 gm infused over 24 hours for 15 days) with yttrium 90 (estimated to deliver 10,000 rad to the liver). They obtained a 35 to 40% objective response rate and a median survival of 12 to 14 months.[200] Mantravadi and colleagues noted three responses in 15 previously treated patients using yttrium microspheres alone and did not observe radiation hepatitis.[201] It is not clear that these response rates are superior to hepatic infusional therapy alone, but the need for further studies is definitely indicated.

Local Tumor Destruction Plus Regional Chemotherapy

Several groups have tried to combine the focal destruction of tumor nodules (in order to remove gross disease) with regional chemotherapy in order to maintain a disease-free status within the liver. Kemeny et al. have reported using surgical removal of multiple metastases combined with intraarterial FUDR.[202] She found superior local control of tumor when patients had surgery plus intraarterial FUDR as compared with intraarterial FUDR alone. Steele and colleagues have used liver cryosurgery in order to destroy bulk disease in the liver.[203] The extent of tumor destruction in the liver was monitored with intraoperative ultrasound.[204] Other groups have used the instillation of absolute alcohol into a tumor mass to achieve a focal destruction of malignant disease.[203–205] Dritschillo and co-workers have used interstitial radiation therapy surgically positioned in the center of a tumor nodule to bring about its destruction.[174] The highly active radiation was left in place long enough to destroy tumor and a small margin of surrounding tissue. This modality promises to have few complications resulting from abscess formation or infection of metastases. These combined approaches to control hepatic metastases may lead to increased survival. Cure is unlikely even with complete control of intrahepatic tumor because of systemic spread of cancer.

References

1. Michaels NA: *Blood Supply and Anatomy of Upper Abdominal Organs with Descriptive Atlas.* Philadelphia, JB Lippincott Co, 1955.
2. August DA, Sugarbaker PH, Schneider PD: Lymphatic dissemination of hepatic metastases: Implications for the follow-up and treatment of patients with colorectal cancer. *Cancer* 1985; 55:1490–1494.
3. Hollinshead WH: *Anatomy for Surgeons.* New York, Harper & Row Publishers Inc, 1971, vol 2, p 319.
4. Bismuth H: Surgical anatomy and anatomical surgery of the liver. *World J Surg* 1982; 6:3–9.
5. Couinaud C: Controlled hepatectomies and exposure of the intrahepatic bile ducts: Anatomical and technical study. Paris, France, 1981.
6. Pickren JW, Tsukada Y, Lane WW: Liver metastases, analysis of autopsy data, in Weiss L, Gilbert GA (eds): *Liver Metastases.* Boston, GH Hall, 1982, pp 2–18.
7. Sugarbaker PH, Reinig JW, Hughes KS: Diagnosis of hepatic metastases, in Rosenberg SA (ed): *Surgical Treatment of Metastases.* Philadelphia, JB Lippincott Co, 1987.
8. Wanebo HJ, Rao B, Pinsky CM, et al: Preoperative carcinoembryonic antigen level as a prognostic indicator in colorectal cancer. *N Engl J Med* 1978; 299:448–451.
9. Kemeny MM, Sugarbaker PH, Smith TJ, et al: A prospective analysis of laboratory test and imaging studies to detect hepatic lesions. *Ann Surg* 1982; 195:163–176.
10. Smith TJ, Kemeny MM, Sugarbaker PH, et al: A prospective study of hepatic imaging in the detection of metastatic disease. *Ann Surg* 1982; 195:486–491.
11. Matsui O, Kadoya M, et al: Work in progress: Dynamic sequential computed tomography during arterial portography in the detection of hepatic neoplasms. *Radiology* 1983; 146:173–178.
12. Bernardino ME, Erwin BC, Steinberg HV, et al: Delayed hepatic CT scanning: Increased confidence and improved detection of hepatic metastases. *Radiology* 1986; 159:71–74.
13. Reinig JW, Dwyer AJ, Miller DL, et al: Liver metastases detection: Comparative sensitivities of MR imaging and CT scanning. *Radiology* 1987; 162:43–47.
14. Hogg L Jr, Pack GT: Diagnostic accuracy of hepatic metastases at laparotomy. *Arch Surg* 1966; 72:251–252.
15. Gray BN: Surgeon accuracy in the diagnosis of liver metastases at laparotomy. *Aust NZ J Surg* 1980; 50:524–526.
16. Harbin WP, Wittenberg J, Ferrucci JT Jr, et al: Fallibility of exploratory lap-

arotomy in detection of hepatic and retroperitoneal masses. *AJR* 1980; 135:115–121.
17. Finlay IG, Meek DR, Gray HW, et al: Incidence and detection of occult hepatic metastases in colorectal carcinoma. *Brit Med J* 1982; 284:803–805.
18. Igwa SI, Sakai K, Kinoshita H, et al: Intraoperative sonography: Clinical usefulness in liver surgery. *Radiology* 1985; 156:473–478.
19. Gozzetti G, Mazziotti A, Bolondi L, et al: Ultrasonography in surgery for liver tumors. *Surgery* 1986; 99:523–529.
20. Castaing D, Kunstlinger F, Habib N, et al: Intraoperative ultrasonographic study of the liver. *Am J Surg* 1985; 149:676–682.
21. Hughes KS, Simon RM, Songhorabodi S, et al: Hepatic Metastases Registry: Resection of the liver for colorectal carcinoma metastases: A multi-institutional study of indications for resection. *Surgery* 1988; 103:278–282.
22. Wagner JS, Adson MA, van Heerden JA, et al: The natural history of hepatic metastases from colorectal cancer. *Ann Surg* 1984; 19:502–508.
23. Pestana C, Reitemeir RJ, Moertel CG, et al: The natural history of carcinoma of colon and rectum. *Am J Surg* 1964; 108:826–829.
24. Jaffe BM, Donegan WL, Watson F, et al: Factors influencing survival in patients with untreated hepatic metastases. *Surg Gynecol Obstet* 1986; 127:1–11.
25. Oxley EM, Ellis H: Prognosis of carcinoma of the large bowel in the presence of liver metastases. *Br J Surg* 1969; 56:149–152.
26. Bengmark S, Hafstrom L: The natural history of primary and secondary malignant tumors of the liver. *Cancer* 1969; 23:198–202.
27. Baden H, Anderson B: Survival of patients with untreated liver metastases from colorectal cancer. *Scand J Gastroenterol* 1975; 10:221–223.
28. Wood CB, Gillis CR, Blumgart LH: A retrospective study of the natural history of patients with liver metastases from colorectal cancer. *Clin Oncol* 1976; 2:285–288.
29. Boey J, Choi TK, Wong J, et al: Carcinoma of the colon and rectum with liver involvement. *Surg Gynecol Obstet* 1981; 153:864–868.
30. Goslin R, Steele G, Zancheck N, et al: Factors influencing survival in patients with hepatic metastases from adenocarcinoma of the colon or rectum. *Dis Colon Rectum* 1982; 25:749–754.
31. Wilson SM, Adson MA: Surgical treatment of hepatic metastases from colorectal cancers. *Arch Surg* 1976; 111:330–334.
32. Foster JH, Berman MM: *Solid Liver Tumors*. Philadelphia, WB Saunders Co, 1977.
33. Morrow CE, Grage TB, Sutherland DER, et al: Hepatic resection for secondary neoplasma. *Surgery* 1982; 92:610–614.
34. Aldrete JS, Agdemir D, Laws HL: Major hepatic resections: Analysis of 51 cases. *Am Surg* 1982; 48:118–122.
35. Blumgart LH, Allison DJ: Resection and embolization in the management of secondary hepatic tumors. *World J Surg* 1982; 6:32–45.
36. Thompson HH, Tompkins RK, Longmire WP Jr: Major hepatic resection: A 25 year experience. *Ann Surg* 1983; 197:375–388.
37. Fortner JG, Silva JS, Golbey RB, et al: Multivariate analysis of a personal series of 247 consecutive patients with liver metastases from colorectal cancer. *Ann Surg* 1984; 199:306–316.
38. Cady B, McDermott WV: Major hepatic resection for metachronous metastases from colon cancer. *Ann Surg* 1985; 201:204–209.

39. Adson MA, van Heerden JA, Adson JH, et al: Resection of hepatic metastases from colorectal cancer. *Arch Surg* 1984; 119:647–651.
40. Gennari L, Doci R, Bignami P: Surgical treatment of hepatic metastases from colorectal cancer. *Ann Surg* 1985; 203:49–54.
41. August DA, Sugarbaker PH, Bianola FJ, et al: Hepatic resection of colorectal metastases: Influence of clinical factors and adjuvant intraperitoneal 5-fluorouracil via Tenckhoff catheter on survival. *Ann Surg* 1985; 201:210–218.
42. Petrelli NJ, Nambisan RN, Herrera L, et al: Hepatic resection for isolated metastases from colorectal carcinoma. *Am J Surg* 1985; 149:205–209.
43. Coppa GF, Eng K, Ranson JHC, et al: Hepatic resection for metastatic colon and rectal cancer: An evaluation of preoperative and post-operative factors. *Ann Surg* 1985; 202:203–208.
44. Gall FP, Scheele J, Altendorf A: Typical and atypical resection techniques of hepatic metastases, in *Recent Results in Cancer Research*. New York, Springer-Verlag, pp 212–220.
45. Iwatsuki S, Esquivel CO, Gordon RD, et al: Liver resection for metastatic colorectal cancer. *Surgery* 1986; 100:804–809.
46. Ekberg H, Tranberg KG, Anderson R, et al: Determinants of survival in liver resection for colorectal secondaries. *Br J Surg* 1986; 73:727–731.
47. Butler J, Attiyeh FF, Daly JM: Hepatic resection for metastases of the colon and rectum. *Surg Gynecol Obstet* 1986; 162:109–113.
48. Hughes KS, Sugarbaker PH: Treatment of hepatic metastases, in Rosenberg SA (ed): *Disease*. Philadelphia, JB Lippincott Co, 1987.
49. Hughes KS: Hepatic Metastases Registry: Resection of the liver for colorectal carcinoma metastases: A multiinstitutional study of patterns of recurrence. *Surgery* 1986; 100:278–284.
50. Griffith K, Chang AE, Sugarbaker PH: Repeat hepatic resections in patients with liver metastases from colorectal cancer, in progress.
51. Steel G Jr, Olsteen RT, Wilson RE, et al: Patterns of failure after surgical cure of large liver tumors: A change in the proximate cause of death and a need for effective systemic adjuvant therapy. *Am J Surg* 1984; 147:554–559.
52. Hughes KS, August DA, Ottow RT, et al: Hepatic resection for colorectal carcinoma metastases: Present status and future prospects, in Mastromarino AJ (ed): *Biology and Treatment of Colorectal Cancer Metastasis*. Boston, Martinus Nijhoff, 1986, pp 159–178.
53. Martin JK, Moertel CG, Adson MA, et al: Surgical treatment of functioning metastatic carcinoid tumors. *Arch Surg* 1983; 118:537–541.
54. Norton JA, Sugarbaker PH, Doppman JL, et al: Aggressive resection of metastatic disease in selected patients with malignant gastrinoma. *Ann Surg* 1986; 203:352–359.
55. Galland RB, Blumgart LH: Carcinoid syndrome, surgical management. *Br J Hosp Med* 1986; 35:168–170.
56. Garre C: Beitraege zur Leber-Chirurgie. *Bruns Deitr Klin Chir* 1888; 4:181.
57. Keen WW: Report of a case of resection of the liver for the removal of a neoplasm, with a table of seventy-six cases of resesction of the liver for hepatic tumors. *Ann Surg* 1899; 30:267.
58. Pringle JH: Notes on the arrest of hepatic hemorrhage due to trauma. *Ann Surg* 1908; 48:451.
59. Wendel W: Beitraege zur Chirurgie der Leber. *Arch Klin Chir* 1911; 95:887.
60. Lortat-Jacob JL, Robert HG: Hepatectomie droite reglee. *Presse Med* 1952; 60:549.

61. Healey JE: Vascular anatomy of the liver. *Ann NY Acad Sci* 1970; 170:8–17.
62. Lin TY, Hsu KY, Hsieh CM, et al: Study on lobectomy of ports on three cases of primary hepatoma treated with left lobectomy of the liver. *J Formosan Med Assoc* 1958; 57:742.
63. Couinaud C: Principes directeurs de hepatectomies reglees. *Chirurgie* 1980; 106:8–10.
64. Storm KF, Longmire WP Jr: A simplified clamp for hepatic resection. *Surg Gynecol Obstet* 1971; 133:103.
65. Starzl TE, Bell RH, Beart RW, et al: Heptic trisegmentectomy and other liver resections. *Surg Gynecol Obstet* 1975; 141:429.
66. Hodgson WJB, Aufses A Jr: Surgical ultrasonic dissection of the liver. *Surg Rounds* 1979; 2:68.
67. Fortner JG, MacLean BJ, Kim DK, et al: The seventies evolution in liver surgery for cancer. *Cancer* 1981; 47:2162.
68. Starzl TE, Iwatsuki S, Shaw BW Jr, et al: Left hepatic trisegmentectomy. *Surg Gynecol Obstet* 1982; 155:21.
69. Lefor AT, Hughes KS, Shiloni E, et al: Intraabdominal intrahepatic disease in patients with colorectal hepatic metastases. *Dis Colon Rectum* 1988; 31:100–103.
70. Huget C, Nordlinger B, Galopin JJ, et al: Normothermic hepatic vascular exclusion for extensive hepatectomy. *Surg Gynecol Obstet* 1978; 147:689–693.
71. Hodgson WJB, Delguercio LRM: Preliminary experience in liver surgery using the ultrasonic scalpel. *Surgery* 1984; 95:230–234.
72. Ottow RT, Barbieri SA, Sugarbaker PH, et al: Liver transection: A controlled study of four different techniques in pigs. *Surgery* 1985; 97:596–601.
73. Tranberg K, Rigotti P, Bracket KA, et al: Liver resection: A comparison using the Nd-Yag laser, an ultrasonic surgical aspirator, or blunt dissection. *Am J Surg* 1986; 151:368–373.
74. Tabuse K, Katsumi M, Kobayashi Y, et al: Microwave surgery: Hepatectomy using microwave tissue coagulator. *World J Surg* 1985; 9:136–143.
75. Joffe SN, Brackett KA, Sankar MY, et al: Resection of the liver with the ND.YAG laser. *Surg Gynecol Obstet* 1986; 163:437–442.
76. Andrus CH, Kaminski DL: Segmental hepatic resection utilizing the ultrasonic dissector. *Arch Surg* 1986; 121:515–521.
77. Carter SK: Single and combination nonhormonal chemotherapy in breast cancer. *Cancer* 1972; 30:1543–1555.
78. Mattsson W, Arwidi A, von Eyben F, et al: Phase II study of combined vincristine, Adriamycin, cyclophosphamide, and methotrexate with citrovorum factor rescue in metastatic breast cancer. *Cancer Treat Rep* 1977; 61:1527–1531.
79. Muss HB, White DR, Richards F II, et al: Adriamycin vs methotrexate in five-drug combination chemotherapy for advanced breast cancer. *Cancer* 1978; 42:2141–2148.
80. Kennealey GT, Boston B, Mitchell MS, et al: Combination chemotherapy for advanced breast cancer: Two regiments containing Adriamycin. *Cancer* 1978; 42:27–33.
81. Tranum B, Hoogstraten B, Kennedy A, et al: Adriamycin in combination for the treatment of breast cancer. *Cancer* 1978; 41:2708–2083.
82. Jones SE, Durie BG, Salmon SE: Combination chemotherapy with Adria-

mycin and cyclophosphamide for advanced breast cancer. *Cancer* 1975; 36:90–97.
83. Chauvergne J, Garr-Bobo J, Klein T, et al: Polychimiotherapie des cancers mammaires en phase avancee. Association ternaire avec doxorubicine: Analyse de 209 observations. *Bull Cance* 1977; 64(4):667–680.
84. Russell JA, Baker JW, Dady PJ, et al: Combination chemotherapy of metastatic breast cancer with vincristine, Adriamycin and prednisolone. *Cancer* 1978; 396–399.
85. Smalley RV, Carpenter J, Bartolucci A, et al: A comparison of cyclophosphamide, Adriamycin, 5-fluorouracil (CAF) and cyclophosphamide, methotrexate, 5-fluorouracil, vincristine, prednisone, (CMFVP) in patients with metastatic breast cancer: A Southeastern Cancer Group Study project. *Cancer* 1977; 40:625–632.
86. Canellos GP, DeVita VT, Gold GL, et al: Combination chemotherapy for advanced breast cancer: Response and effect on survival. *Ann Intern Med* 1976; 84:89–392.
87. George SL, Hoogstraten B: Prognostic factors in the initial response to therapy by patients with advanced breast cancer. *JNCI* 1978; 60:731–736.
88. Abrams HL, Spiro R, Goldstein N: Metastases in carcinoma: Analysis of 1000 autopsied cases. *Cancer* 1950; 3:74–85.
89. Bross IDJ, Viaadana E, Pickren J: Do generalized metastases occur directly from the primary? *J Chron Dis* 1975; 28:149–159.
90. Wasserman T, Comis RL, Goldsmith M, et al: Tabular analysis of the clinical chemotherapy of solid tumors. *Cancer Chemother Rep* 1975; 6:399.
91. Moertel CG, Reitemeier RJ: *Advanced Gastrointestinal Cancer: Clinical Management and Chemotherapy.* New York, Harper & Row Publishers Inc, 1969.
92. Baker LH, Talley RW, Maiter R, et al: Phase II comparison of the treatment of advanced gastrointestinal cancer with bolus weekly 5-Fu vs methyl CCNU plus weekly 5-FU. *Cancer* 1976; 38:1.
93. Siefert P, Baker LH, Reed MD, et al: Comparison of continuously infused 5-Fluorouracil with bolus injection in treatment of patients with colorectal adenocarcinoma. *Cancer* 1975; 36:123.
94. Grage TB, Vassilopoulos P, Shingleton WW, et al: Results of a prospective randomized study of hepatic artery infusion with 5-fluorouracil vs intravenous 5-fluorouracil in patients with hepatic metastases from colorectal cancer: A Central Oncology Group Study. *Surgery* 1979; 86:550–555.
95. Moertel CG, Schutt AJ, Hahn RG, et al: Brief communications: Therapy of advanced colorectal cancer with a combination of 5-fluorouracil, methyl-1, 3-cis (2-chlor-ethyl) -1- nitrosourea and vincristine. *JNCI* 1975; 54:69–71.
96. MacDonald JS, Kisner DF, Smythe T, et al: 5-fluorouracil (5-FU), methyl CCNU and vincristine in the treatment of advanced colorectal cancer: Phase II study utilizing weekly 5-FU. *Cancer Treat Rep* 1976; 60:1597.
97. Buroker J, Kim PN, Groppe C, et al: 5-FU infusion with methyl-CCNU in the treatment of advanced colon cancer. *Cancer* 1978; 42:1228.
98. Kemeny N, Yagoda A, Golbey RB: A randomized study of two different schedules of methyl CCNU, 5-FU and vincristine for metastatic colorectal carcinoma. *Cancer* 1979; 43:78.
99. Kemeny N, Yagoda A, Braun D: Metastatic colorectal carcinoma: A prospective randomized trial of Methyl CCNU, 5-fluorouracil (5-FU) and vincristine

(MOF) versus MOF plus streptozotocin (MOF-strep). *Cancer* 1983; 51:20–25.

100. Kemeny N, Yagoda A, Braun D, et al: Therapy for metastatic colorectal carcinoma with a combination of methyl-CCNU, 5-fluorouracil, vincristine, and streptozotocin (MOF-strep). *Cancer* 1980; 45:876–881.
101. Machover D, Goldschmidt E, Chollet P, et al: Treatment of advanced colorectal and gastric adenocarcinomas with 5-fluorouracil and high-dose folinic acid. *J Clin Oncol* 1986; 4:685–696.
102. Kemeny N, Ahmed T, Michaelson R, et al: Activity of low dose methotrexate and fluorouracil in advanced colorectal carcinoma: Attempted correlation with tissue and blood levels of phosphoribosylpyrophosphate. *J Clin Oncol* 1984; 2:311–315.
103. Pandya KJ, Chans AYU, Qazi R, et al: Combination chemotherapy for advanced colorectal cancer: A pilot study. *Am J Clin Oncol* 1986; 9:31–34.
104. Loehrer PJ Sr, Einhorn LH, Williams SD, et al: Cisplatin plus 5-FU for the treatment of adenocarcinoma of the colon. *Cancer Treat Rep* 1985; 69:1359–1363.
105. Kemeny N, Reichman B, Botet J, et al: Continuous infusion 5-fluorouracil (5-FU) and bolus cisplatin (DDP) for metastatic colorectal cancer. *Proc ACO* 1987; 6:86.
106. Moertel CG: The natural history of advanced gastric cancer. *Surg Gynecol Obstet* 1968; 126:1071–1074.
107. Franks CR: Adriamycin and methotrexate in metastatic gastric cancer: A pilot study. *Clin Oncol* 1980; 6:309–315.
108. Bitran JD, Desser RK, Kozloff MF, et al: Treatment of metastatic pancreatic and gastric adenocarcinomas with 5-fluorouracil, Adriamycin, and mitomycin-C (FAM). *Cancer Treat Rep* 1979; 63:2049–2052.
109. MacDonald JS, Schein PS, Woolley PV, et al: 5-Fluorouracil, doxorubicin and mitomycin (FAM) combination chemotherapy for advanced gastric cancer. *Ann Intern Med* 1980; 93:533–536.
110. Seligman M, Bukowski RM, Groppe CS, et al: Chemotherapy of metastatic gastrointestinal neoplasms with 5-flourouracil and streptozotocin. *Cancer Treat Rep* 1977; 61:1375–1377.
111. Wooley PV III, MacDonald Smuthe TS, et al: A phase II trial of ftorafur, Adriamycin and mitomycin-C (FAM II) in advanced gastric cancer. *Cancer* 1979; 44:1211–1214.
112. The Gastrointestinal Tumor Study Group: Phase II-III chemotherapy studies in advanced gastric cancer. *Cancer Treat Rep* 1979; 63:1871–1876.
113. Bunn PA Jr, Nugent JL, Ihde DC, et al: 5-fluorouracil, methyl CCNU, Adriamycin and mitomycin C in the treatment of advanced gastric cancer. *Cancer Treat Rep* 1987; 62:1287–1293.
114. Cunningham D, Soukop M, McArdle CS, et al: Advanced gastric cancer: Experience in Scotland using 5-fluorouracil, adriamycin and mitomycin-c. *Br J Surg* 1984; 71:673–676.
115. Moertel CG, Lavin PT: Phase II-III chemotherapy studies in advanced gastric cancer. *Cancer Treat Rep* 1979; 63:1863–1869.
116. Kemeny N: The systemic chemotherapy of hepatic metastases. *Semin Oncol* 1983; 10:148–59.
117. Breedis C, Young C: The blood supply of neoplasms in the liver. *Am J Pathol* 1954; 30:969.

118. Sigurdson ER, Ridge JA, Kemeny N, et al: Tumor and liver drug uptake following hepatic artery and portal vein infusion. *J Clin Oncol* 1987; 5:1836–1840.
119. Chen HSG, Gross JF: Intra-arterial infusion of anti-cancer drugs: Theoretic aspects of drug delivery and review of responses. *Cancer Treat Rep* 1980; 64:31–40.
120. Ensminger WD, Rosowsky A, Raso V: A clinical pharmacological evaluation of hepatic arterial infusions of 5-fluoro-2-deoxyuridine and 5-fluorouracil. *Cancer Res* 1978; 38:3784–3792.
121. Ensminger WD, Gyves JW: Clinical pharmacology of hepatic arterial chemotherapy. *Semin Oncol* 1983; 10:176–183.
122. Collins JM: Pharmacologic rationale for regional drug delivery. *J Clin Oncol* 1984; 2:498–504.
123. Collins JM: Pharmacologic rationale for hepatic arterial therapy. *Rec Res Can Res* 1986; 100:140–148.
124. Tandon RN, Bunnel IL, Copper RG: The treatment of metastatic carcinoma of the liver by percutaneous selective hepatic artery infusion of 5-fluorouracil. *Surgery* 1973; 73:118.
125. Ansfield FJ, Ramirez G, Davis HL Jr, et al: Further clinical studies with intrahepatic arterial infusion with 5-fluorouracil. *Cancer* 1975; 36:2413–2417.
126. Buroker T, Samson M, Correa J, et al: Hepatic artery infusion of 5-FUDR after prior systemic 5-fluorouracil. *Cancer Treat Rep* 1976; 60:1277–1279.
127. Oberfield RA, McCaffrey JA, Polio J, et al: Prolonged and continuous percutaneous intra-arterial hepatic infusion chemotherapy in advanced metastatic liver adenocarcinoma from colorectal primary. *Cancer* 1979; 44:414–423.
128. Watkins E Jr, Khazei AM, Nahra KS: Surgical basis for arterial infusion chemotherapy of disseminated carcinoma of the liver. *Surg Gynecol Obstet* 1970; 130:581.
129. Cady B, Oberfield RA: Regional infusion chemotherapy of hepatic metastases from carcinoma of the colon. *Am J Surg* 1974; 127:220–227.
130. Cady B: Hepatic arterial patency and complications after catheterization for infusion chemotherapy. *Ann Surg* 1973; 178:145–161.
131. Massey WH, Fletcher WS, Judkins MP: Hepatic artery infusion for metastatic malignancy using percutaneously placed catheters. *Am J Surg* 1971; 121:160–164.
132. Petrek JA, Minton JP: Treatment of hepatic metastases by percutaneous hepatic arterial infusin. *Cancer* 1979; 43:2182–2188.
133. Reed ML, Vaitkevicius VK, Al-Sarraf M, et al: The practicality of chronic hepatic artery infusion therapy of primary and metastatic hepatic malignancies. *Cancer* 1981, pp 47–402.
134. Smiley S, Schouten J, Chang A, et al: Intrahepatic arterial infusion with 5-FU for liver metastases of colorectal carcinoma. *Proc Am Soc Clin Oncol* 1981; 22:391.
135. Buchwald H, Grage TB, Vassilopoulos PP, et al: Intraarterial infusion chemotherapy for hepatic carcinoma using a totally implantable infusion pump. *Cancer* 1980; 45:866–869.
136. Ensminger W, Niederhuber J, Dakhil S, et al: Totally implanted drug delivery system for hepatic arterial chemotherapy. *Cancer Treat Rep* 1981; 65:393.
137. Kemeny N, Daly J, Oderman P, et al: Hepatic artery pump infusion toxicity

and results in patients with metastatic colorectal carcinoma. *J Clin Oncol* 1984; 2:595–600.
138. Hohn DC, Stagg RJ, Price DC, et al: Avoidance of gastroduodenal toxicity in patients receiving hepatic arterial 5-fluoro-2′-deoxyuridine. *J Clin Oncol* 1985; 3:1257–1260.
139. Ensminger W, Niederhuber J, Gyves J, et al: Effective control of liver metastases from colon cancer with an implanted system for hepatic arterial chemotherapy. *Proc ASCO* 1982; 1:94.
140. Niederhuber JE, Ensminger W, et al: Regional chemotherapy of colorectal cancer metastatic to the liver. *Cancer* 1984; 53:1336.
141. Balch CM, Urist MM: Intraarterial chemotherapy for colorectal liver metastases and hepatomas using a totally implantable drug infusion pump. *Rec Res Can Res* 1986; 100:123–147.
142. Shepard KV, Levin B, Karl RC, et al: Therapy for metastatic colorectal cancer with hepatic artery infusion chemotherapy using a subcutaneous implanted pump. *J Clin Oncol* 1985; 3:161.
143. Cohen AM, Kaufman SD, Wood WC, et al: Regional hepatic chemotherapy using an implantable drug infusion pump. *Am J Surg* 1983; 145:529–533.
144. Weiss GR, Garnick MB, Osteen R, et al: Long-term hepatic arterial infusion of 5-fluorodeoxyuridine for liver metastases using an implantable infusion pump. *J Clin Oncol* 1983; 1:337–344.
145. Schwartz SI, Jones LS, McCune CS: Assessment of treatment of intrahepatic malignancies using chemotherapy via an implantable pump. *Ann Surg* 1985; 201:560–567.
146. Johnson LP, Wasserman PB, Rivkin SE: FUDR hepatic arterial infusion via an implantable pump for treatment of hepatic tumor. *Proc Am Soc Clin Oncol* 1983; 2:119.
147. Kemeny MM, Goldberg D, Beatty JD, et al: Results of a prospective randomized trial of continuous regional chemotherapy and hepatic resection as treatment of hepatic metastases from colorectal primaries. *Cancer* 1986; 57:492.
148. Ramming KP, O'Toole K: The use of the implantable chemoinfusion pump in the treatment of hepatic metastases of colorectal cancer. *Arch Surg* 1986; 121:1440–1444.
149. Hohn DC, Melnick J, Stagg R, et al: Biliary sclerosis in patients receiving hepatic arterial infusions of fluorodeoxycridine. *J Clin Oncol* 1985; 3:98–102.
150. Doria MI Jr, Shepard KV, Levin B, et al: Liver pathology following hepatic arterial infusion chemotherapy. *Cancer* 1986; 58:855–861.
151. Guck WI, Akwari OE, Kelvin FM, et al: A reversible enteropathy complicating continuous hepatic artery infusion chemotherapy with 5-fluoro 2-deoxyuridine. *Cancer* 1985; 56:424.
152. Kemeny N, Daly J, Oderman P, et al: Prognostic variables in patients with hepatic metastases from colorectal cancer: Importance of medical assessment of liver involvement. *Proc ASCO* 1985; 4:88.
153. Kemeny N, Braun DW: Prognostic factors in advanced colorectal carcinoma: The importance of lactic dehydrogenase, performance status, and white blood cell count. *Am J Med* 1983; 74:786–794.
154. Chang AE, Schneider PD, Sugarbaker PH: A prospective randomized trial of regional versus systemic continuous 5-fluorodeoxyuridine chemotherapy in the treatment of colorectal liver metastases. *Ann Surg* 1987; 206:685–693.

155. Niederhuber JE: Arterial chemotherapy for metastatic colorectal cancer in the liver. Conference Advantages in Regional Cancer Therapy. Giessen, West Germany, 1985.
156. Kemeny N, Daly J, Reichman B, et al: Intrahepatic or systemic infusion of fluorodeoxyuridine in patients with liver metastases from colorectal carcinoma. *Ann Intern Med* 1987; 107:459–465.
157. Hohn D, Stagg R, Friedman M, et al: The NCOG randomized trial of intravenous (IV) vs hepatic arterial (IA) FUDR for colorectal cancer metastatic to the liver. *Proc ASCO* 1987; 6:85.
158. Reed GB, Cox AJ: The human liver after radiation injury. *Am J Pathol* 1966; 46:597–611.
159. Ingold JA, Reed GB, Kaplan HS, et al: Radiation hepatitis. *AJR* 1965; 93:200–208.
160. Prasad B, Lee M, Hendrickson FR: Irradiation of hepatic metastases. *Int J Radiat Oncol Biol Phys* 1977; 2:129–132.
161. Borgelt BB, Gelber R, Brady LW, et al: The palliation of hepatic metastases: Results of Radiation Therapy Oncology Group pilot study. *Int J Radiat Oncol Biol Phys* 1981; 7:587–591.
162. Sherman DM, et al: Palliation of hepatic metastases. *Cancer* 1978; 41:2013–2017.
163. Barone RM, Calabro-Jones P, Thomas TN, et al: Surgical adjuvant therapy in colon carcinoma: A human tumor spheroid model for evaluating radiation sensitizing agents. *Cancer* 1981; 47:2349–2357.
164. Moertel DG, Childs PS, Reitmeier PJ, et al: Combined 5-fluorouracil and supervoltage radiation therapy of locally unresectable gastrointestinal cancer. *Lancet* 1969; 2:865–867.
165. Webber BM, Sodergerg CH, Leone LA, et al: A combined treatment approach to management of hepatic metastases. *Cancer* 1978; 42:1087–1095.
166. Raju PI, Maruama Y, DeSimone P, et al: Treatment of liver metastases with a combination of chemotherapy and hyperfractionated external radiation therapy. *Am J Clin Oncol* 1987; 10:41–43.
167. Barone RM, Byfield JE, Goldfarb PB, et al: Intra-arterial chemotherapy using an implantable infusion pump and liver irradiation for the treatment of hepatic metastases. *Cancer* 1982; 50:850–862.
168. Herbsman H, Gardner B, Harshaw D, et al: Treatment of hepatic metastases with a combination of hepatic artery infusion chemotherapy and external radiotherapy. *Surg Gynecol Obstet* 1978; 147:13–17.
169. Rothman M, Kuruvilla AM, Choi K, et al: Response of colorectal hepatic metastases to concomitant radiation therapy and intravenous infusion 5-fluorouracil. *Int J Radiat Oncol Biol Phys* 1986; 12:2179–2187.
170. Lokich K, Kinsella T, Perri J, et al: Concomitant hepatic radiation and intra-arterial fluorinated pryimidine therapy: Correlation of liver scan, liver function tests, and plasma CEA with tumor response. *Cancer* 1982; 48:2569–2574.
171. Gansl RC, Hippolito J, Cutait R, et al: Treatment of liver metastatic colorectal carcinoma with sequential methotrexate (MTX), fluorouracil (5-FU) and external hepatic radiation. *Proc ASCO* 1986; 5:94.
172. Friedman MA, Cassidy MJ, Levine M, et al: Combined modality therapy of hepatic metastases. *Cancer* 1979; 44:906–913.
173. Yablonski-Peretz T, Freund H, Chisin R, et al: Toxic hepatitis: A complication of intra-arterial chemotherapy (IAC) and radiotherapy (XRT) for liver metastases. *Eur Soc Ther Radiol Oncol* Sept 9–15, 1984, p 307.

174. Dritschillo A, Grant EG, Harter KW, et al: Interstitial radiation therapy for hepatic metastases: Sonographic guidance for applicator placement. *AJR* 1986; 147:275–278.
175. Markowitz J: The hepatic artery. *Surg Gynecol Obstet* 1952; 95:644–646.
176. Almersjo O, Bengmark S, Rudenstam CM: Evaluation of hepatic dearterialization in primary and secondary cancer of the liver. *Am J Surg* 1972; 124:509.
177. Balasegaram M: Complete hepatic dearterialization for primary carcinomas of the liver: Report of 24 patients. *Am J Surg* 1972; 124:340–345.
178. Larmi TKI, Karkola P, et al: Treatment of patients with hepatic tumors and jaundice by ligation of the hepatic artery. *Arch Surg* 1974; 108:178–183.
179. Petrelli NJ, Barcewicz PA, Evans JT, et al: Hepatic artery ligation for liver metastasis in colorectal carcinoma. *Cancer* 1984; 53:1347–1353.
180. Didoklar MS, Elias EG, Whitley NO, et al: Unresectable hepatic metastases from carcinoma of the colon and rectum. *Surg Gynecol Obstet* 1985; 160:429–436.
181. Ramming KP, Sparks FC, Eilber FR, et al: Hepatic artery ligation and f-fluorouracil infusion for metastatic colon carcinoma and primary hepatoma. *Am J Surg* 1976; 132:236–242.
182. Sparks FC, Mosher MB, Hallauer WC, et al: Hepatic artery ligation and postoperative chemotherapy for hepatic metastases: Clinical and pathophysiological results. *Cancer* 1975; 35:1074–1082.
183. Koudahl G, Funding J: Hepatic artery ligation in primary and secondary hepatic cancer. *Acta Chir Scand* 1972: 138:289–292.
184. Zike WL, Safaie-Shirazi S, Gluesserian HP, et al: Hepatic artery ligation and cytoxic infusion in treatment of liver neoplasms. *Arch Surg* 1975; 110:641–643.
185. Fortner JG, Mulcare RJ, Solis A, et al: Treatment of primary and secondary liver cancer by hepatic artery ligation and infusion chemotherapy. *Ann Surg* 1973; 178:162–172.
186. Cuschieri A, Swain C: Hepatic artery ligation and prolonged cytotoxic therapy in advanced primary and secondary liver tumors. *Proc Soc Med* 1975; 68:678–680.
187. Laufman LR, Nims TA, Guy JT: Hepatic artery ligation and portal vein infusion for liver metastases from colon cancer. *J Clin Oncol* 1984; 12:1382–1389.
188. Carrasco H, Cuang VP, Wallace S: Apudomas metastatic to the liver: Treatment by hepatic artery embolization. *Radiology* 1983; 149:79–83.
189. Maton PN, Camilleri M, Griffin G: Role of hepatic arterial embolization in the carcinoid syndrome. *Br J Med* 1983; 287:932–935.
190. Moertel CG, May GR, Martin JK, et al: Sequential hepatic artery occlusion (HAO) and chemotherapy for metastatic carcinoid tumor and islet cell carcinoma (ICC). *Proc ASCO* 1985; 4:80.
191. Allison DJ, Modlin IM, Jenkins WJ: Treatment of carcinoid liver metastases by hepatic artery embolization. *Lancet* 1977; 2:1323–1325.
192. Aronsen KF, Hellenkant C, Holmberg J, et al: Controlled blocking of hepatic artery flow with enzymatically degradable microspheres combined with oncolytic drugs. *Eur Surg Res* 1979; 11:99–106.
193. Ziessman HA, Thrall JH, Ensminger WD, et al: Quantitative hepatic arterial perfusion scintigraphy and starch microspheres in cancer chemotherapy. *J Nucl Med* 1983; 24:871–875.

194. Lindell B, Aronsen KF, Nosslin B, et al: Studies in pharmacokinetics and tolerance of substances temporarily retained in the liver by microsphere embolization. *Ann Surg* 1978; 187:95–99.
195. Aronsen KF, Teder H: Indications and therapeutic possibilities using degradable microspheres in liver malignancies: Recent results in cancer research. 1986; 100:283–288.
196. Gyves JW, Ensminger WD, Van Harken D, et al: Improved regional selectivity of hepatic arterial BCNU with degradable microspheres. *Clin Pharmacol Ther* 1983; 34:259–265.
197. Parker G, Regelson W: Treatment of primary and secondary liver cancers with intra-arterial chemotherapy mixed with biodegradable starch microspheres. *Proc ASOC* 1985; 4:90.
198. Dakil S, Ensminger W, Cho K, et al: Improved regional selectivity of hepatic arterial BCNU with degradable microspheres. *Cancer* 1982; 50:631–635.
199. Grady ED, McLaren J, Auda SP, et al: Combination of internal radiation therapy and hyperthermia to treat liver cancer. *South Med J* 1983; 76:1101–1105.
200. Ariel IM, Padula G: Treatment of symptomatic metastatic cancer to the liver from primary colon and rectal cancer by the intra-arterial administration of chemotherapy and radioactive isotopes. *J Surg Oncol* 1978; 10:327–335.
201. Mantravadi RVP, Spigos DG, Tan WS, et al: Intra-arterial yttrium 90 in the treatment of hepatic malignancy. *Radiology* 1982; 142:783–786.
202. Kemeny MM, Goldberg D, Beatty JD, et al: Results of a prospective randomized trial of continuous regional chemotherapy and hepatic resection as treatment of hepatic metastases from colorectal primaries. *Cancer* 1986; 57:492–498.
203. Ravikumar TS, Kane R, Jenkins RL, et al: Hepatic cryosurgery with intraoperative ultrasound monitoring for metastatic colon carcinoma. *Arch Surg* 1987; 122:403–409.
204. Onik G, Kane R, Steele G, et al: Monitoring hepatic cryosurgery with sonography. *AJR* 1986; 147:665–669.
205. Livraghi T, Festi D, Monti F, et al: US-guided percutaneous alcohol injection of small hepatic and abdominal tumors. *Radiology* 1986; 161:309–312.

The Surgical Management of AIDS and HIV-Infected Patients

Anthony A. Meyer, M.D., Ph.D.

Associate Professor of Surgery, University of North Carolina; Director, Surgical Intensive Care Unit, Medical Director of Critical Care, North Carolina Memorial Hospital, Assistant Director, North Carolina Jaycees Burn Center, Chapel Hill, North Carolina

The disease complex known as acquired immunodeficiency syndrome (AIDS) has had unprecedented effects on physicians, their patients, and society in general. The incidence of cases and deaths from the disease has increased unrelentingly and thus made this one of our major health problems. Increasing amounts of patient care and research resources are being committed to this problem. Despite the technological capabilities that have provided so much information about this disease, little has been achieved to control it. This has been complicated by political and social considerations that turned attention away from the medical aspects of this serious problem. The public and even some physicians pay more attention to sensationalized reports and the social and moral implications of some groups at high risk for the disease than they do to the facts. It is essential to understand this new disease, its biology, patterns of infection, and methods to limit its spread, if it is to be dealt with successfully. Surgeons have specific reasons to acquire an understanding about AIDS and all its related states. They need this understanding to treat their patients responsibly while protecting themselves and their fellow health care workers.

Acquired Immunodeficiency Syndrome: A Definition

Acquired immunodeficiency syndrome is the most severe expression of immunocompromise following infection with human immunodeficiency virus (HIV). Acquired immunodeficiency syndrome was first diagnosed as a clinical entity in 1981 after several reports of Kaposi's sarcoma and pneumocystis pneumonia in homosexual men and intravenous (IV) drug users without other explanation.[1] Retrospective review of clinical cases and some blood and tissue samples have documented the disease in the United States at least as early as 1978.[2] Occasional earlier cases have been de-

Adv Surg 22:57–74, 1989

0065-3411/89/22-057–074-$04.00

scribed, but AIDS, in its epidemic form in the United States, started in the late 1970s.

The epidemiology of AIDS and its near confinement to groups at greatly increased risk for hepatitis led investigators to look for an infectious agent as its cause. In 1983 Montagnier et al. at the Pasteur Institute in Paris described a virus isolated from lymph tissue from an AIDS patient and named it lymphadenopathy-associated virus (LAV).[3] In 1984 Gallo et al. at the National Institutes of Health described a virus cultured from AIDS patients that was related to human T-cell lymphotropic virus and identified it as HTLV-III.[4] The initial name given for the virus accepted to be the cause of AIDS was HTLV-III/LAV. Claims and accusations over who discovered the virus continued in the press and the courts until a joint French/United States committee ascribed discovery rights to both teams. The decision has not totally laid the issue to rest. The name of the virus was changed by the International Committee for the Taxonomy of Viruses to human immunodeficiency virus (HIV), the accepted scientific name.[5]

Human immunodeficiency virus is a retrovirus, an RNA virus that infects cells and achieves its reproduction by synthesis of DNA template from its RNA. This is accomplished with the reverse transcriptase coded in the viral genome. In this respect HIV is similar to other tumor viruses. The mechanisms of cell-to-cell transmission of virus are unknown, but must be elucidated to determine if a vaccine is possible.[6]

Human immunodeficiency virus selectively attacks the helper/inducer (T_4) lymphocytes by binding the T_4 cellular antigen with the major envelope glycoprotein gp 120.[7, 8] These T_4 cells die when HIV replication occurs, leading to progressive depletion of this important cellular subgroup. Without the helper/inducer cells, cellular immunity is impaired. The clinical state of immunosuppression is expressed by susceptibility to uncommon tumors and infections.[9, 10] Other immune functions, such as antibody synthesis, are relatively unaffected.[11]

A great deal of the molecular and cellular events that follow HIV infection remain unknown. Estimates of the period between infection and clinical manifestation of disease have continued to change. Estimates of this incubation period have ranged from 27 months in clinical series to 54 months by mathematical models.[12, 13]

Patients infected by HIV do not always present clinically with a diagnosis of AIDS. Lesser stages of immunosuppression such as diffuse adenopathy have been classified as AIDS-related complex (ARC). Present data suggest that all patients with ARC will eventually progress to a diagnosis of AIDS.[20]

The time period between infection with HIV and development of AIDS can also be associated with lesser states of immunodeficiency. The Walter Reed Staging Classification was designed to provide a system to identify these intermediate stages following HIV infection.[14] Furthermore, this system sought to correlate clinical states with specific laboratory diagnoses based upon the number of T_4 lymphocytes in the peripheral blood. Unfortunately, the laboratory results did not consistently correlate with the clinical stages in the Walter Reed Staging Classification.

The definition of AIDS has continued to evolve from its initial reliance on clinical diagnoses to a flexible system that takes into account laboratory evidence of HIV infection.[10] This revised case definition is presented in Table 1. This new definition can be fitted into the existing classification system for the stages of immunosuppression reported by the Centers for Disease Control (CDC) and listed in Table 2.[15] Group III patients represent ARC, while group IV patients are generally those with diseases diagnostic of AIDS, described in more detail in Table 1. Although these definitions and classification systems may change as new information is obtained, they provide a framework to identify patients and follow their disease. The number of HIV-infected patients who will eventually develop AIDS appears to be at least 70%. Continued follow-up of HIV-infected patients and a strict definition of AIDS is needed to better evaluate the natural history of infection with this virus.

Acquired immunodeficiency syndrome has been recognized as a universally fatal disease. However, as in other fatal diseases, the longevity of individual patients varies considerably, and appears to have increased.[16] Survival is directly related to the disease manifestation of AIDS in each patient. In all patients once AIDS has been diagnosed, one-year survival is 49% and five-year survival is 15%.[16] The length of survival may eventually be increased further by new drugs such as AZT, which are antiviral agents.[17] Successful treatment of the infections and malignancies that make up the spectrum of AIDS, along with correction of antiviral therapy, is the present goal for treatment of this disease.

There is some evidence that patients in different high-risk groups have different incubation periods as well as different frequencies of clinical problems related to immunodeficiency.[18] Hemophiliacs have a lower incidence of *Pneumocystis carinii* pneumonia than homosexuals.[19, 20] Additional studies have revealed some relationship between expression of specific proteins, antibody response to those proteins, and the severity of immunosuppression of T_4 cells.[18]

Diagnosis of AIDS and HIV Infection

Infection with this virus leads to antibody synthesis against envelope and core antigens. Detection of such antibody by an enzyme-linked immunosorbent assay (ELISA) technique has provided the test presently used to screen patients. The sensitivity of the test varies with the manufacturer, but the percentage of false negatives is less than 1%. The relative specificity of the test, however, is dependent on the prevalence of infection in the population. False positives are a more fixed number, so if the prevalence of infection is only 0.2%, 72% of ELISA positives will be false positives. If the prevalence is 2%, only 20% will be false positive.[21, 22]

TABLE 1.
Case Definition for AIDS (Revised 1987)

I. No HIV test or inconclusive results
   A. In the absence of HIV tests or if the results of HIV tests are inconclusive, and the patient had none of the following:
      1. Steroids or other immunosuppressive therapy in the last 3 months
      2. A primary lymphoreticular or histiocytic malignancy (except brain lymphoma)
      3. Congenital or an acquired immunodeficiency not typical of that induced by HIV infection
   B. The diagnosis of AIDS is made by definitive diagnosis of one of the following *indicator diseases.*
      1. Infections
         a. *Pneumocystis carinii* pneumonia
         b. Extrapulmonary cryptococcosis
         c. Candidiasis of the esophagus, trachea, bronchi, or lungs
         d. *Mycobacterium avium* or *kansasii* in a site outside the lungs, skin, or cervical lymph nodes
         e. Cryptosporidiosis with diarrhea lasting more than 1 month
         f. In patients greater than 1 month of age
            1) Toxoplasmosis of the brain
            2) Herpes simplex infection with bronchitis, esophagitis, or pneumonitis; or mucocutaneous ulcer for more than 1 month's duration
      2. Tumors
         a. Kaposi's sarcoma in a patient less than 60 years old
         b. Primary brain lymphoma in a patient less than 60 years old
      3. Other
         a. Progressive multifocal leukoencephalopathy
         b. Lymphoid interstitial pneumonia or pulmonary lymphoid hyperplasia in a child younger than 3

II. Laboratory evidence of HIV infection
   A. With laboratory evidence of HIV infection, definitive diagnosis of one of the following indicator diseases is diagnostic of AIDS:
      1. *Infections*
         a. Recurrent or multiple bacterial infections by *Hemophilus, Streptococcus,* or other pyogenic bacteria causing septicemia, meningitis, pneumonia, bone or joint infection, or abscess of an internal organ or body cavity
         b. Recurrent *Salmonella* septicemia (nontyphoid)
         c. Mycobacteria infection outside the lungs (except for atypical mycobacteria in the cervical or hilar lymph nodes or the skin)
         d. Histoplasmosis, disseminated beyond the lungs and cervical or hilar lymph nodes coccidioidomycosis, disseminated

2. *Tumors*
    a. Kaposi's sarcoma at any age
    b. Lymphoma of the brain (primary)
    c. Non-Hodgkin's lymphomas of the Burkitt or immunoblastic sarcoma type
3. *Other*
    a. HIV encephalopathy (or dementia)
    b. HIV-wasting syndrome

B. With laboratory evidence of HIV infections, even presumptive diagnosis of any of the following is considered diagnostic of AIDS:
1. Infection
    a. *Pneumocystis carinii* pneumonia
    b. Candidiasis of the esophagus
    c. Cytomegalovirus retinitis
    d. Mycobacterial infection (disseminated)
    e. Toxoplasmosis of the brain in a patient older than 1 month of age
2. Tumor
    a. Kaposi's sarcoma
3. Other
    a. Lymphoid interstitial pneumonia or pulmonary lymphoid hyperplasia in a child under 13 years of age

III. Laboratory evidence against HIV infections

A. If laboratory tests fail to show any evidence of HIV infection, the diagnosis of AIDS may still be made if the following are present:
1. All other causes of immunodeficiency have been excluded, *and*
2. The patient has *Pneumocystis carinii* pneumonia, *or*
3. The patient has a T-helper/inducer lymphocyte count of less than 400/cu mm *and* has any of the indicator diseases listed in first section of table.

Because of the high incidence of false positives, laboratory diagnosis of infection by HIV is not made without a Western blot test. This involves testing serum for antibody to specific protein components of HIV separated on a polyacrylamide gel. Presently, antibody to protein 24 (p24) and glycoprotein 41 (gp41) are considered diagnostic of HIV infection. The incidence of false positives using the Western blot assay is less than 0.3%, even with a prevalence of only 0.2% infection in the population.[22]

Unlike other infections where antibody identifies patients who have recovered from infection and are immune to further problems from that virus, antibody to HIV confers no immunity. In fact, the presence of antibody identifies a person who is infectious.

Although most patients develop antibody to HIV within 12 weeks of infection, some patients may not have positive tests for a year; some even develop AIDS before they become seropositive.[23] This has limited the ability to rely on a negative HIV test as evidence of absence of HIV infection.

TABLE 2.
Classification System for HIV Infection

GROUP I: Acute infection (will eventually move to another group)
GROUP II: Asymptomatic infection
GROUP III: Persistent generalized lymphadenopathy
GROUP IV: Other diseases (outlined and updated in Table 1)

Subgroup A.—Constitutional disease (fever, weight loss, or diarrhea for more than 1 month without other disease)

Subgroup B.—Neurologic disease (dementia, myelopathy, or peripheral neuropathy without other cause)

Subgroup C.—Secondary infectious disease (moderately indicative of a defect in cell-mediated immunity)

Category C1.—Infectious disease presently accepted as diagnostic of AIDS (see Table 3)

Category C2.—Symptomatic or invasive oral hairy leukoplakia, multidermatomal herpes zoster, recurrent salmonella bactermia, nocardiosis, tuberculosis, or oral candidiasis (thrush)

Subgroup D.—Secondary cancers (see Table 3)

Subgroup E.—Other conditions in HIV infection (disease not previously listed, suggestive of impaired cell-mediated immunity, such as chronic lymphoid interstitial pneumonitis)

New tests are being developed and tested, including a test for HIV antigen, which would be positive earlier and would not rely on generation of antibodies to HIV.

Additional concern over present testing systems arises from mutation of HIV. Alternation in antigenic expression may occur without a change in virulence. Such an event could allow infectious cases to be falsely identified as noninfectious. Continued study of the virus and its mutations will assist in limiting the likelihood of such an event.

Epidemiology of HIV Infection

From the initial distribution of AIDS cases, it was apparent that the disease had an infectious component. Like hepatitis B and other sexually transmitted diseases, AIDS most often occurred in patients exposed percutaneously to blood or to body fluids from many different individuals. Because of this pattern, people at high risk of AIDS fell into several groups (Table 3). These are the same groups at high risk of hepatitis B. Practices that place individuals at increased risk include unprotected sexual intercourse with an HIV-infected partner, sharing needles from HIV-infected

TABLE 3.
Groups at High Risk for HIV Infection and AIDS

Homosexual and bisexual men
Intravenous drug users
Children of HIV-infected mother
Persons transferred with HIV-contaminated blood or blood products
Heterosexual contacts of HIV-infected partners

drug users, infusion of blood or blood products from HIV-infected donors, or parturition from an HIV-infected mother. It is important to remember, however, that infection does not occur by casual contact. Multiple studies of people living with AIDS victims have identified no infection without blood exposure or sexual contact.[12, 24, 25] Fortunately, HIV is not a highly infectious agent.

The number of known AIDS cases in the United States as of October 1987 is over 35,000 and the number of HIV-infected individuals is estimated at 1 to 1.5 million. Over 95% of these cases involve persons in the high-risk groups shown in Table 3. Initial concern about rapid spread of HIV into the general population, exaggerated by media attention, has not been documented. Although heterosexual transmission accounts for a significant percentage of new HIV infection in Haiti and Africa, the rate remains low in the United States. Furthermore, the increases in heterosexual transmission in the United States are associated with sexual partners of IV drug users. Unreported IV drug use and prostitution cannot be ruled out as another possible means of HIV transmission in many of these cases. There will always be a percentage of cases where high-risk practices, which may actually be the cause of infection, are denied.

Evidence to support limited infectivity through heterosexual exposure is found in the long-term sexual partners of HIV-infected hemophiliacs. Despite exposure through unprotected intercourse for at least one year, HIV infection occurred in only 16% of sexual partners.[26]

Close monitoring of heterosexual transmission of HIV will have to continue.[12] Since many of our projections are based on a new and evolving disease, future facts may permit correction of present assumptions.

Another area of intense epidemiologic concern involves infection of HIV through occupational exposure to AIDS and HIV-infected patients. Occupational exposure to health care workers presents a considerable problem, but the degree of risk has not been adequately determined. Health care workers most likely to be at risk would be those most frequently exposed to body fluids, especially blood. Even greater risk would be encountered if such exposure would occur in uncontrolled situations. As was seen with AIDS, such risk would generally follow the degree of risk of infection with hepatitis B virus. Groups of health care workers most likely to be at risk for occupational infection with HIV are listed in Table 4. Concern about occupational exposure to HIV has prompted recent articles for clinicians in fields where such risk might be increased.[27–29]

Fortunately, HIV transmission is much less likely than that of hepatitis B. Accidental percutaneous exposure to blood from an individual with infectious hepatitis B results in transmission in at least 15% of cases.[30] Three studies of nearly 800 health care workers with injury by needles from HIV-positive patients have identified seroconversion in four who denied other risk factors.[22] In addition, infection of health care workers has occurred without needlestick injury when infected blood came in contact with open lesions.[31]

These infrequent but well-documented cases do confirm the concern that HIV can infect health care workers through occupational transmission. Although very uncommon (a less than 0.6% chance of infection with needlestick injury), the risk is real and the fears are understandable. Furthermore, there is no doubt that additional cases of occupational HIV infection will occur. One to 1.5 million people in the United States are infected with HIV. All actively working health care personnel will be involved in the management of these patients. In order to minimize these risks, the role of the surgeon in management of AIDS and HIV-infected patients and means of limiting risk of occupational infection by HIV will be reviewed.

Direct Surgical Concerns in AIDS and HIV-Infected Patients

The goals for surgeons in the management of patients in this era of AIDS and HIV infection should be provision of optimal care while limiting risks to the patients and health care workers, including themselves. In order to meet those goals surgeons must know the role they play in the treatment of AIDS and HIV-infected patients; as well as the measures available to protect patients and hospital staff.

Protection of patients has been dramatically improved by screening blood donations by testing for antibody to HIV. This has decreased the risk of infection of units of blood to approximately 1:50,000. The rapid development and adoption of this test have largely eliminated blood transfusions as a risk for HIV transmission. The inability to identify HIV in some units because of delay in antibody response is a problem. This is presently addressed by excluding all high-risk groups from donation. The development of a test for HIV antigen may further limit the likelihood of transmission by blood products by eliminating the need for antibody response in the donor.

TABLE 4.
Health Care Workers at Greatest Risk for Occupational HIV Infection

Frequent blood exposure
Dialysis nurses and technicians
Laboratory technicians who handle blood samples
Exposure to blood in uncontrolled situations
Emergency room personnel
Trauma, vascular and cardiac surgeons, and obstetricians

Patients receiving organ transplants have also been at some risk for HIV from the organ or tissue. This has been addressed by using the same procedures used for blood transfusion to screen organ donors.

A final area of patient risk is infection from blood or body fluids of a health care worker during an invasive procedure. Such infection has not been documented, nor is it likely to occur. Still, CDC recommendations suggest that health care workers infected by HIV refrain from patient care procedures that might put a patient at risk for infection. Legislation has been proposed, but not passed, that would require all health care workers to be tested periodically for HIV infection to protect patients against possible infection from them.[32]

The role of surgeons in the management of AIDS patients can be separated into diagnostic, provision of supportive care, and management of complications requiring surgical evaluation and treatment.[33] With the availability of serologic tests for HIV, the diagnosis of AIDS does not usually require a surgical procedure. However, it may be necessary to identify the disease that is the result of severe immunosuppression in order to provide appropriate treatment of specific malignancies and certain infections. Such procedures are indicated when the diagnosis will alter treatment or provide important, useful information that cannot be obtained by other methods. The decision to do such diagnostic procedures should involve attending-level surgeons and physicians who can best appreciate the potential risks and benefits.

Patients with AIDS may require supportive care to assist medical treatment of their immunosuppression-associated diseases. Chronic venous access is often needed for long-term antifungal and antibiotic therapy for infections, and occasionally for chemotherapy. The efficacy of such treatment in improved survival with quality of life is unknown, but will be determined with further studies. Selection of patients to undergo such procedures must always be preceded by the consideration of whether or not the treatment will truly benefit the patients. Presently, clinical judgment and common sense must be used for these decisions. Again, such a decision should be made by physicians and surgeons at the attending level.

Patients with AIDS also develop complications that require surgical management. These may include simple cutaneous abscesses, life-threatening injuries, or intraabdominal catastrophes. Treatment of the complications is no different than for any patient. However, as would be done in the case of a patient with metastatic cancer, some consideration should be given to the likelihood of the procedure to affect the ultimate outcome. If a patient with AIDS has no realistic chance of short-term survival from his or her primary disease, treatment of a life-threatening complication may be a disservice to the patient, besides exposing health care personnel to a risk with no real chance of patient benefit. As in the other scenarios, attending involvement in such decision-making is crucial. Too frequently, such decisions are put off because they are uncomfortable to make, and then they are not made when acute problems arise because of rapid evolution of events.

Surgeons will also have a role in the treatment of HIV-infected patients without AIDS, frequently without knowing it. The majority of HIV-infected patients do not have AIDS and will not be easily separated from noninfected patients. Despite attempts to screen patients and avoid contact with HIV-infected patients, it is likely that all clinically active surgeons will treat them. These patients will often be seen for treatment of routine problems, or problems associated with the risk factors that led them to be infected with HIV, such as subcutaneous abscesses in an IV drug user or degenerative joint disease from bleeding in a hemophiliac. These standard operations on HIV-infected patient without AIDS will probably constitute the greatest number of procedures on all patients in the infectious population.

Some surgeons have recently been criticized publicly for refusing to operate on HIV-positive patients. This arbitrary denial of care is contrary to guidelines described by the American Medical Association (AMA) and the CDC.[22, 34] Such a broad inflexible position does not seem ethically tenable given the surgeon's commitment to patients and their care; and yet every surgeon who knows about AIDS and HIV infection must be concerned. Although initial studies did not document occupational infection, the risk, though very small, is irrefutable. Assurance that these risks are small by physicians who are at no risk of occupational infection because they do not have much patient contact and do not do invasive procedures may seem hollow at best to those who have such exposure, especially in locales with increased incidence of HIV infection in the patient population. As surgeons we must understand there is a small degree of risk and employ means to minimize it rather than flee our responsibility or ignore the risks. Furthermore, adopting a posture of not operating on AIDS or HIV-positive patients is an ostrich approach to a serious problem. Surgeons who adopt this attitude are deluding themselves if they think they can eliminate HIV-infectious patients from their practice. Because of the variable incubation periods and lack of 100% accuracy in testing, a small but real number of patients will be infectious despite negative results. False assumptions that their patients are "safe" may lead those surgeons to put themselves and others at unnecessary increased risk because of inadequate adherence to recommended safety measures.

Another concern regarding surgery on AIDS and HIV-infected patients is that such procedures might be assigned to the most junior members of the surgical group or service. Concentration of the risk to an individual or small group cannot be justified. Furthermore, assignment of a case to a resident not sufficiently skillful at that procedure increases the risk of injury and occupational infection. In cases where the patient is known to be HIV-infected, the surgery should be performed by someone with adequate experience to limit risk for everyone.

Methods of Avoiding Occupational Infection By HIV

Infection by HIV does not occur by casual contact.[12, 24, 25] Examining or talking to a patient infected by HIV does not put physicians or other health care personnel at risk of infection. Occupational infection, like all other situations of infection by HIV, result from exposure to blood or body fluids. Preventing occupational infection, therefore, centers on avoiding such exposure. Since most of the documented cases of occupational transmission of HIV have involved blood exposure, greater care should be taken when dealing with blood.

Transcutaneous infection with HIV through existing open skin wounds in health care personnel has been documented.[31] This is most likely to occur in situations where there is accidental exposure to significant amounts of blood or other body fluids in an uncontrolled setting, such as during emergency patient care or a laboratory accident.

Percutaneous infeciton with HIV has also been documented.[12, 22, 35, 36] The group of studies following health care workers with needlestick injuries involving HIV-infected patients has identified at least four cases of transmission, an approximately 0.5% risk. Although this is low, as is the relative percentage of HIV-infected individuals in this country, there will be continued episodes of occupational HIV infection.

Presently 33 health care workers with AIDS have been found to have no other identifiable risks; five of these were physicians, three of whom are surgeons.[22] None of these cases has been traced to known exposure to AIDS or HIV-infected patients, but such exposure cannot be ruled out. Unfortunately, no major survey of health care workers at greatest risk for hepatitis B (and therefore HIV) infection has been performed. Such a survey is being planned and will hopefully provide some better estimate of the degree of risk to health care workers, and identify locales and situations most likely to result in occupational infection by HIV.

The precautions and methods to limit risk of occupational infection by HIV have been outlined and updated.[22, 37, 38] These are not new or elaborate ideas. They are not significantly different from those used for hepatitis or other viral infections, since the routes of transmission are the same. These precautions, recommended by the CDC, are outlined in Table 5.[22] Specific precautions for health care personnel participating in invasive procedures are listed in Table 6.[37] These guidelines seem simple and limited given the consequences of infection with HIV. However, rigid adherence

TABLE 5.
Universal Precautions to Prevent Transmission of HIV

Use appropriate barrier to prevent skin or mucous membranes from contact with patient blood or body fluids. These barriers include gloves, gowns, protective eyewear, and masks.
Hands should be thoroughly washed after removal of gloves, and any skin contacting patient blood or body fluid should be washed *immediately*.
Great care should be taken to avoid injury by needles or other sharp objects that have been used on patients. Protocols for handling disposables should be rigidly followed.
Equipment for emergency ventilation should be available where resuscitation is most likely to occur to avoid mouth-to-mouth contact.
Health care workers with open skin lesions should avoid direct patient contact or handling of patient care equipment.
Pregnant health care workers must follow guidelines strictly.

TABLE 6.
Precautions for Health Care Workers Involved With Invasive Procedures to Prevent Transmission of HIV (In Addition to Universal Precautions)

During invasive procedures all personnel involved should wear protective barriers that may include gowns, gloves, protective eyewear, and masks.
If a glove is damaged, it should be discarded immediately, as should be any instruments that may have caused or been associated with the damage.

to these guidelines is the most likely means of avoiding occupational infection by HIV.

A question that arises frequently is how to identify those patients in whom such precautions should be taken. Mandatory screening of all hospitalized patients and even the public in general has been proposed to facilitate such identification. Given the previously described incubation period during which patients are infectious but negative by present HIV testing, the small chance of false-negative testing, and the need for repeated testing to identify all the patients who may have become infected since their last test, reliance on such a system to implement precautionary guidelines would be prohibitively expensive and generally unsafe. The CDC has recommended testing for HIV for those patients in whom infection is likely, or the risks of transmission is increased if infection is present (persons planning marriage, or women of childbearing age). The groups recommended for testing by the CDC are summarized in Table 7. Another problem with relying on testing to identify infectious patients is that test results are not available immediately. Patient care and invasive procedures frequently cannot wait for such results. Furthermore, the percentage of HIV-positive patients needing emergency care is increased, especially in trauma patients.[39] Because of this and the above-mentioned limitations of testing, precautionary measures should be used on *all* patients. However, it is realistically impossible to maintain maximum precautionary measures on all cases; attention to detail will subside. Hopefully, adequate education, adherence to guidelines, and continued reminders will limit the relaxation of precautionary measures. Identification of known patients with HIV-infection to health care workers involved in their care will permit rigorous adherence to protective measures without implying a false sense of security in those patients with negative or unknown HIV status.

TABLE 7.
Individuals for Whom the CDC Recommended Testing for HIV

Persons with sexually transmitted diseases
Intravenous drug users
Persons who consider themselves at risk for HIV infection
Women of childbearing age
Persons planning marriage
Persons undergoing medical evaluation
Persons admitted to hospitals
Persons in correctional facilities
Prostitutes

Implications of AIDS and HIV Infection for Medicine and Society

The impact of AIDS on this society is extraordinary, considering the disease did not exist ten years ago. In some population subgroups, it is the most common cause of productive years-of-life lost.[40] Projections to the year 1991 include continued exponential rise of HIV infection and AIDS cases and a cost in health care money that is staggering.[41]

AIDS has also produced a level of fear and panic in society even greater than the significant concern it merits. Furthermore, this frenzied reaction is not even directed into appropriate and established methods to address the problem. This is due to the moral and social implications of the disease; the immediate assumption that a person infected with HIV has been involved with illicit drug use or homosexuality. The increased number of cases due to blood transfusion, heterosexual, maternal, and occupational exposure may reduce this prejudgment, but it will remain a major obstacle to preventing the disease and treating its victims compassionately. Control of this epidemic will be delayed until people recognize it as an infectious disease instead of a social disease.

Education has been described as one of the principal means of controlling the spread of HIV.[42] Public service announcements and printed information have been effective in increasing public awareness of the disease and methods to avoid infection. Some changes in behavior have been identified and used as examples of how education can be effective.[43, 44] Unfortunately, many persons at high risk are far more concerned about continuing their high-risk practices than they are about avoiding HIV infection.[45] As these populations become maximally infected, there may actually be a decrease in the rate of HIV transmission, if the incidence risk of infection by heterosexual or occupational exposure remains low.

Education is an essential part of the coordinated plan to deal with AIDS and HIV infection. Programs in schools and those targeted at high-risk groups and locales may be the most important aspect of the education program. This also includes frequent updates to health care workers. Monitoring the effectiveness of these programs by anonymous testing of those being educated will identify programs that work. Hopefully, such programs will be ultimately effective in curbing the spread of HIV infection.

Acquired immunodeficiency syndrome and HIV infection has had significant impact on government. Unfortunately, early attention focused on considerations identified as a threat to individuals' civil liberties, rather than on society as a whole. Consequently, standard measures of infection control were not initiated. Even before HIV was identified as the cause of AIDS, the methods of transmission were known. Despite their identification as places where transmission would occur to a large number of people, bath houses in San Francisco remained open. One attempt to close them was blocked by a court order from the owners and political pressure by the homosexual community, whose members were most likely to benefit by decreased transmission.[46] Initial legislation also was aimed at protection of civil liberties of victims of AIDS and HIV infection without also addressing legitimate public health concerns. Protection of victims of this epidemic is necessary; but protection of society by trying to limit its spread is also necessary.

Present state legislation is concentrating on both concerns. Many bills include antidiscrimination clauses to protect victims from unreasonable housing or employment actions against them, while permitting standard infection reporting and follow-up used for other sexually transmitted diseases.[32, 46] Action by these state bodies are essential, since many federal groups such as the CDC can only provide information and have no legal authority in infection control in individual states.

The federal government has responded to this problem with some inconsistency. Despite present significant commitments for research, the delays in making funds available have been justly criticized. A major concern at present will be how to pay for care of AIDS patients, since private insurers and state agencies want to limit their fiscal commitments. Progress toward a solution has been limited, but will be a problem of major proportion in a short period of time.

Summary

The consequences of AIDS and HIV infection on society, medical care in general, and surgery in particular are considerable, and will continue to grow. Major problems facing surgeons will be how and when to provide appropriate care for AIDS patients, and protection of themselves and all health care personnel from occupational infection by the highly lethal HIV. Strict adherence to guidelines to prevent such occupational infection is paramount, and these should be observed in all patients, since it is impossible to always identify patients who are infectious. A sound understanding of the clinical problem and attention to this evolving epidemic are also essential for surgeons and all other health care personnel.

With respect to society in general, control of AIDS and HIV can only be achieved by a joint effort of education, individual responsibility, and a coordinated governmental commitment to the problem.

References

1. CDC: Kaposi's sarcoma and pneumocystis pneumonia among homosexual men in New York City and California. *MMWR* 1981; 25:305–308.
2. CDC: Update: Acquired immunodeficiency syndrome—United States. *MMWR* 1986; 35:17–21.
3. Montagnier L: Lymphadenopathy-associated virus: From molecular biology to pathogenicity. *Ann Intern Med* 1985; 103:689–693.

4. Gallo RC, Wong-Staal F: A human T-lymphotropic retrovirus (HTLV-III) as the cause of the acquired immunodeficiency syndrome. *Ann Intern Med* 1985; 103:679–689.
5. Coffin J, Hasse A, Levy JA, et al: Human immunodeficiency viruses (letter). *Science* 1986; 232:697.
6. Francis DP, Petricciani JC: The prospects for and pathways toward a vaccine for AIDS. *N Engl J Med* 1985; 313:1586–1590.
7. McDougal JS, Kennedy MS, Sligh JM, et al: Binding of HTLV-III/LAV to T4 and T cells by a complex of the 110 K viral protein and the T4 molecule. *Science* 1986; 231:382–385.
8. Ho DD, Pomerantz RJ, Kaplan JC: Pathogenesis of infection with human immunodeficiency virus. *N Engl J Med* 1987; 317:278–286.
9. CDC: Revision of the case definition of acquired immunodeficiency syndrome for national reporting—United States. *MMWR* 1985; 34:373–375.
10. CDC: Revision of the CDS surveillance case definition for acquired immunodeficiency syndrome. *MMWR* Aug 14, 1987, pp 35–145.
11. Huang KL, Ruben FL, Rinaldo CR Jr, et al: Antibody responses after influenza and pneumococcal immunization in HIV-infected heterosexual men. *JAMA* 1987; 257:2047–2051.
12. Friedland GH, Klein RS: Transmission of the human immunodeficiency virus. 1987; 317:1125–1135.
13. Lui KJ, Lawrence DN, Meade Morgan W, et al: A model-based approach for estimating the mean incubation period of transfusion-associated acquired immunodeficiency syndrome. *Proc Natl Acad Sci* 1986; 83:3051–3055.
14. Redfield RR, Wright DC, Tramont EC: The Walter Reed Staging Classification for HTLV-III/LAV infection. *N Engl J Med* 1986; 314:131.
15. CDC: Classification system for human T-lymphotropic virus type III/lymphadenopathy associated virus infection. *MMWR* 1986; 35:334–339.
16. Rothenberg R, Woelfel M, Stoneburner R, et al: Survival with the acquired immunodeficiency syndrome: Experience with 5833 cases in New York City. *N Engl J Med* 1987; 317:1297–1302.
17. Yarchoan R, Broder S: Development of antiretroviral therapy for the acquired immunodeficiency syndrome and related disorders: A progress report. *N Engl J Med* 1987; 316:557–564.
18. Allan JP, Laurain Y, Paul DA, et al: Long-term evaluation of HIV antigen and antibodies to p24 and gp41 in patients with hemophilia: Potential clinical importance. *N Engl J Med* 1987; 317:1114–1121.
19. Valle S, Saxinger C, Ranki A, et al: Diversity of clinical spectrum of HTLV-III/LAV infection. *Lancet* 1985; 1:301–304.
20. Volberding PA: The clinical spectrum of the acquired immunodeficiency syndrome: Implication for comprehensive patient care. *Ann Intern Med* 1985; 103:729–733.
21. Carlson JR, Bryant ML, Hinrichs SH, et al: AIDS serology testing in low and high risk groups. *JAMA* 1985; 253:3405–3408.
22. CDC: Recommendations for prevention of HIV transmission in health care settings. *MMWR* Aug 21, 1987, pp 35–185.
23. CDC: Public Health Service Guidelines for counseling and antibody testing to prevent HIV infection and AIDS. *MMWR* 1987; 36:509–515.
24. Friedmand GH, Saltzman BR, Rogers MF, et al: Lack of transmission of HTLV-III/LAV infection to household contacts of patients with AIDS or AIDS related complex with oral candidiasis. *N Engl J Med* 1986; 314:344–349.

25. Curran JW, Morgan WM, Hardy AM, et al: The epidemiology of AIDS: Current status and future prospects. *Science* 1985; 229:1352–1357.
26. Smiley L, White GC, Macik G, et al: Transmission of human immunodeficiency virus from hemophiliacs to their sexual partners. Presented at the Third International Conference on Acquired Immunodeficiency Syndrome, Washington, DC, June, 1987.
27. Weber DJ, Redfield RR, Lemon SM: Acquired immunodeficiency syndrome (AIDS): Epidemiology and significance for the obstetrician and gynecologist. *Am J Obstet Gynecol* 1986; 155:235–240.
28. Seek M, Weber DJ, Mattern WD: AIDS, renal disease, and dialysis. *AKF Nephrol* 1985; 4:29–36.
29. Kunkel SE, Warner MA: Human T-cell lymphotropic virus type III (HTLV-III) infection: How it can affect you, your patients, and your anesthesia practice. *Anesthesiology* 1957; 66:195–207.
30. Werner BG, Grady GF: Accidental hepatitis-B surface-antigen-positive inoculations: Use of e antigen to estimate infectivity. *Ann Intern Med* 1982; 97:367–369.
31. CDC: Update: Human immunodeficiency virus infections in health care workers exposed to blood of infected patients. *MMWR* 1987; 36:285–289.
32. Lewis HE: Acquired immunodeficiency syndrome: State legislative activity. *JAMA* 1987; 258:2410–2414.
33. Meyer AA: AIDS: The disease and its relevance to surgeons. *Bull Am Coll Surg* 1986; 71:11–17.
34. AIDS—Board of Trustees: Prevention and control of acquired immunodeficiency syndrome: An interim report. *JAMA* 1987; 258:2097–2103.
35. McCray E, et al: Occupational risk of acquired immunodeficiency syndrome among health care workers. *N Engl J Med* 1986; 314:1127–1132.
36. Stricof RL, Morse DL: HTLV-III/LAV seroconversion following deep intramuscular needlestick injury (letter). *N Engl J Med* 1986; 314:1115.
37. CDC: Recommendations for preventing transmission of infection with human T-lymphotropic virus type III/lymphadenopathy associated virus during invasive procedures. *MMWR* 1986; 35:221–223.
38. CDC: Summary: Recommendations for preventing transmission of infection with human T-lymphotropic virus type III/lymphadenopathy-associated virus in the workplace. *MMWR* 1985; 34:682–686, 691–695.
39. Baker JL, Kelen GD, Siverston KT, et al: Unsuspected human immunodeficiency virus in critically ill emergency patients. *JAMA* 1987; 257:2609–2611.
40. Kristal AR: The impact of the acquired immunodeficiency syndrome on patterns of premature death in New York City. *JAMA* 1986; 255:2306–2310.
41. Francis DP, Chin J: The prevention of acquired immunodeficiency syndrome in the United States: An objective strategy for medicine, public health, business and the community. *JAMA* 1987; 257:1357–1374.
42. Bowen OR: The war against AIDS. *J Med Educ* 1987; G2:543–548.
43. McKusick L, Horstman W, Coates TJ: AIDS and sexual behavior reported by gay men in San Francisco. *Am J Public Health* 1985; 75:493–496.
44. Van der Groaf MJ, Diepersloot RJA: Transmission of human immunodeficiency virus (HIV/HTLV-III/LAV): A review. *Infection* 1986; 14:203–211.
45. Osborn JE: The AIDS epidemic: Multidisciplinary trouble. *N Engl J Med* 1986; 314:779–782.
46. Mills M, Wofsy CB, Mills J: The acquired immunodeficiency syndrome: Infection control and public health law. *N Engl J Med* 1986; 314:931–936.

Current Status of Blood Therapy in Surgery

John A. Collins, M.D.

Professor of Surgery, Stanford University School of Medicine, Stanford, California

The scientific era of blood transfusion, and with it the beginnings of safe transfusion, began in 1900 with the discovery of the ABO red cell antigen system by Landsteiner. During World War I, several groups discovered citrate as an effective and relatively safe anticoagulant for whole blood and plasma. Not until the early 1930s was it demonstrated that special care in preparing the glass bottles and rubber tubing used for transfusion would decrease the incidence of the then almost universal febrile reactions. The first centralized blood service functioned in Barcelona during the Spanish Civil War and soon after, in 1937, was established at Cook County Hospital in the United States by Fantus, who popularized the term blood bank. The anticoagulant used for storage of whole blood was markedly improved in 1943 to acid citrate dextrose (ACD). In the 1950s the system in the United States converted to plastic equipment, which was safer for the recipient and allowed for the harvesting of components from donated whole blood. In the 1960s and 1970s the anticoagulant was further refined to citrate phosphate dextrose (CPD), component therapy became the rule, and the donor system changed to an almost exclusively voluntary basis. In the 1980s, adenine was added to the anticoagulant to extend storage time of red cells, more components were developed as separate products, better screening of the products for safety was developed, and a dramatic, deadly new disease was identified as transmissible by transfusion.[1, 2]

Currently, there are a number of concerns regarding blood banking among surgeons and among patients. Surgeons often express concern about the near total conversion to a component system of blood banking, usually expressed as the disappearance of whole blood as a readily available product. Red cell concentrates ("packed red cells") contain only about one third of the plasma component of whole blood. The missing two thirds is usually not needed, however. The amount of albumin and other protein involved is rather small in terms of the total body economy, and contained in the missing plasma are antigenic and metabolic products that are potentially harmful to the recipient. The real defense of the component approach, however, is the principle of the greatest good for the greatest number. A single donation of blood can now supply needed material to several different patients. With storage as whole blood, these ele-

Adv Surg 22:75–104, 1989

0065-3411/89/22-075-104-$04.00

ments would be given where not needed. Even worse, most would be lost so no one would benefit. Platelets in a donation of whole blood become pretty worthless within a day, and factor V and factor VIII deteriorate steadily during storage.[3] By separating them off soon after collection and treating them differently, they can be made useful. Most surgeons understand the waste in burying transplantable organs with the dead; the same thing occurs with storage of whole blood. This is so compelling that even elective presurgical donations for autologous use should be separated into components with only the red cells targeted for the donor.

The medical community and especially prospective patients are alarmed by the possibility of transmitting human immunodeficiency virus (HIV) by transfusion, thereby giving the recipient a fatal disease. Nearly constant media attention keeps this possibility in the forefront of patient's concerns. The best available data indicate that a transfused patient is several times as likely to die of non–A, non–B hepatitis (NANB) as of HIV. For the public, the concern over HIV in transfused blood is too great. For the profession, the concern over NANB after transfusion is much too little. Ironically, it is the concerns of the public over the less likely event rather than the informed practice of professionals because of the more likely event that has led to a significant tightening of transfusion practices. Some responses have been largely ineffective, such as directed donations, but some have been excellent. Patients and families are questioning physicians about whether transfusions are really needed, prospective patients are informing surgeons that the likelihood of requiring transfusion is influencing their decision of whether to have an operation and by which surgeon, and a surge of interest in elective autotransfusion has been driven primarily by patient interest. This has been beneficial in reducing the risks of transfusion and in forcing the medical profession to become better informed of the risks and benefits of transfusion.

In the space allotted I cannot review the entire field of blood therapy in surgery. I have chosen instead to focus on recent developments and concerns and to approach these in the following sequence: products and their use, problems associated with these products, and possible solutions to these problems. Where pertinent the reader is referred to existing reviews in various areas. Several excellent brief[2–4] and more comprehensive references exist.[1]

Products

Red Blood Cells

Over 90% of the red blood cells (RBCs) issued by the major blood banking systems in the United States are in the form of red cell concentrates ("packed red cells").[3, 4] This product contains the amount of red cells found in a normal donation of 450 ml of whole blood plus about 63 ml anticoagulant. From this mixture, two thirds of the plasma-anticoagulant supernatant is removed. The resulting product has a volume of approximately 300 ml and a hematocrit of about 70%. This high hematocrit makes the product more difficult to administer rapidly. Adding saline dilutes the mixture to a lower hematocrit and allows more rapid administration. The fluid added should not contain glucose or calcium, should be isotonic, and should not be added until just before administration. Problems with RBC concentrates are the same as those with whole blood except, of course, that the volume of fluid administered is less, and the plasma and anticoagulant component are less, meaning less citrate, potassium, and organic acid, and less protein and coagulation factors. All stored RBC products are essentially without functioning platelets. The risk of transmitting disease is the same for RBC concentrates as for whole blood.

The anticoagulant most commonly used for storing red cells in the United States is a mixture of citrate, phosphate, dextrose, and adenine (CPD-A). This produces a product that has a higher glucose, citrate, and phosphate content and organic acid load than the donor blood. With time in liquid storage, potassium and ammonium also increase significantly in the plasma phase and microaggregates consisting of leukocyte and platelet clumps with some fibrin are formed. The RBCs retain a survival of at least 75% 24 hours after transfusion with a normal life span of the surviving red cells. Concentrated RBCs in CPD-A can be stored for five weeks at 4°C.

Red cells are used to restore oxygen carrying capacity to the circulation of the recipient. Given time, an active marrow, and the needed nutritional factors, recipients will do this for themselves without the hazards of transfusion. The transfused cells are mostly gone in several weeks. Transfusion of red cells, then, is a temporary boost in oxygen carrying capacity at significant risk. When is this warranted?

There is a truly vast literature on the effects of anemia under different circumstances. Some of the observations seem contradictory, and there are conflicting theories regarding such issues as the optimal hematocrit for stressed individuals. At one of the recent Olympics, for example, there were charges of "blood doping," that is, raising the athletes' hematocrit level before competition by transfusion. Some of the most vociferous complainers were athletes who had had the financial support to train for long periods at high altitude to achieve the same effects; obviously, they believed in the effectiveness of higher hematocrit readings even if the niceties of even handed competition escaped them. At almost the same time, teams of mountain climbers were attempting very high altitude climbs without supplemental oxygen. Their special approach was to have phlebotomies at the high base camps to keep their hematocrits below normal because of their belief that lower hematocrits were advantageous during physical stress. It seems apparent that both of these groups could not have been correct, yet both consisted of world-class competitors completely convinced that they gained a significant edge in physical performance by manipulating their hematocrit levels—in opposite directions! These were not mere faddists. Both camps were supported by sophisticated studies in exercise physiology and by the weight of significant scientific opinion.

When looked at for broad patterns, the picture does not seem quite as confusing as the above circumstances seem to indicate. Lowering hematocrit lowers the oxygen carrying capacity of blood, but also makes the blood easier to pump around. The product of flow times content determines the amount of oxygen delivered by the circulation. Therefore, manipulating the hematocrit produces simultaneous opposing changes. The relationship between hematocrit and oxygen content is linear. The relationship between hematocrit and resistance to flow is much less clear.[5] Older studies on acute hemodilution in intact animals indicated maximal oxygen delivery at hematocrit levels near normal, but there were exceptions.[6–8] Well-controlled and sophisticated studies in patients, however, indicated little detectable impairment of physical or mental performance at hematocrits reduced to near half normal.[9] The discrepancy between these observations was explained by the discovery of the role of 2,3-diphosphoglyceric acid. This red cell product of glycolysis lowers the affinity of hemoglobin for oxygen, thereby making hemoglobin much more efficient at off-loading oxygen in the tissues, especially when increased demand is manifested by a lower tissue oxygen tension.[10] Studies in severely anemic patients showed that this response can nearly double the amount of oxygen delivered by hemoglobin at physiologic gas tensions, nicely explaining the above observations.[11] This marvelous compensatory response is independent of cardiac output, synthesis of new RBCs, or changing oxygen tensions; it occurs at the cost of some extra glucose.

Not so easily explained are more recent observations showing a relationship between concentration of hemoglobin and work performance by agricultural field workers.[12–15] There are several such studies, but they share certain characteristics. The settings were all in economically poor parts of the world in a semi-industrialized agricultural system, the workers and their families were living at subsistence level, pay was doled out on a daily basis and was related to the amount of product produced that day (tea leaves, raw latex for rubber, various food crops, etc.). This constituted a maximum incentive system. End points were actual product produced or simple field tests of work capacity performed for rewards (step tests, etc.). There were control groups treated with iron-free supplements and test groups treated with iron-enriched supplements. Performance improved as hemoglobin was restored toward normal. In some control groups, however, performance improved in groups given iron-free supplements without effect on hemoglobin levels. In all these studies the subjects were characterized by multiple health problems and almost certainly by poor nutrition and barely adequate caloric intake. In that setting, the concentration of hemoglobin in blood may well relate closely to work capacity up to near normal levels of hemoglobin; the studies referred to earlier with intact work capacity down to half normal levels of hemoglobin were all done in otherwise healthy, well-nourished European and North American subjects. There is a lot more different between those populations than just the levels of hemoglobin. An interesting gap in the studies on the field agricultural workers is the lack of measurement for compensating response in oxyhemoglobin dissociation, but even if present it is possible that their many other deficiencies make the concentration of hemoglobin a performance-limiting factor.

In the absence of significant other disease, it seems from several studies in animals and in patients that detrimental levels of hematocrit occur in the range above about 60%, beyond which oxygen delivery clearly declines because of impaired perfusion. The harmful low range is the hotly debated question. Several studies indicate that the healthy heart converts from a lactate consumer to a lactate producer at hematocrits about 20%.[16] Heart failure had been reported experimentally and clinically at hematocrits around 10% in individuals with otherwise seemingly normal hearts.[17, 18] In other studies, individuals supported by ventilators begin dying at hematocrits around 10%.[19] In some instances, if the patient is paralyzed and given high concentrations of inspired oxygen, death can be deferred until hematocrits around 5%. Ability to withstand any additional challenges or work demands is almost certainly totally absent at such levels, and even at 20% the ability to meet unexpected demands is likely significantly impaired. There is little in these studies, however, to indicate that hematocrit levels of 30% should be significant triggers for transfusion. Quite the opposite, increasing experience in trauma centers and in other settings indicates that hematocrit levels in the mid to low 20s can be well tolerated by patients recovering normally even from major injuries and operation. One must be confident at these low levels, however, that significant and sudden blood loss is unlikely to occur. Allowing a patient with intestinal bleeding of uncertain status to remain at such low levels would not be good practice. The claims that hematocrits in the very low ranges, for example, the mid-20s, are actually more advantageous than those in the normal range must be viewed with skepticism. One such study found a higher tissue oxygen tension in skeletal muscle of animals brought to low hematocrit levels, but such animals had a higher mortality than the controls at normal hematocrits.[20] The authors concluded that the lower hematocrit levels were beneficial!

All of the above applies to patients who are otherwise intact. If one adds significant vascular disease, the situation may be quite different. Over 30 years ago it was shown that banding the coronary arteries to prevent dilation in response to anemia creates a situation in which acute decrements in hematocrit significantly below normal result in decreased performance by the left ventricle.[21] This important principle has been confirmed in many ways, most importantly by patients with coronary artery disease and concomitant anemia. Such patients develop angina pectoris and/or signs of congestive heart failure at certain levels of anemia, which can be corrected by raising the hematocrit level by transfusion. Deliberate hemodilution to "improve flow" to areas perfused by diseased arteries is a questionable and hazardous practice. A recent study of this approach in men with stable claudication illustrates this point well.[22] The opposite is more likely to be true: stressed patients with coronary artery disease will require a higher hematocrit if anemic than comparable patients without coronary artery disease. The same may be true for cerebrovascular disease, but the evidence is lacking.

Fresh Frozen Plasma

Fresh frozen plasma[3, 4] is about the only form of blood plasma available as a separate product for therapeutic use. It is produced by separating most of the plasma fraction from freshly collected whole blood, removing the platelets, and freezing the remaining plasma, which is then stored frozen for up to one year. The volume is usually about 250 ml, each unit represents a different donor, the product must be thawed before use, and it should be ABO (red cell antigen) compatible with the recipient. Because of freezing soon after collection, fresh frozen plasma contains all of the coagulation components in nearly normal concentrations. It contains no coagulation components in concentrated form. All of the viral diseases transmitted by whole blood can be transmitted by fresh frozen plasma with the same risk; whether there is less risk for the primarily intraleukocytic viruses is not clear, but the product can transmit these viruses.

The recent consensus conference of the National Institutes of Health (NIH) on fresh frozen plasma came to the conclusion that this is currently the most overused product available in the field of blood banking.[23] The data on nationwide use show an almost logarithmic increase in use over the past ten years. There is nothing known clinically to account for such an increase nor for the current high levels of use.

Fresh frozen plasma should be used to correct deficiencies in coagulation factors that are clinically significant. Even then it is inefficient because nothing is in concentrated form. Cryoprecipitate is a single donor product that contains some coagulation factors in concentrated form and is a more effective and rational choice for replenishing those factors. For several coagulation factors, however, the only concentrated products available carry a very high risk of transmitting disease, so fresh frozen plasma is a better choice. The conditions in which it is needed are very limited. Significant bleeding or the immediate need for a major operation in a patient taking coumadin is a clear example. Even then, the coagulation factors specifically saved by freezing are not effected by coumadin, but no other whole plasma products are available. Most coagulation factors work satisfactorily at circulating levels 20 to 50% of normal, so the dose of fresh frozen plasma can be estimated on that basis; at times it may be necessary to remove some of the patient's deficient plasma so as not to overload the circulation. If there is sufficient time, vitamin K is a safe way to restore the needed factors. Patients with severe liver disease often have deficiencies in multiple coagulation factors. As with coumadin, significant bleeding or the need to perform an invasive procedure are indications to try to correct the deficiencies by giving fresh frozen plasma. Vitamin K is much less likely to be effective in such patients. Critically ill patients sometimes develop severe coagulopathies on the basis of intravascular consumption. The efficacy of fresh frozen plasma in these disorders is less evident as they carry high mortality rates regardless of treatment. Replacement is a reasonable approach, however, and fresh frozen plasma is a good choice because factors V and VIII are usually depleted in such patients. Fresh frozen plasma and fresh whole blood are the only available sources of factor V for treatment. Correction of the underlying cause is essential for reversing the coagulopathy. Thrombotic thrombocytopenic purpura and other rare conditions may also be associated with multiple factor depletion and require fresh frozen plasma as part of treatment.

The above clear-cut indications for fresh frozen plasma account for only a small part of its use. Much more common is the highly questionable practice of prophylactic administration, and even worse, administration for as yet unidentified but "probably helpful factors." The latter is best described as a search for magic, and is perhaps most evident in settings like neonatal intensive care units where the error is compounded by giving the material frequently in small amounts in such a way as to maximize exposure to donors.

Prophylactic use in adults, though, probably accounts for the greatest single use (and abuse) of the product. Far too often, one sees several units of fresh frozen plasma given because a bleeding patient has received, or even might receive, 3 or 4 units of blood. This is clearly harmful practice, as there is nothing in theory or actual experience to support such an intervention. Similarly, slight abnormalities of a screening coagulation test, especially prothrombin time or partial thromboplastin time, are sometimes "treated" with fresh frozen plasma. Such abnormalities are usually clinically insignificant and often not even reproducible on repeat testing. Less clear is the use of prophylactic fresh frozen plasma in truly massively transfused patients (at least one blood volume in less than 12 hours). Stored blood is deficient in factors V and VIII, completely lacking functioning platelets, and in the case of packed RBCs lacking two thirds of all other circulating coagulation factors. Washout or dilutional coagulopathy is unlikely to occur even in such circumstances, however, as the mathematics of exchange transfusion under the conditions that must apply if the patient survived the event indicate.[24] Under the worst likely scenario, exchange transfusion of one blood volume results in one third of the original blood elements still circulating in the recipient, even if there is no endogenous replacement and the transfused fluid is completely deficient, neither of which applies.[25, 26] Even with two blood volumes transfused, at least one eighth of the patient's blood elements remain. Levels of 20% are probably sufficient for hemostasis with almost all coagulation factors, although studies with multiple simultaneous deficiencies are rare.

More important are the actual measurements in patients. Although many of the studies are confusing because of the multiple and different tests and assays done and because of the inherently uncontrolled nature of the clinical setting, certain patterns may be discerned. Some massively transfused patients bleed abnormally, and some do not. Those who do bleed abnormally tend to show levels of depletion of coagulation factors that are greater than can be accounted for by dilutional effects and show abnormalities that do not relate to the blood transfused, e.g., the presence of fibrin-split products. In the casualties we studied in Vietnam, some of those who subsequently bled abnormally had significant coagulation abnormalities before they were transfused, the abnormalities improved during transfusion, then worsened again after transfusion.[27] These observations do not support a simple dilutional mechanism as the explanation. Rather, they suggest an underlying consumption of coagulation factors as is seen in disseminated intravascular coagulation (DIC). Important confirmation of such an interpretation has come from a study of heavily transfused patients in Germany.[28] Within that population, laboratory abnormalities of coagulation did not correlate with the amount of blood transfused. When the patients were grouped according to the duration of time spent hypotensive, a strong correlation with coagulation abnormalities was evident. The group in Seattle prospectively studied 27 patients massively transfused with modified whole blood (platelets and cryoprecipitate removed).[29] Despite large amounts of hemorrhage and transfusion it was very unusual for the measured coagulation factors to decrease to dangerous levels. Those who bled abnormally seemed to do so because of thrombocytopenia and/or DIC. These researchers saw no justification for routine use of fresh frozen plasma in transfused patients. Confirmatory, if less significant, evidence was reported from a study in dogs treated with RBC concentrates with or without supplemental fresh frozen plasma.[30]

Platelets

Platelets[1, 3] are harvested from freshly donated whole blood with an average yield of about 5 to 6×10^{10} per donor in a volume of anticoagulant of about 30 to 50 ml. Occasionally, larger numbers are collected from a single donor by a process called plateletpheresis; this product is usually called single-donor platelets, which implies that a therapeutic dose of platelets has been harvested from a single donor. The more common form of platelet donation is pooled with that from other donors to provide a therapeutic dose. The product is usually referred to by the number of such donors (six pack, eight pack, etc.). The product is stored at room temperature for up to five days. Dosage is approximate at best. A general rule of thumb is that one usual donor pack per 10 kg of body weight will raise the recipient's platelet count by 30,000/cu mm. The response to infused platelets, however, is very dependent on the status of the recipient. Any platelet destructive or consumptive disorder will obviously lessen the expected increment, but so also will fever, sepsis, large recent wounds, continued active bleeding, and splenomegaly. Platelets are probably more antigenic than RBCs, so unnecessary use is even more likely to result in immunization of the recipient against future reception of the product. Platelets unavoidably contain some RBCs and white cells, so RBC compatibility is required. Platelets transmit all the viral diseases transmitted by blood and are usually a multi-donor product.[31]

The indications for the use of platelets are not quite clearly established. There are several excellent reviews.[32] A significantly bleeding patient with thrombocytopenia or thrombocytopathy should be given platelets. The problems as with fresh frozen plasma arise in the area of prophylactic use. Prospective studies show better results in leukemic patients transfused prophylactically for platelet counts of 20,000/cu mm or less, but lower levels were not tested.[33, 34] In thrombocytopenic patients, bleeding times begin to prolong at platelet counts between 50,000 to 100,000/cu mm, but do not reach potentially dangerous levels until much lower. The relationship between platelet count and bleeding time is effected among other factors by the mechanism of thrombocytopenia.[32] Platelet destructive disorders with normal production result in a circulating population of young platelets, which are functionally superior. Patients with idiopathic thrombocytopenic purpura, for example, rarely need to be transfused with platelets, and certainly do *not* routinely need platelets for splenectomy. The need for administering platelets to such patients is best judged by the bleeding observed after removal of the spleen, and should be present in a small minority of such patients. Several controlled studies have shown no benefit from the prophylactic use of platelets in patients undergoing cardiopulmonary bypass.[35, 36]

Again, patients receiving massive transfusion form an interesting test case for the prophylactic administration of platelets. This use seems logical as stored red cells are essentially platelet-free and thrombocytopenia has been very well documented as a consequence of massive transfusion.[37] The problem is that very few patients develop platelet counts below 50,000/cu mm, a level that is not dangerous. Fortunately, there is an excellent study in this area, again from Seattle.[38] Patients who were bleeding rapidly were randomly assigned to receive 6 units of platelets for every 12 units of RBCs transfused (17 patients) or 2 units of fresh frozen plasma for every 12 units of RBCs transfused (16 patients). This made an interesting control, because platelets come in fresh plasma, so the fresh frozen plasma was a true control (same volume of carrier lacking the element being tested). The results were unequivocal: there was no clinical difference between the two groups, and the differences in platelet counts were remarkably small. The authors also found what others had shown: the platelet counts predicted by exchange mathematics were far less than the platelet counts observed.[39, 40] In other words, the recipients had a resilient and effective system for maintaining platelet counts despite injury and massive replacement. Those patients who did bleed abnormally were distributed equally in both groups and most showed evidence of DIC.

Another interesting if less momentous recent study followed platelet counts in patients undergoing laparotomy for peritonitis.[41] These patients developed significant thrombocytopenia bottoming out on the fourth post-operative day. There was no abnormal bleeding associated with these counts down to 50,000/cu mm, and no evidence that administration of platelets was needed or would have been helpful.

Other Coagulation Products[1–3]

Cryoprecipitate is obtained from freshly harvested plasma by controlled cold precipitation with reconstitution in about 10 ml saline just before use. It can transmit all of the viral diseases that whole blood can. It contains in concentrated form factors VIII and XIII, fibrinogen (factor I), fibronectin, and von Willebrand factor in amounts of 25 to 75% of that found in the donor plasma. Its primary use is for correction of factor VIII deficiency (hemophilia A) by a single donor product. Such patients should have factor VIII levels raised to therapeutic ranges and checked by appropriate laboratory tests before undergoing invasive procedures and as soon as possible after significant injuries, including soft-tissue injuries considered minor in other patients. Most such patients are quite knowledgeable in their own requirements and have well-informed physicians who provide care.

Cryoprecepitate is now the only available form of concentrated fibrinogen in the United States. Fibrinogen is rarely needed as such. Disastrous obstetrical complications or acute DIC from other causes may sometimes be associated with profound hypofibrinogenemia, but often this aspect of the disorder is covered by the fibrinogen present in fresh frozen plasma.

Cryoprecipitate is the preferred agent for prophylaxis and treatment of patients deficient in von Willebrand's factor. In such patients, replacing von Willebrand's factor is accompanied by a more sustained increment of factor VIII than in patients with hemophilia A and also by correction of the prolonged bleeding time without giving platelets. As with hemophilia, relatively small wounds require treatment and correction should be carried out before performing invasive procedures.

Deficiency of factor XIII is rare. Only small amounts are needed for full effect and administered factor XIII lasts a relatively long time.

Concentrated, pooled factor VIII is available in lyophilized form and has become popular because of the ease of use. Unfortunately, it is a product pooled from the plasma of many donors and therefore carries a very high risk of transmitting viral diseases. Recently, carefully controlled heating has been used to apparently eliminate the risk of transmitting HIV[42], but the risk of hepatitis remains.

Concentrated, pooled factor IX was developed as an analagous product for the treatment of hemophilia B. It is also very prone to transmit viral diseases and is also now provided in a heat-treated form, which seems to have eliminated HIV but not hepatitis. The product was characterized by the development of fatal thromboembolic complications in some recipients. Changes in manufacturing and screening several years ago seem to have at least lessened the probability of this event. In addition to factor IX, the product contains factors II, VII, and X in concentrated form. This makes it particularly effective in reversing the effects of coumadin, but the risks of transmitting hepatitis are quite high. It is occasionally also useful in patients with severe liver disease and multiple coagulation defects, but some of these patients have developed fatal thromboembolism after use. The older forms with activated coagulant components sometimes proved effective in treating patients with factor VIII deficiency who were resistant to simple replacement because of antibodies to factor VIII.

Fibronectin

As noted, cryoprecipitate contains plasma fibronectin in a moderately concentrated form and it is the most readily available source for this material. Fibronectin is an interesting substance, which in its circulatory form seems to function primarily as an opsonin, that is, it facilitates phagocytosis by the reticuloendothelial system of certain gram-positive bacteria, fibrin particles, and possibly certain other foreign bodies. It also binds quickly to collagen and may be important in wound healing. Fibronectin levels in plasma decrease significantly after operations, injury, burns, and DIC, and are low in certain chronic wasting diseases. All these conditions are characterized by increased susceptibility to infection. In survivors, the levels come back to normal, but remain low in nonsurvivors. All of this led to great expectations regarding the therapeutic benefits of administering fibronectin to certain acutely ill surgical patients. The results have been unclear at best, and perhaps disappointing. Congenital deficiencies also seem not to be associated with disastrous consequences.[43] A recent, prospective, well-done study, however, detected a possible beneficial effect on survival in certain critically ill surgical patients.[44] The results were carefully and cautiously analyzed, and there may be something there. Clearly, more evaluation is needed, and uncontrolled use at the present would be very premature. Cryoprecipitate transmits disease and in some animal models appears to make worse what it was hoped to make better.

Antithrombin III

Antithrombin III[45] is not yet a licensed product in the United States, but may soon be available. Antithrombin III[45] is the main thrombin antagonist in plasma; it also helps neutralize a number of activated coagulation components. It thus appears to be a key factor in the balance between hemorrhage and clotting. Antithrombin III is reduced after major injuries, large operations, sepsis, DIC, severe cirrhosis, and immediately after extensive venous thrombosis. All of these states are characterized by the recent occurence of or increased susceptibility to extensive intravascular coagulation. Heparin works as an anticoagulant primarily through its effect on antithrombin III, which was formerly called heparin cofactor. With deficient levels, heparin resistance is apparent, that is, large doses of heparin produce little or no effect on laboratory tests of clotting. Such patients also appear to be more prone to severe thromboembolic events. Antithrombin III needs to be present at levels well above 50% by the currently used assay. Levels below 50% in fact are rarely found. This suggests that an inactive form is also being measured by this assay as such a low margin of reserve is very uncharacteristic of such an important circulatory protein. Congenital deficiency states are characterized by thromboembolic events beginning early in life. The material now available is being tested in various appropriate clinical circumstances. It may have a special role in the prevention of thromboembolic complications after injury and operation. Little has been published yet concerning its hazards. Presumably, it will also transmit at least hepatitis.

Problems

For the infectious diseases transmitted by transfusion, one of the clinically important but unclear aspects is that of a dose-response relationship. It would be helpful, especially educationally, to know the risk of transmitting a disease with the first unit transfused, the fifth, the 20th, etc. If the risk becomes negligible for incremental exposure beyond a certain level, therapeutic decisions for the heavily transfused patient can be made in a different context. Unfortunately, it is not clear what those relationships are, but some reasonably informed guesses can be made.

Part of the problem in obtaining more precise knowledge is the inherently uncontrolled nature of the experiment. Patients are not, nor should they be, transfused randomly. The exposure itself and the dose involved is determined by other factors. In most studies the pretransfusion status of the recipient with regard to the transmissible disease is not known. For some of the most important transmitted diseases (especially non–A non–B hepatitis) there are no direct diagnostic tests available and the diagnosis is made by implication with all the uncertainty inherent in that approach. Finally, the pattern of exposure is not at all evenly spread over a reasonable dose range. Very few patients are exposed to a single donor, so that important datum is very difficult to establish. Exposure in the United States clusters heavily around four to five donors per recipient.

An additional problem, not often discussed, is that of possible protection conferred by an occasional donor. For many of these diseases, antibody is used as a marker for infectivity rather than protection. For HIV, there is very little to suggest that antibody can be protective; for cytomegalovirus (CMV) and hepatitis B, donors with antibody seem more likely to be infective than protective, but the possibility of occasional protection exists. If donors are screened for antibody by an effective test, presumably the chance of having a protective donor disappears. (For hepatitis A, antibody is protective, but hepatitis A is very rarely if ever transmitted by tranfusion.) The effect(s) of NANB antibody(s) is unknown because there is no way of identifying such antibody.

For some of these diseases, then, some of the recipients may be already protected or doomed by exposure prior to transfusion; for them, transfusion has no impact on the disease in question. Most donors are probably neutral with respect to the disease; some will be infective, a few may be protective. If this scenario applies, then the dose-response relationship can be complex. This is possibly the situation with NANB. There are some data to support an incidence of NANB of 4% in recipients after exposure to a single donor. There is much more evidence to support an incidence of 7 to 8% after exposure to four donors, and some evidence in patients after cardiopulmonary bypass indicating an incidence of 15 to 20% after exposure to ten to 20 donors. Some of these studies were at different times and places, however, so they are not strictly comparable to each other. Nevertheless, to the extent that they are interpretable they suggest a complex relationship with a significant risk for the first exposure that seems to progressively decrease with subsequent exposures, but not to the point of absent incremental risk. Some recipients, however, will probably never be infected by transfusion.

At the other end of the spectrum is HIV. This is a relatively rare disease in the general population of recipients, and distinctly rare in the population of donors. When contracted it is probably uniformly fatal, so the end point is clear. There is no protection conferred by donors. Under these circumstances, the dose-response relationship remains essentially a straight line through very large exposures, i.e., the 30th unit is almost as likely to be fatal as the first, and 30 units are almost 30 times likely to be fatal as one.

Hepatitis

Hepatitis A is rarely if ever transmitted by transfusion. The incidence of hepatitis B transmitted by transfusion has been reduced to a low level because of better laboratory screening for markers of infectivity and because of the extensive conversion to a truly volunteer donor system. The incidence is not zero, however, as the screening tests are not yet sufficiently sensitive. Probably less than 1% of transfused patients now contract hepatitis B as a result of transfusion.

The most serious infectious disease transmitted by transfusion is NANB.[46–50] It is the most serious because current evidence indicates it will cause the death of more patients than any other transmitted disease. According to the studies in the mid-1970s, about 7% of transfused patients develop evidence of NANB (significantly abnormal liver tests, especially enzymes, within a few months after transfusion).[46] The alarming data now emerging are that half of these patients will have these abnormalities persist for over a year. In carefully studied cohorts, these chemical abnormalities are accompanied by structural abnormalities in the liver seen on biopsy that parallel in degree the chemical abnormalities. As many as half of these patients with persistent hepatitis may progress to serious hepatic impairment after an interval of ten to 15 years. Thus NANB appears to be an initially bland but eventually disabling and even fatal disease in a significant percentage of transfused patients. Exactly what percentage eventually becomes disabled and killed by this disease remains to be established. Careful long-term studies are in progress, but the results to date are cause for alarm. Unless these studies are somehow seriously flawed, far more patients will die of NANB than of HIV transmitted by transfusion. They will die later and more slowly, but the chances are they will stay just as dead.

There are two possible improvements in this picture. More extensive surrogate testing is becoming common and may soon be required of blood banks in the United States. Alanine amino transferase has been evaluated in several studies; high levels in donors are associated with a much higher incidence of NANB in recipients.[46] Unfortunately, like most surrogate tests it lacks both sensitivity and specificity. Some seemingly safe blood will be eliminated and most of the NANB will remain in the donor pool. The incidence in recipients should be lessened, but not to a great degree. Testing for hepatitis B core antigen will also be included; it may also serve as a surrogate for HIV. The other hopeful development is early evidence that human alpha-interferon produced by recombinant DNA technology can suppress the chemical and structural abnormalities of chronic NANB for at least a year or longer.[51] If so, this may provide a way of controlling the progression of this disease in at least some recipients.

Acquired Immunodeficiency Syndrome

Human immunodeficiency virus can be transmitted by blood transfusion and by at least some plasma products. This is a pertinent distinction because the virus seems to reside primarily in cells and not in plasma. Pooled plasma products, however, have unquestionably transmitted the disease in the hemophiliac population. Ironically, HIV is the easiest to eliminate from plasma of all the major infectious agents, and this appears to have been accomplished by gentle controlled heating for the pooled products used by hemophiliacs.[42] Such an approach does not work for products that are cellular, such as blood, and is not feasible because of problems of cost and quality control in single donor products such as fresh frozen plasma and cryoprecipitate. There are no good data on the infectivity of extensively washed red cells for HIV.

The story of HIV in transfusion is well known. The disease seemed to appear in significant numbers in the donor population a bit less than ten years ago. Because of the long interval between exposure and clinical manifestation, the lack of diagnostic markers until recently, and the initial very low incidence of transmission by transfusion, it was not clear for several years that transmission by transfusion could occur in any but an already immunosuppressed recipient population. It has been clear for at least five years now that such transmission does occur, that it can occur in minimally transfused patients, and that the infective blood could easily pass the then applied screening procedures. Two changes have occurred since then to make the supply of blood safer: donors have been asked to exclude themselves if they fall into groups at high risk for carrying the virus, and a test of antibody to the virus is being applied to all donor blood (the use of surrogate testing referred to above is more likely to alter the incidence of NANB, but may effect the transmission of HIV also). The programs aimed at educating donors to exercise voluntary exclusion are difficult to assess. In some areas, there appears to have been good cooperation and effectiveness,[52] but not so in other locations, at least at the times assessed. More reliance has been placed on the tests for HIV antibody. These indicate prior exposure. Antibody is believed to be minimally if at all protective in this disease, so the presence of antibody is presumably a marker of infectivity. In that respect, HIV parallels the situation for another intraleukocytic virus transmitted by transfusion, CMV. The problems with the antibody test are, again, specificity and sensitivity. There are false positive reactions that are in themselves unusual, but against a very low rate of expected true positive reactions they become significant. They are certainly distressing, at times devastating to the donors who may be told incorrectly that they have a soon-to-be fatal condition. Western blot analysis is believed to be much more specific, and "positive" antibody tests should be confirmed by this method in seemingly healthy donors. The Western blot test is expensive and prolonged, and availability is limited.

Because of the long interval between exposure and clinical changes, it is not clear what impact these measures have had on the transmission of HIV by transfusion. Certainly, some early public statements that "the nations blood supply is now completely safe" were premature and almost certainly incorrect. There are already several well-studied instances of recipients developing antibody after receiving blood that did not contain antibody, and with no other detectable risks of infection. In some of these instances, the donors were traced and had developed antibody after donating the blood. It was originally thought that the interval between exposure and the development of antibody was relatively brief, that is, a few weeks. This may be so in many instances, but there are now well studied examples of intervals up to six months or more between exposure and the development of antibody. Apparently at least some of these individuals can be infective during this interval.

The incidence of HIV in the population still donating blood is not clear. Early studies using Western blot confirmation are few and scattered, so conclusions are hazardous. The numbers reported so far indicate something between 1/10,000 and 1/100,000. The more important question, the incidence of HIV infective units still entering the system, cannot be answered clearly for several years. The answer will not be zero.

Clinical manifestations of HIV after exposure to blood products varies. For some there is a febrile adenopathy soon after exposure with development of antibody within a few weeks. This usually fades gradually and seeming good health returns. After several years, the later stages of the disease with the characteristic opportunistic infections begins. In others, the interval after exposure seems uneventful and typically lasts several years. In at least some of these patients, antibody appears late and monitoring within a few months of exposure may yield incorrect information. It is not certain but appears likely that most people infected with the virus will die within five to ten years. Most major transfusion agencies now offer testing for antibody in patients transfused since 1978 at reduced cost. Concerned patients should be offered these tests if the transfusion occurred at least six months before proposed testing.

The disease has become worldwide, but the incidence of infected individuals still varies greatly. Some of the spread can be traced to the international commerce in blood products. The worst area by far appears to be central Africa, where major fractions of the young adult population are infected. Transfusion of blood in those areas will be extraordinarily hazardous. In the United States, as noted, NANB is a much greater threat to life. Other retroviruses are beginning to appear in donor populations, and testing for HTLV-1 has recently been proposed. Given the extremely labile nature of the genetic material in some of these viruses, the situation could change rather quickly.[53, 54]

Immunosuppression

The logical assumption had been made in transplantation circles that exposure of recipients to similar antigenic material prior to transplantation of an allograft would worsen the results of transplantation by making rejection of the allograft more likely. Patients in renal failure requiring transfusion were treated with extensively washed red cells to minimize exposure to transplantation-related antigens if those patients were potential candidates for receiving a renal allograft. It came as quite a surprise when retrospective analysis of the results of renal transplantation showed exactly the opposite: prior transfusion seemed to improve the results of transplantation and there may have been a beneficial dose-response relationship.[55] After initial skepticism, many other analyses confirmed this observation and deliberate exposure to the antigens on leukocytes in stored blood became part of experimental protocols and accepted treatment regimens.

The understanding of this phenomenon is very incomplete. Some prospective recipients do indeed become immunized by prior exposure and become more difficult to treat, but the majority seem to be easier to manage after transplantation. The effect of transfusion seems to be more than simply a way of selecting weak reactors for transplantation, however. Many other mechanisms have been considered, but none proven.

Most of the viral diseases transmitted by transfusion are at least temporarily immunosuppressive.[56] Human immunodeficiency virus is the extreme example, but CMV, hepatitis B, Epstein-Barr virus, and probably NANB are also lymphopathic and immunosuppressive. Immunologic abnormalities are characteristic of populations exposed to many donors over long periods receiving blood products that can transmit these diseases.[57] Noteworthy for the subsequent discussion, a marked decrease in natural killer cells has been reported in these populations. Other mechanisms may also be involved. Donor lymphocytes can be detected in the circulation of recipients for days after transfusion.[58] Immunologically normal recipients may have cytologically "abnormal" lymphocytes in their peripheral circulation for several weeks after transfusion.[59] Graft-versus-host disease is a specific condition in which immunologically competent donor cells in the transfusion colonize and attack the recipient. This has been well documented in animals and in humans.[60, 61] The recipients are severely immunosuppressed and it is common practice now to irradiate blood before transfusing it into such recipients. Worsened immunosuppression is characteristic of graft-versus-host disease. Other possible explanations of immunosuppression after transfusion include the fortuitous production of blocking antibodies that serve to protect the graft and stimulation of T-suppressor cells in the recipient. To make the situation more confusing, it may be that prior transfusion impairs rather than improves success after bone marrow transplantation.

Experimental work in animal models has not yielded consistent or easily interpreted results. Allogenic transfusion suppressed the response of lymphocytes to mitogen stimulation and enhanced the growth of transplanted tumors in rodents.[62, 63] Transfusion of syngeneic blood was without effect. In other similar experiments, plasma had the greatest effect, washed red cells were without effect, and leukocytes were intermediate, and the effect was apparent only when donor and recipient differed at the H_2 locus.[64] In other experiments in rodents, however, prior transfusion of donor specific blood led to prolongation of organ grafts but accelerated rejection of both antigenically strong and weak transplanted tumors.[65] Other studies have also reported a suppression of tumor growth in transfused rodents, but the results varied with the donor-recipient combinations tested.[66] The effect was observed with transfused leukocytes alone or with whole blood, and could not be prevented by measures effective against graft-versus-host disease, implying that proliferation and persistence of donor cells after transfusion were not necessary. Allogenic blood transfusion partially restored the ability of burned mice to reject allogenic skin grafts.[67] In a very interesting study in dogs, however, allogenic transfusion after hemorrhage impaired the ability of the animals to clear intravenously injected bacteria.[68] The impairment was greater with stored blood than with fresh blood, which showed little effect. This suggests that in that particular study, immunologic phenomena may not have been prominent.

Prompted by the apparent identification of a lasting immunosuppressive effect of transfusion in patients in renal failure, concerns were expressed about possible related adverse effects of transfusion in patients being treated for cancer.[69] Considerable evidence supports the importance of immune defenses in determining outcome in patients treated for cancer. Immunosuppressed patients seem to have a higher incidence of many kinds of malignancy and to have a poorer outlook for cure by standard methods of treatment. A moderate number of studies have been published over the past five years on the relationship between transfusion and outcome in patients treated for cancer. All have been retrospective and all have been uncontrolled. Nevertheless, some conclusions have been drawn and implications regarding treatment made.

The most extensively studied relationship involves cancer of the colon. Burrows and Tartter in 1982 reported a series of 58 transfused and 65 nontransfused patients who underwent colectomy between 1978 and 1981 for cancer of the colon.[70] In patients with comparable stage of tumor, transfused patients had significantly more recurrences of cancer. The series was expanded one year later to 177 transfused, 118 nontransfused.[71] Transfused patients still did less well, although the difference may have been greater for left-sided tumors in the expanded series. Neither report has appeared in detail: the first was a letter to the editor, the second a published abstract. Blumberg et al. reported a series of 129 transfused and 68 nontransfused patients treated surgically for cancer of the colon and followed six months to 11 years.[72] Within each pathologic stage, transfused patients had a much higher rate of recurrence than nontransfused patients. Transfusion was associated with increasing age, increasing duration of operation, tumors in the rectum, and preoperative anemia. At least some of these variables are associated with poorer outcome. Transfusion stood out as independently significant on multivariate analysis, but the variables were all tested in binary form only. Furthermore, in the nontransfused group, the results for Dukes' C_2 stage was no worse than for A and B combined and there was an amazingly low rate of recurrence overall in the nontransfused patients (9%). Clearly, there was something strange about that series. Foster et al. reported 65 transfused and 81 nontransfused patients resected for cure of cancer of the colon excluding rectum from 1974 to 1979.[73] Transfused patients did less well. Again, transfusion was associated with increasing age, anemia, and right-sided tumors (which in this series were of more advanced stage).

Several different approaches at multivariate analysis yielded differing results; by at least some methods, transfusion stood out as an independently significant variable for right sided tumors, but not for other locations. A group of 74 patients treated for rectal cancer during the same period were independently evaluated; no effect of transfusion on outcome was detected. Thus, the only group in which transfusion seemed to be associated with a poorer outcome was the group that was older, more anemic, had more advanced stage of disease, and had fewer nontransfused patients. The strongest support for the hypothesis that transfusion impairs the survival of patients treated for cancer of the colon comes from a study at Newcastle.[74] Transfused (373) and nontransfused (144) patients followed for one to 11 years were compared within similar pathologic stages. Transfused patients had more recurrences, but also had longer operations, more operative blood loss, lower preoperative hemoglobin levels, and more rectal cancers. Even when rectal cancers, which have a poorer outlook for similar pathologic stage, were eliminated (180 transfused, 111 not transfused) the other differences remained statistically significant.

Contrary evidence came first from a study by Ota and colleagues on 162 transfused and 45 nontransfused patients age 65 or less treated for cancer of the colon (rectum excluded).[75] Overall, no effect of transfusion was found. When examined according to the number of units transfused there was a tendency toward poorer outcome at large volumes of transfusion. These same patients had more extensive operations, however, because of greater local spread of the tumor. The authors also used the number of nodes reported in the resected specimens as an index of the adequacy of resection. The numbers of nodes reported were the same for the transfused and nontransfused groups. Thus, with the elderly patients and rectal tumors excluded, the only differences found related to the local extent of the tumor. This seems to be the first of these studies to evaluate the apparent reasons for intraoperative transfusions and to relate these to the subject of the study. A subsequent study from Seattle showed no difference within similar pathologic stages for the incidence of recurrence or time to recurrence of 75 transfused vs. 47 not transfused patients followed up five to six years.[76] A series from New Zealand of 103 transfused and 71 not transfused patients followed up for three to four years reported that the recurrence rate was not different within similar pathologic stages.[77] A study from Australia of 60 transfused and 49 nontransfused patients followed one to eight years found no difference in recurrence rates within similar pathologic stages.[78] A study from Detroit of 199 transfused vs. 167 not transfused patients treated by six different surgeons and followed up for seven to 13 years found no difference in recurrences within similar pathologic stages.[79] There was a trend toward poorer results with very large volumes transfused, but the numbers of patients were small. Significantly, the authors stated there was no difference between those transfused with RBCs vs. "plasma" (? whole blood or fresh frozen plasma). A somewhat different study from St. Mark's hospital used as the end point dead from disease by five years after treatment and classified 301 patients according to intraoperative transfusion only.[80] There were no differences in survival of patients in stages A and B. Transfused patients in stage C had better survival statistics than those not transfused.

Thus, the early reports of a correlation between transfusion and poor outcome for the treatment of cancer of the colon had some inconsistencies and some odd features. Most of the recent analyses do not support such an association. The evident correlation in most of those studies between transfusion and other prognostically active variables indicates caution in assigning an independent role to transfusion itself.

Two studies deal with the same question in patients treated surgically for cancer of the lung. The series reported by Tartter et al. is unusual because all the patients were operated on by the same surgeon, thereby eliminating a potentially important variable.[81] Patients operated on for stage I non–oat cell cancer of the lung and followed up at least two years were evaluated according to whether transfused (59) or not transfused (106). By multivariate analysis, the extent of the operation was by far the most significant variable relating to outcome, but transfusion was also significantly related. When pneumonectomies were excluded the effect of transfusion was not quite significant. The authors did not comment on the likely correlation between transfusion and the extent of operation. Hyman et al. reported patients resected for primary cancers of the lung, stages I and II, 33 transfused and 72 nontransfused.[82] The transfused patients did less well, but no comment was made about the need for transfusion and the extent of the operation.

Both studies indicate that transfusion is associated with poorer outcome when patients with primary cancer of the lung are treated surgically. Cancer of the lung does not typically bleed significantly, however, so it seems likely that the need for transfusion is associated with prognostically poor variables such as hilar location, invasion of neighboring structures, and so on.

Two studies have examined the association between transfusion and outcome in patients treated for cancer of the breast. Foster et al. reported on patients followed up for one to seven years after surgical treatment. Stage of tumor and nodal involvement were similar for those transfused (65) and those not transfused (161).[83] There was no effect of transfusion on outcomes. The authors comment that the use of transfusion varied widely among the 11 surgeons represented in the study, but they did not evaluate results by surgeon. Tartter et al. reported 39 transfused and 130 nontransfused patients treated for cancer of the breast and followed up for five to 13 years.[84] The transfused patients did less well within each stage and the results were significantly different when all stages were combined. It does not appear that this combined contrast was weighted for stage, however, and the transfused patients were disproportionally represented in the locally advanced stage. "Adjuvant" therapy (not specified, but presumably local radiation therapy) was given to significantly more of the transfused patients. The results were also evaluated for 89 patients operated on by the same surgeon and the effects of transfusion were still significant, but no details were given.

The results were conflicting in those two studies on cancer of the breast. The study that found a detrimental effect of transfusion, however, gave abundant evidence of a correlation between transfusion and more advanced stage of disease. Of additional interest in these two series is the very high percentage of patients transfused for surgical treatment of cancer of the breast, 29% and 23%. One hopes this is not a common pattern.

Other malignancies have also been considered for this relationship between transfusion and the success of treatment. Rosenberg et al. found that transfusion was associated with earlier and more frequent recurrence of tumor in patients treated for high-grade, soft-tissue sarcomas of the extremities and assigned to different treatment protocols.[85] The effect of transfusion was found only in the group given adjuvant chemotherapy. In this study also there was a correlation between increased size of tumor and transfusion during treatment. The authors attempted to correct for this in their statistical analysis. Blumberg, whose study of patients with cancer of the colon contained such odd results, suggested improved survival of patients treated for cancer of the uterine cervix who were not transfused compared with those who were transfused.[86] The data in the table accompanying the abstract are quite unconvincing, however: recurrences of cancer in those transfused vs. not transfused by stage: 6/42 vs. 6/25 in stage I; 7/17 vs. 4/19 in stage II; 6/9 vs. 6/13 in stage III. Blumberg et al. have recently reported one of the more interesting observations.[87] Reviewing patients treated for cancer of the colon, rectum, cervix, or prostate, there was no impairment of survival of those transfused 3 units or less of RBC concentrates. Those transfused more than 3 units of red cell concentrates or any amount of whole blood had impaired survival. Nathanson in the study from Detroit cited earlier seemed to find no such difference, but the statement is a bit cryptic.

In all of those studies on the relationship between transfusion and outcome in patients treated surgically for cancer several problems remain. First, it appears that the more studies that are done, the more the results are inconsistent. Second, all of these studies are retrospective and uncontrolled. Indeed, a prospective controlled trial in which transfusions were administered randomly would not be acceptable because of the other known risks of transfusion. Third, transfusion is not only not a random event, it is in most instances related to other prognostically unfavorable variables. This indicates caution in trying to identify the role of transfusion as an independent variable, and the probable need for large numbers of patients before being able to draw valid statistical conclusions. The hypothesis of Blumberg regarding red cell concentrates versus whole blood should, however, be evaluable and such a study is now being considered in England.

The relationship between transfusion and outcome has also been evaluated in nonmalignant conditions. In a retrospective study of 565 patients undergoing large abdominal operations, Maetani et al. reported that transfusion was the variable most strongly associated with multiple organ failure.[88] The statistical methods seem a bit obscure, however, and only five other specific organ risks factors were considered, all treated as binary. Tartter et al. compared 43 transfused with 16 nontransfused patients operated on for inflammatory bowel disease.[89] The groups seemed comparable at the time of operation. At six to 18 months after operation, T-cell counts and total lymphocyte counts were significantly lower in the transfused patients, and the effect was proportional to the amount transfused. There was no difference in clinical outcome. Tartter et al. subsequently reported a higher incidence of postoperative infections in patients transfused during hospitalization for resection of colon cancer (69 transfused, 99 not transfused).[90] The authors did not comment on stomas vs. anastamoses, left side vs. right, obstruction, coexistent diabetes, etc. Strangely, patients with lower preoperative hematocrits had significantly *fewer* infections. This implies that transfusion was related to intraoperative blood loss and not to preoperative anemia.

For the nonmalignant conditions, some of the same types of problems apply. More transfusion presumably results from more blood loss, which in turn usually means more hypoperfusion or bigger operations. Hemorrhage itself seems associated with impaired antibacterial defenses and multiorgan impairment. Interpretation of simple correlation must therefore be very cautious.

Solutions

Solutions to the problems arising from the use of blood and blood products are partially at hand and partially in an uncertain future.

The major problem in the current use of these products is the transmission of disease. Several approaches are possible and are not mutually exclusive. Better testing for the infective agents will improve the safety of the products in proportion to the efficacy of the tests. The current tests for hepatitis B are not quite sufficiently sensitive, those for HIV do not detect part of the infective period in donors, tests for Epstein-Barr virus are expensive, and there are no usable tests for NANB. Other viruses of clinical significance may be entering the system and will certainly do so in the future and some may already be there but are currently not suspected. No test will ever be perfect. There will always be problems of sensitivity and specificity, and the proliferation of tests when available will inexorably increase the cost of the products.

The next level of approach would be inactivation of the agents in the collected blood. Several approaches to this have been taken in the past, but have usually been ineffective or impractical. Given the delicate nature of the desired product, there is not much hope for this approach in the short term. Immunization of the recipient population may be a more efficient strategy. This may not be effective against some of the infectious agents; however, HIV and retroviruses may be difficult as a class to control by immunization.

Effective methods of treating the patient after infection are less desirable than prevention, and usually less effective. The recent trials with alpha interferon in patients with NANB offer some hope for that problem, but at very considerable expense and uncertain long-term efficacy.

An immediately available and largely effective approach is to eliminate unnecessary exposure of patients to the risks of transfusion. This has the further beneficial effect of extending the supply of product and of decreasing the expenses of treatment. There is probably not a single blood product that is not overused, some of them extraordinarily so. Such overuse is based largely in the ignorance of the ordering physicians and is therefore correctable. It is amazing how few physicians who order blood are aware of the data regarding risk, and how few know of the controlled studies bearing on the use of different components. Consider each of the major products in turn.

Red blood cells are often given to treat numbers rather than patients. It would be quite revealing to know what fraction of RBC use in the United States occurred in order to raise the hematocrit level above 30% regardless of the status of the patient. This is one of the truly damnable "magic numbers" in clinical medicine. It serves as a wretchedly poor replacement for thinking. As if it weren't pernicious enough by itself it is usually coupled with a truly awesomely ignorant concept: "if you need one, you need two." Many patients in fact are exposed to the risks of two donors because their hematocrit levels are below 30%, when they don't need to be exposed to any. It's difficult to know where this concept began. The scientific principle that should apply is to give blood only when it is needed, and then to give the least amount necessary. A practice arose years ago of investigating single unit transfusions by committee. The result was the use of double unit transfusions, which were ignored. If any monitoring is needed now, it is of two unit transfusions. A sign of return to rationality would be the reappearance of the occasional single unit transfusion (under the proper circumstance). Another area of excessive use in surgery is the operating room where some anesthesiologists often without discussing the decision administer blood because the operative field looks red. Most studies on intraoperative transfusion show patients emerging with hematocrit levels far higher than requiring to be supported by transfusion.[91] The recent development and successful testing of recombinant human erythropoietin promise to reduce one category of need, the patients with end stage renal disease. Unfortunately, it is doubtful that many other anemic conditions will be corrected by additional erythropoietin.[92]

The other side of the RBC coin is iatrogenic hemorrhage. The amount of blood drawn for diagnostic purposes turns up as a continually astonishing amount in repeated studies.[93, 94] Restraint, reason, and better use of other monitoring methods could reduce this significantly.

Fresh frozen plasma, as already noted, is considered the most overused of all blood bank products.[23, 95] There are good indications for its use, but most of its use appears to be in questionable or outright ineffective prophylactic adventure. The use of fresh frozen plasma for tuning up, for nutritional supplementation, and for mystical hoped-for effects is particularly irrational. It is quite likely that the population of hospitalized patients in the United States would on balance be better off without this product, given its level of overuse and its disease causing potential.

Platelets have also had a rapid increase in use, but usually with better documentation of at least somewhat reasonable circumstances. The weight of evidence from controlled trials, however, also points to significant overuse for prophylactic purposes. Sometimes, simply rewarming the patient may suffice.[96] Reports on the efficacy of desmopressin and of conjugated estrogens in reducing bleeding after cardiopulmonary bypass and in patients in renal failure if confirmed may lead to decreased use of disease-transmitting components.[97, 98]

Some patients will unequivocably require transfusion. The safest blood to receive is one's own.[99] Emergency autotransfusion has had a number of problems relating to equipment and safety. The newer devices provide washed RBCs in a reasonably short time. Washing eliminates some of the potentially harmful debris and thromboplastic material collected from wounds. Even with frequent and experienced use, however, such autologous transfusion usually supplies only about 25% of total transfusion needs in severely bleeding patients. In patients undergoing elective operations in which 1 to 2 L blood loss is anticipated, autologous predonation can avoid exposure to allogenic products and donors. Many elective surgical patients who are transfused fall into this category. Unfortunately, the method is not used nearly frequently enough. One recent study of 18 teaching hospitals documents the shamefully poor use of this method in suitable elective surgical patients.[100] In that study, had the method been used exposure to non–self donors could have been avoided in about 60% of the transfused patients. This superb alternative to hepatitis and other diseases needs much wider application. It also extends the supply of blood and blood products.

Every time a patient with modest blood loss is treated with electrolyte solution and not transfused, a blood substitute has been used. The search for substitutes now extends to agents capable of replacing a major fraction of blood volume. The development of usable coagulation factors from recombinant DNA technology still seems to be rather remote. Substitutes for red cells, however, have been developed. The first product to be tested based on halogenated hydrocarbons has proven disappointing. The rather small amount that can be safely given and the limited oxygen carrying capacity of the product result in a minimal impact on oxygen delivery.[101] More promising at the moment are developments with stroma free hemoglobin. Some of the early problems with this approach have been solved, and various cross-linked products now show sufficient intravascular persistence and oxygen-delivering capability to be promising.[102] Clinical trials may start soon for some of these products. Properly used, they can potentially minimize RBC transfusion in some patients and avoid them altogether in others. Artificial substitutes for platelets seem very unlikely at the moment.

Finer mesh microfilters were developed to prevent pulmonary injury from microembolization caused by transfusion, especially of large volumes of blood. These special filters in controlled trials have shown very little effect on pulmonary function. What they do seem to accomplish is to reduce the transfusion of white cells and platelet clumps and thereby reduce immunization and febrile transfusion reactions.[103]

Warming blood for transfusion remains an annoying problem. Hypothermia in severely injured patients and in those extensively transfused during operations still occurs frequently and probably contributes to many other problems, including impaired hemostasis. Various devices to warm blood during transfusion all must deal with the same problem: the contact heating surface cannot be warm enough to damage red cells, flow must be rapid, and too large a dead space is impractical. Direct microwave heating devices are unsafe because of the problems of "hot spots" and subsequent hemolysis. The search continues.

Of all the problems with blood and blood products, the worst should it occur would be not to have blood available when it is truly needed. A safe national blood supply is the culmination of many acts of personal sacrifice without monetary gain by the true volunteer blood donors. They constitute a small fraction of those capable of donating blood, and the balance between supply and demand sometimes becomes precarious, especially around major holidays. More rational use of blood will preserve this precious resource for times of true need. The general public also needs to be better informed about the importance of donating blood. Physicians and surgeons can help substantially by occasionally talking to community groups and by mentioning this when appropriate to patients and their families. A safe blood supply is a voluntary effort.

References

1. Mollison PL: *Blood Transfusion in Clinical Medicine,* ed 7. Oxford, Blackwell Scientific Publications, 1983.
2. Oberman H, Chaplin H, Polesky HF, et al: *General Principles of Blood Transfusion,* ed 2. Chicago, American Medical Association, 1985.
3. Snyder EL, Kennedy MS: *Blood Transfusion Therapy: A Physician's Handbook.* Arlington, Va, American Association of Blood Banks, 1983.
4. *The Collection, Fractionation, Quality Control, and Uses of Blood Products.* World Health Organization, Geneva, 1981.
5. Chien S: Role of blood cells in microcirculatory regulation. *Microvasc Res* 1985; 29:129–151.
6. Murray JF, Gold P, Johnson BC: Systemic oxygen transport in induced normovolemic anemia and polycythemia. *Am J Physiol* 1962; 203:720–724.
7. Smith EE, Crowell JW: Influence of hematocrit ratio on survival of unacclimatized dogs at simulated high altitude. *Am J Physiol* 1963; 205:1172–1174.
8. Crowell JW, Smith EE: Determinant of the optimal hematocrit. *J Appl Physiol* 1967; 22:501–504.

9. Vellar OD, Hermansen L: Physical performance and hematological parameters. *Acta Med Scand* 1971, suppl, p 522.
10. Finch CA, Lenfant C: Oxygen transport in man. *N Engl J Med* 1972; 286:407–415.
11. Duhm J: Effects of 2,3-diphosphoglycerate and other organic phosphate compounds on oxygen affinity and intracellular pH of human erythrocytes. *Pflugers Arch* 1971; 326:341–356.
12. Bosta SS, Soekirman MS, Karyadi D, et al: Iron deficiency anemia and the productivity of adult males in Indonesia. *Am J Clin Nutr* 1979; 32:916–925.
13. Edgerton VR, Gardner GW, Ohira, Y, et al: Iron-deficiency anaemia and its effect on worker productivity and activity patterns. *Br Med J* 1979, pp 1548–1549.
14. Viteri F, Torien B: Anaemia and physical work capacity. *Clin Haematol* 1974; 3:609–626.
15. Edgerton VR, Ohira Y, Hettiarachchi J, et al: Elevation of hemoglobin and work tolerance in iron-deficient subjects. *J Nutr Sci Vitaminol* 1981; 27:77–86.
16. Delano BG, Nacht R, Friedman EA, et al: Myocardial anaerobiosis in anemia in man. *Circulation* 1970; 42:(suppl 3):148.
17. Varat MA, Adolph RJ, Fowler NO: Cardiovascular effects of anemia. *Am Heart J* 1972; 83:415–426.
18. Johansen SH, Laver MB: Cardiovascular effects of severe anemic hypoxia. *Acta Anaesth Scand* 1966; 24(suppl):63–68.
19. Crowell JW, Ford RG, Lewis VM: Oxygen transport in hemorrhagic shock as a function of the hematocrit ratio. *Am J Physiol* 1959; 196:1033–1038.
20. Sunder-Plassmann L, Klovekorn WP, Messmer K: Limited hemodilution in hemorrhagic shock in dogs: Effects on central hemodynamics and the microcirculation in skeletal muscle. *Res Exp Med* 1973; 159:167–182.
21. Case RB, Berglund E, Sarnoff SJ: Ventricular function: VII. Changes in coronary resistance and ventricular function resulting from acutely induced anemia and the effect thereon of coronary stenosis. *Am J Med* 1955; 18:397–405.
22. Wolfe JHN, Waller DG, Chapman MB, et al: The effect of hemodilution upon patients with intermittent claudication. *Surg Gynecol Obstet* 1985; 160:347–351.
23. Tullis JL, Alving B, Bove JR, et al: *Fresh Frozen Plasma: Indications and Risks*. NIH Consensus Development Conference Statement. Bethesda, Md, US Dept HHS, 1984, vol 5, No. 5.
24. Collins JA: Problems associated with the massive transfusion of stored blood. *Surgery* 1974; 75:274–295.
25. Domen RE, Kennedy MS, Jones LL, et al: Hemostatic imbalances produced by plasma exchange. *Transfusion* 1984; 24:336–339.
26. Flaum MA, Cuneo RA, Appelbaum FR, et al: The hemostatic imbalance of plasma-exchange transfusion. *Blood* 1979; 54:694–702.
27. Simmons RL, Collins JA, Heisterkamp CA, et al: Coagulation disorders in combat casualties, II, III. *Ann Surg* 1969; 169:463–470, 471–482.
28. Harke H, Rahman S: Haemostatic disorders in massive transfusion. *Bibl Haematol* 1980; 46:179–188.
29. Counts RB, Haisch C, Simon TL, et al: Hemostasis in massively transfused trauma patients. *Ann Surg* 1979; 190:91–99.

30. Martin DJ, Lucas CE, Ledgerwood AM, et al: Fresh frozen plasma supplement to massive red blood cell transfusion. *Ann Surg* 1985; 202:505–511.
31. Aster RH, Bartolucci AA, Collins JA, et al: *Platelet Transfusion Therapy.* Consensus Development Conference Statement. Bethesda, Md, US Dept HHS, Oct 1986, vol 6, no. 7.
32. Slichter SJ: Controversies in platelet transfusion therapy. *Ann Rev Med* 1980; 31:509–540.
33. Higby DJ, Cohen E, Holland JF, et al: The prophylactic treatment of thrombocytopenic leukemic patients with platelets: A double blind study. *Transfusion* 1974; 14:440–446.
34. Murphy S, Litwin S, Herring LM, et al: Indications for platelet transfusion in children with acute leukemia. *Am J Hematol* 1982; 12:347–356.
35. Harding SA, Shakoor MA, Grindon AV: Platelet support for cardiopulmonary bypass surgery. *J Thoracic Cardiovasc Surg* 1975; 70:350–353.
36. Simon TL, Abel BF, Murphy W: Controlled trial of routine administration of platelet concentrates in cardiopulmonary bypass surgery. *Ann Thoracic Surg* 1984; 37:359–364.
37. Harrigan C, Lucas CE, Ledgerwood AM, et al: Serial changes in primary hemostasis after massive transfusion. *Surgery* 1985; 98:836–843.
38. Reed RL, Heimbach DM, Counts RB, et al: Prophylactic platelet administration during massive transfusion. *Ann Surg* 1986; 203:40–48.
39. Miller RD, Robbins TO, Tong MJ, et al: Coagulation defects associated with massive blood transfusions. *Ann Surg* 1971; 174:794–801.
40. Cote CJ, Liu LM, Szyfelbein SK, et al: Changes in serial platelet counts following massive blood transfusion in pediatric patients. *Anesthesiology* 1985; 62:197–201.
41. Iberti TJ, Benjamin E, Berger ER, et al: Thrombocytopenia following peritonitis in surgical patients. *Ann Surg* 1986; 204:341–345.
42. Daenen S, Hoogeveen Y, Smit JW, et al: Risk of transmission of human immunodeficiency virus (HIV) by heat-treated factor VIII concentrates in patients with severe hemophilia A. *Transfusion* 1987; 27:482–484.
43. Shirakami A, Shigekiyo T, Hirai Y, et al: Plasma fibronectin deficiency in eight members of one family. *Lancet* 1986; 1:473–474.
44. Lundsgaard-Hansen P, Doran JE, Rubli E, et al: Purified fibronectin administration to patients with severe abdominal infections. *Ann Surg* 1985; 202:745–759.
45. Blick RL: Clinical relevance of antithrombin III. *Semin Thromb Hemost* 1985; 8:276–287.
46. Aach RD, Szmuness W, Mowsley JW, et al: Serum alanine aminotransferase of donors in relation to the risk of non-A, non-B hepatitis in recipients: The transfusion-transmitted viruses study. *N Engl J Med* 1981; 304:989–994.
47. Koretz RL, Stone O, Gitnick GL: The long-term course of non-A, non-B posttransfusion hepatitis. *Gastroenterology* 1980; 79:893–898.
48. Alter HJ, Purcell RH, Feinstone SM, et al: Non-A, non-B, hepatitis: Its relationship to cytomegalovirus, to chronic hepatitis, and to direct and indirect test methods, in Szmuness W, Alter HJ, Maynard JE (eds): *Viral Hepatitis, 1981 International Symposium.* Philadelphia, Franklin Institute Press, 1982, pp 279–294.
49. Dienstag JL: Non-A, non-B hepatitis: I. Recognition, epidemiology, and clinical features. *Gastroenterology* 1983; 85:439–462.

50. Alter HJ, Hoofnagle JH: Non-A, non-B: Observations on the first decade, in Vyas GN, Dienstag JL, Hoofnagle JH (eds): *Viral Hepatitis and Liver Disease.* Orlando, Fla, Grune & Stratton Inc, 1984, pp 345–354.
51. Hoofnagle JH, Mullen KD, Jones DB, et al: Treatment of chronic non-A, non-B hepatitis with recombinant human alpha interferon. *N Engl J Med* 1986; 315:1575–1578.
52. Kalish RI, Cable RG, Roberts SC: Voluntary deferral of blood donations and HTLV-III antibody positivity. *N Engl J Med* 1986; 314:1115–1116.
53. Melief CJ, Goudsmit J: Transmission of lymphotropic retroviruses (HTLV-1 and LAV/HTLV-III) by blood transfusion and blood products. *Vox Sang* 1986; 50:1–11.
54. Perrault RA, Derrick JB, Mankikar SD: Retroviruses and blood transfusion workshop. *Vox Sang* 1986; 51:75–78.
55. Opelz G, Terasaki PI: Improvement of kidney-graft survival with increased numbers of blood transfusions. *N Engl J Med* 1978; 299:799–803.
56. Southern P, Oldstone MBA: Medical consequences of persistent viral infection. *N Engl J Med* 1986; 314:359–367.
57. Cascon P, Zoumbos NC, Young NS: Immunologic abnormalities in patients receiving multiple blood transfusion. *Ann Intern Med* 1984; 100:173–177.
58. Schechter GP, Soehulen F, McFarland W: Lymphocyte response to blood transfusion in man. *N Engl J Med* 1972; 287:1169–1173.
59. Schechter GP, Whang-Peng J, McFarland W: Circulation of donor lymphocytes after blood transfusion in man. *Blood* 1977; 49:651–656.
60. Brubaker DB: Human posttransfusion graft-versus-host disease. *Vox Sang* 1983; 45:401–420.
61. Collins JA, Hechtman HB, Theobald TJ, et al: Treatment by transfusion of severe general radiation injury in dogs. *Transfusion* 1966; 6:134–139.
62. Francis DMA, Shenton BK, Proud G, et al: Tumour growth and blood transfusion. *Eur Surg Res* 1982; 14:124.
63. Francis DMA, Shenton BK: Blood transfusion and tumour growth: Evidence from laboratory animals. *Lancet* 1981; 2:871.
64. Horimi T, Kagawa S, Ninomiya M, et al: Possible induction by blood transfusion of immunologic tolerance against growth of transplanted tumors in mice. *Acta Med* 1983; 37:259–263.
65. Jeekel J, Eggermont A, Heystek G, et al: Inhibition of tumor growth by blood transfusion in the rat. *Eur Surg Res* 1982; 14:124–125.
66. Oilawa T, Hosokawa M, Imamura M, et al: Anti-tumor immunity by normal allogeneic blood transfusion in rat. *Clin Exp Immunol* 1977; 27:549–554.
67. Krob MJ, Shelby J: Immunosuppressive effects of burn injury and nonspecific blood transfusion. *J Trauma* 1986; 26:40–43.
68. Ollodart R, Mansberger AR: The effect of hypovolemic shock on bacterial defenses. *Am J Surg* 1965; 110:302–307.
69. Gantt CL: Red blood cells for cancer patients. *Lancet* 1981; 2:363.
70. Burrows L, Tartter P: Effect of blood transfusions on colonic malignancy recurrence rate. *Lancet* 1982; 2:662.
71. Burrows L, Tartter P: Blood transfusions and colorectal cancer recurrence: A possible relationship. *Transfusion* 1983; 23:419.
72. Blumberg N, Agarwal MM, Chuang C: Relation between recurrence of cancer of the colon and blood transfusion. *Br Med J* 1985; 290:1037–1039.
73. Foster RS, Costanza MC, Foster JC, et al: Adverse relationship between

blood transfusions and survival after colectomy for colon cancer. *Cancer* 1985; 55:1195–1201.

74. Parrott NR, Lennard TWJ, Taylor RMR, et al: Effect of perioperative blood transfusion on recurrence of colorectal cancer. *Br J Surg* 1986; 73:970–973.
75. Ota D, Alvarez L, Lichtiger B, et al: Perioperative blood transfusion in patients with colon carcinoma. *Transfusion* 1985; 25:392–394.
76. Weiden PL, Beam MA, Schultz P, et al: Perioperative blood transfusion does not increase risk of colorectal cancer recurrence. *Blood* 1984; 64(suppl 1):232a.
77. Frankish PD, McNee RK, Alley PG, et al: Relation between cancer of the colon and blood transfusion. *Br Med J* 1985; 290:1827.
78. Francis D, Judson R: Relation between recurrence of cancer of the colon and blood transfusion. *Br Med J* 1985; 291:544.
79. Nathanson SD, Tilley BC, Schultz L, et al: Perioperative allogeneic blood transfusions: Survival in patients with resected carcinomas of the colon and rectum. *Arch Surg* 1985; 120:734–738.
80. Blair SD, Janvrin SB: Relation between cancer of the colon and blood transfusion. *Br Med J* 1985; 290:1516–1517.
81. Tartter PI, Burrows L, Kirschner P: Perioperative blood transfusion adversely affects prognosis after resection of Stage I (subset NO) non-oat cell lung cancer. *J Thorac Cardiovasc Surg* 1984; 88:659–662.
82. Hyman NH, Foster RS, DeMeules J, et al: Blood transfusions and survival after lung cancer resection. *Am J Surg* 1985; 149:502–507.
83. Foster RS, Foster JC, Costanza MC: Blood transfusions and survival after surgery for breast cancer. *Arch Surg* 1984; 119:1138.
84. Tartter PI, Burrows L, Papatestas AE, et al: Perioperative blood transfusion has prognostic significance for breast cancer. *Surgery* 1985; 97:225–230.
85. Rosenberg SA, Seipp CA, White DE, et al: Perioperative blood transfusions are associated with increased rates of recurrence and decreased survival in patients with high-grade soft-tissue sarcomas of the extremities. *J Clin Oncol* 1985; 3:698–709.
86. Blumberg N, Agarwal M, Chuang C: A possible association between survival time and transfusion in patients with cervical cancer. *Blood* 1986; 66(suppl 1):274a.
87. Blumberg N, Heal JM, Murphy P, et al: Association between transfusion of whole blood and recurrence of cancer. *Br Med J* 1986; 293:530–533.
88. Maetani S, Nishikawa T, Hirakawa A, et al: Role of blood transfusion in organ system failure following major abdominal surgery. *Ann Surg* 1986; 203:275–281.
89. Tartter PI, Heimann TM, Aufses AH: Blood transfusion, skin test reactivity, and lymphocytes in inflammatory bowel disease. *Am J Surg* 1986; 151:358–361.
90. Tartter PI, Quintero S, Barron DM: Perioperative blood transfusion associated with infectious complications after colorectal cancer operations. *Am J Surg* 1986; 152:479–482.
91. Tartter PI, Barron DM: Unnecessary blood transfusions in elective colorectal cancer surgery. *Transfusion* 1985; 25:113–115.
92. Eschbach JW, Egrie JC, Downing MR, et al: Correction of the anemia of end-stage renal disease with recombinant human erythropoietin. *N Engl J Med* 1987; 36:73–78.

93. Henry ML, Gorner WL, Fabri PJ: Iatrogenic anemia. *Am J Surg* 1986; 151:362–363.
94. Smoller BR, Kruskall MS: Phlebotomy for diagnostic laboratory tests in adults. *N Engl J Med* 1986; 314:1233–1235.
95. Blumberg N, Laczin J, McMican A, et al: A critical survey of fresh-frozen plasma use. *Transfusion* 1986; 26:511–513.
96. Valeri CR, Cassidy G, Khuri S, et al: Hypothermia-induced reversible platelet dysfunction. *Ann Surg* 1987; 205:175–181.
97. Salzman EW, Weinstein MJ, Weintraub RM, et al: Treatment with desmopressin acetate to reduce blood loss after cardiac surgery: A double-blind randomized trial. *N Engl J Med* 1986; 314:1402–1406.
98. Livio M, Mannucci PM, Vigano G, et al: Conjugated estrogens for the management of bleeding associated with renal failure. *N Engl J Med* 1986; 315:731–735.
99. Thurer RL, Hauer JM: Autotransfusion and blood conservation. *Curr Probl Surg* 1982; 19:97–156.
100. Toy PT, Strauss RG, Stehling LC, et al: Predeposited autologous blood for elective surgery. *N Engl J Med* 1987; 316:517–520.
101. Gould SA, Rosen AL, Lakshman RS, et al: Fluosol-DA as a red-cell substitute in acute anemia. *N Engl J Med* 1986; 314:1653–1656.
102. DeVenuto F: Acellular oxygen-delivering resuscitation fluids. *Crit Care Med* 1982; 10:237–245.
103. Hassig A, Collins JA, Hogman C, et al: International forum: When is the microfiltration of whole blood and red cell concentrates essential? When is it superfluous? *Vox Sang* 1986; 50:54–64.

Splenectomy for Hematologic Disease

Peter A. Vevon, M.D.

Department of Surgery, The Ohio State University College of Medicine, Columbus, Ohio

E. Christopher Ellison, M.D.

Clinical Assistant Professor of Surgery, Department of Surgery, The Ohio State University College of Medicine, Grant Medical Center, Columbus, Ohio

Larry C. Carey, M.D.

Clinical Professor of Surgery, Department of Surgery, The Ohio State University College of Medicine, Grant Medical Center, Columbus, Ohio

The role of the spleen in health and disease has been a focus for investigation for more than 2,000 years. Aristotle questioned the necessity of the spleen to maintain life. The spleen was described as an organ for filtering and purifying blood in ancient Babylonia and in the writings of Maimonides in the 12th century. Early modern studies of the spleen were performed mainly by means of splenectomy in animals, and several authors described changes in peripheral blood.[1-3] The first recorded splenectomy was performed in 1549 by Zaccarelli,[1] presumaby for splenomegaly. Several scientists performed splenectomies in animals in the 1600s, without the consequent death of the animal.

The immunologic function of the spleen was first described after experiments on splenectomized rats in the early 1900s by Morris and Bullock, who considered the spleen an aid in "resisting infectious processes." This was both disputed and supported.

The first splenectomies were performed because of trauma, after which the patient was found to live a normal life. This initiated the idea of spleen "expendability." It was subsequently uniformly believed that total splenectomy was the only proper operation on the spleen. This was based on three basic theories regarding the spleen. The first was the fact that splenectomy could be performed without early or delayed sequelae. Second, it was universally believed that death resulted from splenic injury not operated on. And last was the concept of "delayed rupture," which made splenectomy the treatment of choice.[4] It was not until 1952 when King and Schumacher[1, 5] described the high incidence of infection in infants following splenectomy that the expendability of the spleen was reevaluated.

Adv Surg 22:105–140, 1989

0065-3411/89/22-105–140-$04.00

Splenectomy for hematologic disease was first described in 1887 by Spencer Wells, who performed the procedure for hypersplenism. Eventually the condition was recognized as hereditary spherocytosis, but the role of splenectomy in hematologic diseases had begun. Chaufford, in 1907, described splenectomy as a possible treatment of the hematologic disease caused by increased splenic function. Splenectomy as a cure of primary hypersplenism was described by Doan and Wiseman[6] in 1939 in a disease state consisting of neutropenia and splenomegaly. Evans and Duane,[7] in 1949, described a series of patients with autoimmune hemolytic anemia as well as leukopenia or thrombocytopenia treated by splenectomy, although the response was not always complete. Splenectomy in leukemia has always been regarded with skepticism since the first documented splenectomy in June 1966 in a 20-year-old man with massive splenomegaly who died two hours after the operation from intraabdominal hemorrhage.[8, 9] Since the classification of Hodgkin's disease in Rye, New York, in 1965,[3] a staging laparotomy has become one of the most common indications for splenectomy according to Traetow et al.[10] Idiopathic thrombocytopenia purpura was described in 1937 by Wintrobe,[11] who reported a series of untreated patients, more than half of whom had a relapse or remained thrombocytopenic for years. Subsequently, a 1960 study by Doan[12] reported an 85% increase in splenectomy without recurrence. Since this study, splenectomy for idiopathic thrombocytopenic purpura has been universally accepted if response to steroids is poor.

We will describe the role of splenectomy in hemolytic anemia, thrombocytopenia, and hypersplenism, as well as for hematologic malignancy. We will discuss the etiology, pathophysiology, and indications for splenectomy and the results. Finally, we will discuss the complications of splenectomy.

Hemolytic Anemia

Anemia is defined as decreased production or increased destruction of red cells. Anemias for which splenectomy is a therapeutic choice are characterized by increased destruction of red cells, or hemolysis. Hemolysis, which accounts for less than 10% of anemias, occurs in either the intravascular or extravascular spaces. Intravascular hemolysis is lysis of red cells in the vascular spaces with release of free hemoglobin into the plasma. Extravascular hemolysis is destruction of red cells by reticuloendothelial phagocytosis. Since the spleen is not involved in the etiology of intravascular hemolysis, it will not be discussed.

Extravascular hemolysis is characterized by an increase in reticulocyte count as well as elevated bilirubin. Lactic dehydrogenase (LDH) is usually increased but may be normal in mild hemolysis. Some type of inherent hereditary disorder is present in either the red cell membrane or the hemoglobin protein itself, including hereditary spherocytosis, hereditary elliptocytosis, sickle cell disease, and thalassemia—major and minor. Also in the category of extravascular hemolysis are the acquired autoimmune hemolytic anemias, which are described as either primary, or idiopathic, and secondary (Table 1).

Hereditary Spherocytosis

Genetically determined erythrocyte cell membrane abnormalities lead to hemolytic anemia. Hereditary spherocytosis, the most common example, is an inherited autosomal-dominant defect in the erythrocyte cell membrane. The defect is a deficiency in spectrin, which is the component of the red cell membrane skeleton responsible for cell shape, strength, and reversible distensibility. These cells also demonstrate increased osmotic fragility. Lysis occurs at a concentration of saline less hypotonic than those at which normal cells are lysed. The abnormalities are found in marrow precursor cells or reticulocytes.

Symptoms

Jaundice is a universal sign. The disease is characterized by a series of major and minor crises, occasionally hemolytic in nature and accompanied by increasing jaundice, sometimes fever with pronounced anemia, and an enlarging spleen. It is believed that the crises are most commonly the result of hypoproduction of marrow elements, or aplastic anemia. They occur after viral or other flu-like illnesses, usually lasting seven to 14 days, and are self-limited.

Diagnosis

Diagnosis is established from peripheral blood smear; usually 50 to 60% of red cells are spherocytes but may be less in milder forms of the disease.

TABLE 1.
Extravascular Hemolysis

Hereditary spherocytosis
Hereditary elliptocytosis
Sickle cell anemia
Thalassemia
Acquired autoimmune hemolytic anemia
  Primary
    Coombs'-positive
    Coombs'-negative
  Secondary malignancies
    Lymphoma
    Leukemia

Mean corpuscular hemoglobin concentration (MCHC) is usually elevated, as is bilirubin. Reticulocytosis is universally present, and the Coombs' test is negative. Other abnormalities include increased osmotic fragility and splenic sequestration of transfused ^{51}Cr-labeled red cells. Importantly, normal red cells labeled with ^{51}Cr are not sequestered, demonstrating that the defect is in the red cell and not in the spleen.

Treatment

Splenectomy is performed during periods of remission, except in mild forms of the disease. This approach decreases the amount of blood products needed. Although Barker and Martin[13] reported a series of ten patients undergoing splenectomy immediately after crises, this is generally avoided. The optimal time for the surgical procedure is during a period of stable splenic size and peripheral blood counts.

The biliary tract is routinely evaluated before splenectomy. Pigmented gallstones have been found in 30 to 62% of patients. Laurie and Ham,[4] in 1974, described 20 patients with hereditary spherocytosis, 40% of whom had biliary tract symptoms and 40% hematologic symptoms. The remaining 20% were evaluated after family members had been found to have hereditary spherocytosis. The fact that 60% of the patients underwent biliary tract operations stresses the need for preoperative biliary tract evaluation.

In children it is generally recommended that operation be delayed until after the fourth year of life because of possible immunologic complications and an increased risk of overwhelming sepsis. Although Krueger and Burgert[14] reported no deaths in 30 children under 5 years of age, Diamond[15] reported two deaths from sepsis in 140 children under 4 years old undergoing splenectomy. While splenectomy is best avoided in children, it is recommended that splenectomy be performed even in the very young in the presence of severe anemia, symptomatic cholelithiasis (rare under age 10), or recurrent crises.

Results of splenectomy for hereditary spherocytosis are very good. The underlying defect of the erythrocyte membrane is unchanged, but red cell survival becomes normal. Musser et al.,[16] in 1983, reported a 90% response rate among 39 patients undergoing splenectomy for hereditary spherocytosis. A fatal outcome is rare in adults.[4, 16] In children, the risk of death increases. Diamond[15] reported a mortality rate of 1.5% in 140 children under 4 years of age. Morbidity ranges from 5 to 25% in various series. There are no general untoward effects of splenectomy for hereditary spherocytosis other than those commonly associated with benign hematologic disease.

Hereditary Elliptocytosis

Most patients with hereditary elliptocytosis (HE) are asymptomatic, but this autosomally dominant transmitted trait varies in severity. Hereditary elliptocytosis has a reported incidence in the general population of about 0.04% (1 in 2,500) with no special predilection for race or geographic area.

Normally, humans have some oval (elliptical) erythrocytes, varying from 1 to 15% of circulating cells. These cells frequently vary only mildly from the morphology of the normal red cell. The exact factor responsible for the aberrant morphology is uncertain. Several factors of the cytoskeletal matrix have been incriminated. These include membrane cholesterol and permeability, as well as hemoglobin distribution. Spectrin and actin, components of the red cell membrane, have been examined. No exact role has been assigned to any of these factors as causative in HE.

Symptoms

Most patients are asymptomatic, with only 10 to 20% showing varied degrees of anemia. Although some are compensated, red cell indices suggesting a microcytic hypochromic disorder such as those seen in iron deficiencies can occur. In patients with crises, uncompensated anemia, and a large percentage of oval cells, erythrokinetic (^{51}Cr)-labeled red cell studies may show splenic sequestration.

Treatment

Most patients require no treatment, but those with hemolysis usually benefit from folate supplementation (1 mg orally per day). If anemia is severe with evidence of splenic sequestration, splenectomy may be performed. Indications for splenectomy include uncompensated anemia and biliary disease. If significant hemolysis is a problem, splenectomy can be performed to decrease the risk of gallstones.

Results have uniformly been good, since patients are generally in good health, and few are at high risk. Morbidity and mortality data are sparse owing to the infrequency of this disorder, but no major complicating factors of splenectomy for HE have been described. As in hereditary spherocytosis, the erythrocyte morphology is unchanged, but anemia is alleviated after splenectomy because there is no further red cell sequestration.

Sickle Cell Disorders

Sickle cell disorders vary both in hemoglobin defect and the severity of hematologic abnormalities. Sickle cell anemia homozygous for HbS occurs in approximately 0.5% of blacks, while the sickle cell trait (heterozygous for HbS) occurs in about 8% of Afro-Americans. The concentration of HbS varies from disease to trait. Sickle cell disease has a complete absence of HbA with the erythrocytes containing mostly HbS. Sickle cell trait has a combination of HbA and HbS, of which 30 to 50% is HbS.

The hemoglobin moeity of the red cell is abnormal in this disease. In the sickle cell hemoglobin (HbS), valine is substituted for glutamic acid at the sixth position of the beta chain. The sickle cell trait contains a combination of abnormal and normal beta chains, while the hemoglobin is totally abnormal. Another abnormal hemoglobin that contains the sickle cell anomaly is sickle cell HbC disease. In this heterozygous disorder there is no normal beta chain, but the red cell contains a combination of HbS and HbC. Similar to sickle cell-HgC disease is sickle cell beta-thalassemia disease, which is a combination of genes by HbS and the thalassemia hemoglobinopathies.

Diagnosis

These disorders are usually diagnosed by the history, peripheral smear, and hemoglobin electrophoresis. Depending on which disorder is present, there are varying degrees of anemia and reticulocytosis. Anemia is usually microcytic hypochromic as in iron deficiency disease. The peripheral smear shows sickled cells, target cells, and Howell-Jolly bodies. Other abnormalities include renal and hepatic abnormalities characterized by increased bilirubin and elevated liver enzymes. There can also be bony abnormalities. These systemic alterations are usually found in sickle cell disease and are usually lacking in the other three sickle hemoglobin disorders.

The sickle cell trait is present in 8 to 10% of black Americans. Patients are usually asymptomatic, with a normal physical examination and life expectancy. Splenic infarction is rare. No treatment is required, but hemoglobin can become unstable during periods of deoxygenation.

Patients with sickle cell disease totally lacking normal hemoglobin A are susceptible to both acute crises and chronic complications, which include retarded growth and development, hematuria, and bone disease. Other problems include hepatobiliary, genitourinary, and cardiopulmonary disease, and distal extremity ulcerations. Acute crises often result in infarction, which occurs in muscles, bones, lungs, and spleen. The severe abdominal pain of these crises can mimic acute cholecystitis and appendicitis.

Treatment

Treatment is supportive and symptomatic directed to the event causing the crisis, consisting of transfusion when anemia becomes symptomatic or the hemoglobin seriously low. Factors precipitating crises are not always obvious, but events leading to deoxygenation, acidosis, dehydration, or stress may precipitate sickling of red cells. Abnormal erythrocytes may then be sequestered in the spleen. Acute crisis management in children is usually more aggressive. Splenic involvement characterized by sequestration occurs primarily in the very young. Sudden sequestration causes splenomegaly without regard to intravascular volume status, which can lead to shock and death.

Although splenic sequestration occurs, it is not related to splenic function, since most patients are functionally asplenic.

Splenectomy for sickle cell disease is infrequent. In a report of experience from 1956 to 1981, only 1 of 306 patients who underwent splenectomy for hematologic disorders had sickle cell disease.[16] Splenectomy is usually reserved for patients with splenomegaly associated with sequestration, rarely hypersplenism. A more frequent surgical procedure for sickle cell anemia is cholecystectomy, since there is an increased risk of pigment gallstones increasing with age and occurring in approximately 70% of adults.[3]

Sickle Cell Thalassemia

Sickle cell thalassemia is characterized by a heterozygous hemoglobin containing one gene for beta-thalassemia and one for HbS. The relative presence of HbA and HbF dictate the severity of the associated anemia, which is mild to moderate in severity, intermediate between sickle cell trait and sickle cell disease. This is due to the presence of a reduced amount of HbS owing to the heterogeneity of the sickle disease, but also the presence of the beta thal gene, decreasing the amount of HbA present.

Diagnosis is made as in other hemoglobinopathies, and treatment varies with the severity of the anemia. Splenectomy is usually not indicated.

Thalassemia

The thalassemia syndromes are inherited hemolytic anemias seen in persons of Mediterranean origin or descent, such as Greeks and Italians. They are also seen in Oriental people, especially those of Southeast Asia. The disorders are due to errors in globin synthesis. There are various combinations of homozygous and heterozygous alpha- and beta-thalassemias, but thalassemia minor, the heterozygous form, usually has a benign course. Homozygous alpha thalassemia is a complete absence of alpha-globulin incompatible with life, resulting in hydrops fetalis and stillbirth.

Homozygous beta-thalassemia is the decreased or absent synthesis of the beta sub-unit of hemoglobin. This is compensated for by increased amounts of Hgb F and Hgb A_2. Hgb F concentration can vary from 40 to 100% of total hemoglobin. The syndromes vary in their impairment of hemoglobin synthesis and associated anemia, hyperbilirubinemia, iron overload, marrow hyperplasia, and shortened life expectancy. The red cell morphologic appearance on peripheral smear is microcytic and hypochromic. The anemia of beta-thalassemia major is usually severe, with clinical manifestations apparent within the first few years of life. Retarded growth, hepatosplenomegaly, and bony abnormalities are present. Bone marrow hyperplasia causes cavitation of erythropoietic centers, predisposing to fractures. Anemia requiring transfusions as well as poor iron utilization cause iron overloading.

Treatment

Treatment is symptomatic, consisting of transfusion for anemia and chelating (deferoxamine) agents to decrease the risk of iron overload. Splenectomy can help by reducing transfusion requirements, thus reducing the effects of hemosiderosis. Splenectomy also serves to remove a symptomatic spleen as well as help significant leukopenia or thrombocytopenia. In children, splenectomy is usually postponed because of the high risk of infection after splenectomy, but life expectancy has been increasing with the use of splenectomy and aggressive medical management. In 1985 Feretis et al.[17] reported prophylactic cholecystectomy in conjunction with splenectomy without increased operative risk. Morbidity (25%) was the same in those treated by splenectomy only and splenectomy with prophylactic cholecystectomy in those with no preoperative or intraoperative evidence of biliary tract disease. There were no deaths.

Death usually results from cardiac failure and is described in the second to third decades, but recent evaluation shows life expectancy to be increasing. No deaths were reported by Freretis et al.,[17] but the mean age of patients undergoing the operative procedure was 24 years. This may suggest an increase in life expectancy in patients with beta-thalassemia.

Acquired Autoimmune Hemolytic Anemia

Acquired autoimmune hemolytic anemia (AIHA) is characterized by the presence of antibodies or complement on the red cell membrane and is classified as primary, or idiopathic, and secondary, occurring with other diseases. The majority of patients (75%) have secondary AIHA due to infection, drugs, malignancies, or other autoimmune diseases such as systemic lupus erythematosus. The remaining 25% have the idiopathic form. Autoimmune hemolytic anemias are classified as warm antibody and cold antibody. Warm-reacting antibodies account for 75% of occurrences, and the remainder are cold-reacting. Antibodies are classified according to their affinity for red blood cells at 37°C or 0°C (Table 2).

Diagnosis

Patients exhibit anemia, splenomegaly, jaundice, or symptoms of the underlying disorder. Laboratory findings include anemia, elevated bilirubin, reticulocytosis, and hyperplastic bone marrow. There can also be abnormalities of leukocytes and platelets. Red cell survival is also decreased. Hemolytic crises may be seen after viral infection. A positive Coombs' test is the key diagnostic feature of AIHA, although 2 to 4% of patients may have a negative Coombs' test.[18] The strength of Coombs' positivity or the amount of antibody on the erythrocyte membrane does not correlate with red cell survival and degree of anemia.

Most warm-reacting antibodies are IgG, although IgM and IgA have also been detected. The antibodies coat the red cells, which are then sequestered and destroyed in the spleen. This is the picture in the idiopathic form, as well as in most drug-induced anemias. Drug-induced anemias are secondary to IgG in penicillin, cephalosporin, and dopa compounds, but IgM seems to mediate the response to quinidine, quinine, and hydralazine.

TABLE 2.
Types of Hemolytic Anemia

	Warm Antibody	Cold Antibody
Definition	Antibody attaches to red cell membrane at core body temperature (37°C)	Antibody attaches to red cell membrane at lower temperatures such as extremities (28°C)
Percent of cases	75%	25%
Type of antibody	IgG/complement (C_3 rare) IgA or IgM	IgM
Site erythrocyte destruction	Splenic sinusoids	Hepatic macrophages
Coombs' reactivity	Positive	Positive
Treatment	Glucocorticoids if refractory to splenectomy	Most self-limited

Complement also plays a role in the hemolytic process, with C_3 usually being present.

Cold-reacting antibodies bind the erythrocyte membrane in the extremities of patients at low temperatures, below 28°C, but do not attach at 37°C. This type of response usually complicates infections or malignancies. The infectious agents can range from mycoplasma to bacterial to viral. IgM is the antibody most often responsible. This process can be seen in association with Reynaud's phenomenon. The IgM cold agglutinins are limited to the intravascular space, with sequestration occurring in the liver. Liver macrophage receptors attack complement on the erythrocyte membrane.

Treatment

Treatment of acquired autoimmune hemolytic anemia varies with the type of antibody present and the cause. Warm-reacting antibodies are sequestered in the spleen, so therapy is directed toward decreasing splenic phagocytosis and sequestration. Cold-reacting antibodies are phagocytized in the liver, and this is primarily an intravascular process.

Warm antibody hemolysis is first treated with steroids at a dose of 40 mg/sq m/day of prednisone. Steroids lower the affinity of reticuloendothelial cells for IgG, thus decreasing phagocytosis. Approximately 70% of patients will respond. Sustained remission with complete withdrawal of steroids occurs in less than 20% of patients with idiopathic disease.[19] Indications for splenectomy include failure of steroids, a requirement for sustained high doses of steroids, or unacceptable side effects. Coon[18] states that in addition to eliminating splenic sequestration, splenectomy will lower antibody production. Steroid requirements usually decrease, and the direct Coombs' test may revert to negative.

Results of splenectomy have been uniformly good; Musser and associates[16] reported a response rate of 83% with no operative deaths and 21% minor complications. Coon[18] reported 64% of patients required no further steroid therapy and decreased prednisone requirements in another 21%.

Evans syndrome reported in 1949 by Evans and Duane[20] is the presence of leukopenia and thrombocytopenia in association with AIHA and responds to splenectomy with a return to near normal levels, but the response has varied. If splenectomy fails, a trial of cytotoxic agents can be undertaken.

Cold-reacting antibodies are usually secondary and self-limiting. Sequestration occurs in the liver, so splenectomy is ineffective and is not indicated. Chronic cold agglutination can be treated with a change of climate and avoidance of cold. If hemolysis requiring transfusions occurs, chlorambucil or cyclophosphamide should be tried. Life-threatening disease can be treated with plasmapheresis.

Coombs'-negative hemolytic anemia occurs in 2 to 4% of patients with AIHA. If a search for secondary causes fails to show toxins, sepsis, or drug toxicity, there may be a favorable response to splenectomy. Clinical and laboratory features are similar to those in AIHA, except for a negative Coombs' test. The disease may be identical to Coombs'-positive hemolytic anemia, but the IgG antibody on red cells does not react with reagent because concentration of IgG may be too low for detection by autoglobulin serum.[18]

Thrombocytopenia

Generally, hemorrhagic disorders are discovered in two settings: (1) in a patient who requires a preoperative screening test, and (2) in a patient who has experienced one or more episodes of spontaneous bleeding, minor or dramatic. Thrombocytopenia (TCP) or a platelet count less than 150,000/cu cm can be caused by four major factors: decreased production, splenic sequestration, dilutional loss, and abnormal destruction. Decreased production involves both hypoproliferation and ineffective platelet production. Hypoproliferation is centered in areas of hematopoiesis, generally the bone marrow. Toxic agents such as alcohol, radiation, or chemotherapy can deplete the marrow. Sepsis as well as processes replacing the marrow can cause lowered production. Myelofibrosis and tumor replacement of marrow cause a failure of hematopoiesis. Aplastic anemia of whatever etiology also may be responsible for thrombocytopenia as well as pancytopenia. Ineffective platelet production is seen with megaloblastic anemia as well as DiGuglielmo's syndrome.

Splenic sequestration of platelets is seen in both idiopathic and secondary disease. Normally about one third of circulating platelets are stored reversibly in the spleen, but this proportion can increase as the spleen size increases. Secondary hypersplenism is usually secondary to hepatic cirrhosis with portal hypertension, myeloid metaplasia, lymphoma, and Gaucher's disease. Hypersplenism also causes sequestration of platelets, but will be discussed later. Sequestration may also occur in giant cavernous hemangiomas.

Abnormal destruction is usually consumptive or immunologically mediated. Consumptive thrombocytopenia may be drug-induced, due to disseminated intravascular coagulation, due to infectious processes, prematurity, and thrombotic thrombocytopenic purpura (TTP). We will discuss TTP, since it is treated by splenectomy. The other causes will not be discussed here.

Immune mechanisms play a major role in thrombocytopenia. Autoimmune thrombocytopenia may be idiopathic (ITP) or secondary. Other causes that are immune-mediated and not to be discussed here are neonatal TCP due to transplacental transfer of maternal autoimmune TCP, drug-induced TCP, and posttransfusion purpura.

Autoimmune Idiopathic Thrombocytopenic Purpura

Autoimmune ITP is a syndrome of low platelet count, normal or increased megakaryocytes in the bone marrow in the absence of any systemic disease, or history of drug ingestion known to produce thrombocytopenia. Also excluded are transfusion complications as etiologic factors. There are two distinct clinical scenarios, the prognosis of which varies with the age and sex of the patient, and whether the disease is acute or chronic (Table 3).

Acute Idiopathic Thrombocytopenic Purpura

Acute ITP has a rapid onset, usually with a history of viral infection within the preceding two to three weeks. There is an even distribution in men and women. Purpura is the most frequent presenting symptom, but a small proportion of patients will have gastrointestinal (GI) or central nervous system hemorrhage. This disease is usually self-limited, with remission within three to four weeks and in 80% within six months. Treatment is usually supportive to avoid trauma and salycilates. Steroids are usually reserved for severe disease, but are generally effective. Splenectomy is contraindicated, except in patients with intracranial hemorrhage.

Chronic Idiopathic Thrombocytopenic Purpura

Chronic ITP is most frequently seen in adults, and 75% of the patients are women. Onset is insidious, with no history of recent viral infections. In

TABLE 3.
Acute vs. Chronic ITP

	Acute	Chronic
Age at onset	80% children Infrequent in adults	20% children Most are adults
Sex predilection	Equal	Females 3:1
Preceding viral infection	Common	Uncommon
Splenomegaly	Rare	Rare
Antiplatelet antibodies	90% (IgG most often)	90% (IgG most often)
Treatment	Protective steroids if severe	Steroids initially if refractory; splenectomy
Complications/fatalities	1% with intracranial hemorrhage	Rare

three studies, the average age at onset in patients requiring splenectomy was 36, 35, and 41 years.[16, 21, 22]

Diagnosis

Most symptoms are related to a bleeding diathesis in which petechiae and purpura are classic. Symptoms include epistaxis, menorrhagia, and GI bleeding. Less frequent are retinal hemorrhage and hematuria. Neurologic symptoms of intracranial hemorrhage (ICH) occur in about 1% of patients, but the majority of these are in acute ITP. Akwari et al.[22] reported that in 17% of patients requiring splenectomy, thrombocytopenia was found incidentally by routine complete blood count.

Physical examination is usually noncontributory, except for signs of petechiae, purpura, or other evidence of bleeding. The spleen is rarely enlarged,[21–23] with 2% of patients having palpable splenomegaly.

Laboratory findings include thrombocytopenia, occasionally with anemia. Peripheral smear shows platelets with megathrombocytes. Bone marrow examination shows an increased number of megakaryocytes. Evaluation should include antinuclear antibody (ANA) and lupus erythematosus preparation to exclude systemic lupus erythematosus. Coombs' antiglobulin test should be performed to evaluate for Evans syndrome if anemia is present.

From the turn of the century it has been suggested that immune factors are implicated in platelet destruction. This theory was suggested by Harrington et al.[24] They demonstrated circulating antibody responsible for platelet destruction in volunteers transfused with serum from patients with ITP. Steroid therapy was employed shortly thereafter. Subsequent to this, a platelet-associated IgG was shown in patients with ITP. Occasionally IgM or IgA may be found in combination with IgG. IgM was found in only 5% of patients,[25] but with increased frequency in acute ITP.[26] Complement has also been found in association with platelet autoantibodies. Up to 90% of patients with both chronic and acute disease have been found to have antibodies adherent to platelets. Higher antibody levels have been correlated with increased platelet destruction.[25]

The spleen is the primary site of platelet destruction as well as antibody production. Reticuloendothelial hepatic sequestration may ocur and is more common in adults with severe disease and high platelet-associated antibody levels. Bone marrow production of antibody has been documented in ITP.[25]

Treatment

Treatment of chronic ITP is corticosteroid therapy and splenectomy. Refractory cases may respond to the administration of immunosuppressive agents such as vincristine and cyclophosphamide. Other therapies described recently include the use of vinca alkaloids and danazol.

Corticosteroids, the mainstay of medical therapy, are instituted at a dose of 1 mg/kg of prednisone. Steroids are believed to interfere with antibody binding to platelets, decreasing phagocytosis. Other effects are inhibition of IgG production and increased IgG catabolism.[27] Steroids do not affect platelet production. Although the first response to steroids may be favorable in nearly 50% of patients, complete and lasting remission after withdrawal is seen in only 20 to 25%.[23, 25]

Splenectomy was performed for ITP as long ago as 1913 by Kaynelson.[28] Splenectomy removes the site of splenic sequestration as well as antibody formation. In patients with evidence of sequestration in the liver or other reticuloendothelial sites, splenectomy still produces a response in up to 40%.[25]

Results of splenectomy have been quite good, with operative morbidity and mortality decreasing as surgical techniques and postoperative care have improved. Indications for splenectomy are failure to respond to corticosteroids, the inability to withdraw steroids during a three- to six-month trial, prolonged requirement of high-dose corticosteroids, toxic side effects, or other contraindications to corticosteroid therapy. Complete response is described as a normal platelet count without steroids. Response to splenectomy is currently 75%. Schwartz et al.[21] reported an 88% complete response rate and 3% partial response. Partial response is described as either an increase in platelets to a subnormal range or a decrease in prednisone requirements. Other studies report similar response rates; Musser[16] described a 77% complete and a 14% partial response. Coon[29] reported a 72% complete and 16% partial response for a total response rate of 98%. Table 4 shows cumulative data for results of splenectomy in the 1980s.

Morbidity and mortality have improved since the initial reports in 1928 of splenectomy for ITP. Spence[30] reported an operative mortality of 21%, but more recent studies place mortality figures between 1 to 2%. Schwartz reported a 4% mortality, which included five deaths, four of which were due to intercerebral hemorrhage. There was no increased incidence of thromboembolic complications or sepsis. More recent studies by Musser et al.[16] in 1983 and Akwari et al.[22] in 1987 report an operative mortality of 2% and 0%, respectively. The only death in the UCLA report occurred in a 5-month old infant with intracerebral hemorrhage. Akwari et al.[22] reported no operative mortality, but three patients died three months after operation, two from pulmonary emboli and one from generalized sepsis.

Morbidity frequency in splenectomy is in the 20 to 25% range. The most frequent complications are atelectasis and pneumonia, accounting for one third to one half of all complications. Other complications in decreasing order of frequency are bleeding, subphrenic abscess, pancreatic fistula, wound hematoma, and infection. In ITP, major morbidity is rare. The spleen is not usually enlarged, with the mean splenic weight in three large series reported to be 130 mg,[34] 147 gm,[36] and 217 gm.[22, 23, 31] In splenectomy for massive splenomegaly (more than 1,500 gm) the complication rate was 56%, but all hematologic disorders were included. Patients with ITP are young (30–40 years) and have small spleens, both favorable factors in reducing the risk of complications.

The incidence of accessory spleens in large autopsy studies is about 10%.[33] The occurrence of accessory spleens in ITP is 18%.[15, 16, 21] Akwari et al.[22] described a 13% incidence of accessory spleens on radionuclide imaging studies. Failure to remove an accessory spleen may result in failure of splenectomy to control thrombocytopenia. A careful search for ac-

TABLE 4.
Splenectomy for ITP in the 1980s

	Coon[32]	Schwartz[21]	Akwari[22]	Musser[16]	Total
No. of patients	216	120	100	65	501
Complete remission	72%	88%	71%	77%	76%
Morbidity	7%	19%	8%	22%	14%
Mortality	2%	4%*	0	2%	1.7%

*80% of these due to intracranial hemorrhage.

cessory spleens should be performed in all patients undergoing splenectomy for ITP.

After failure of corticosteroids and splenectomy, and the exclusion of overlooked accessory spleens, immunosuppressive agents such as cyclophosphamide, azathioprine, and vincristine may be tried. Burns and Saleem[34] state that either 2 to 3 mg/kg/day orally or 300 to 600 mg/kg of intravenous cyclophosphamide may produce a complete remission in 30 to 40% of patients with ITP. Cyclophosphamide is withdrawn four to six weeks after achieving normal platelet count. Azathioprine (1–3 mg/kg/d) in conjunction with corticosteroids will produce adequate platelet levels, but complete remission is rare, and withdrawal of treatment causes a relapse. The administration of vincristine (0.025 mg/kg, with total dose not to exceed 2 mg) produces rapid response, but relapse occurs within three to four weeks in many cases.

Picozzi et al.[35] described long-term follow-up of 15 patients with post-splenectomy recurrences of TCP. Eight of 15 had adequate platelet levels in a three to 12 year period with no therapy. Three had complete response and one a partial response to immunosuppressive therapy. These observations suggest a nonaggressive approach when splenectomy has not produced optimal results in ITP.

Treatment of secondary ITP is directed to the underlying disease and exposure to toxins or drugs must be stopped. Management of infections, whether they be viral, bacterial, or rickettsial must be instituted. Malignant diseases such as lymphoma and leukemia should be treated. Failure to respond after treatment of the cause in secondary ITP is an indication for surgical therapy. In a recent review by Akwari et al.,[22] ten patients who received diazide or quinidine progressed to chronic ITP requiring splenectomy.

In conclusion, good response rates in ITP have been attained with splenectomy. A review of published series (1937–1984)[22] demonstrated a complete remission in 72% of patients with operative mortality of 2%. Because good results are attained with minimum risk, splenectomy continues to be a major treatment for chronic ITP.

Thrombotic Thrombocytopenic Purpura

Thrombotic thrombocytopenic purpura is a poorly understood syndrome comprising a pentad of clinical findings: fever, thrombocytopenic purpura, microangiopathic hemolytic anemia, renal abnormalities, and fluctating neurologic signs and symptoms. Half of patients with TTP will have all five symptoms. Common symptoms include neurologic complaints, including headache, lethargy, aphasia, paresis, paresthesias, paralysis, seizures, and coma. Renal abnormalities are proteinuria, hematuria, abnormal urine sediment, and, less often, oliguria. The pathogenesis of TTP is uncertain, and inciting events are unknown. It is suspected that immune factors play a major role, since the disease occurs in autoimmune disorders such as systemic lupus erythematosus and Graves' disease,[36] but it also can accompany infections and toxic disorders.

Incidence peaks in the third decade, with patients commonly in the third to sixth decades, and more women are affected. The course of the disorder varies from an acute fulminant one to one of chronic, relapsing disease. The death rate in untreated patients approaches 80%, although most reports cite a 50% mortality. Steroids and splenectomy are the therapy of choice. New treatment using plasmapheresis and antiplatelet drugs have produced survival rates approaching 90%.[36, 37] Death results from diffuse thromboses leading to cardiac arrhythmias, cardiorespiratory failure, and hemorrhage.

Clinical and pathologic findings suggest that platelet aggregation, due to immune-mediated factors or endothelial injury, plays a major role in the vaso-occlusive aspect of the disease. Although not pathognomonic, clinical suspicion of TTP can be confirmed by the demonstration of subendothelial and intraluminal deposits of "hyaline" composed of platelet aggregates and fibrin.[38] Although gingival biopsy is used, biopsy of affected skin also gives good results. Biopsies may be negative, but the clinical course of the disorder demands diagnosis and rapid treatment.

Findings include microangiopathic hemolytic anemia, reticulocytosis, and histocytosis with elevated indirect bilirubin without hemolysis. The direct Coombs' test result is negative. Thrombocytopenia resulting from platelet destruction or aggregation usually produces a platelet count of less than 20,000/μL. Screening coagulation test results are normal or mildly elevated. Bone marrow aspirate shows nonspecific hyperplasia.

With the clinical suspicion of TTP and the failure of screening tests to exclude other disorders, treatment should begin. Recent trials using plasmapheresis and antiplatelet agents either together or separately have achieved remission rates approaching 90% with minimal morbidity.[36, 37] The role of splenectomy has changed in recent years. Once the therapy of choice, it has now become an alternative therapy in the treatment of TTP. Even though a review of the literature in 1978 by Rutkow[39] stated that 70% of long-term survivors with TTP had undergone splenectomy, the survival has been improved with plasmapheresis. Schwartz et al.[21] reported a 40% operative mortality in a series with splenectomy. Schneider et al.[37] in 1985 suggested splenectomy should be reserved for cases in which plasmapheresis had failed. Plasmapheresis is the initial therapy of choice in many centers, and may be the only therapy required. Even when plasmapheresis yields a transient response, the surgical risk may be improved. Once medical management fails, splenectomy should be considered.

If medical and surgical treatments are successful, the pentad of symptoms usually resolves, but may require continued therapy with antiplatelet agents, such as aspirin and dipyridamole, for at least six months.

Hyperspenism

Hypersplenism as described at the turn of the century consisted of (1) cytopenia, anemia, leukopenia, and thrombocytopenia; (2) splenomegaly; (3) compensatory bone marrow hyperplasia; and (4) correction of hematologic abnormalities with splenectomy. Hematologic abnormalities are caused by enlargement of the spleen with an increase in splenic function. Abnormal sinusoidal circulation, decreased transit time, and sequestration of blood cells cause cytopenia. There is an increased pool of cells in the spleen, as well as phagocytosis of blood cells. Large numbers of platelets and granulocytes in the spleen decrease these elements in the peripheral blood. Anemia can result from sequestration or phagocytosis of opsonized red cells.

Hypersplenism is considered idiopathic, or primary, when no underlying cause is found, and secondary when another disease is the cause. Secondary hypersplenism can result from inflammation, neoplasatic disease, infection, and infiltrative and congestive splenomegaly. Possible causes of hypersplenism are listed in Table 5.

Hematologic disorders causing secondary hypersplenism are amenable to splenectomy, but indications, results, and complication rates vary remarkably with specific hematologic disorders.

Splenomegaly may be present but is not a requirement for secondary hypersplenism, although they frequently coincide. Splenomegaly is seen in the neoplastic disorders described as well as in inflammatory, myeloproliferative, and congestive disorders. In both primary and secondary hypersplenism, the size of the spleen is not related to the severity of cytopenia or clinical symptoms.

Splenectomy for primary hypersplenism is indicated for cytopenias involving leukocytes, red cells, or platelets. Results are generally good. Musser et al.[16] reported a response rate of 71% in patients with idiopathic hypersplenism. Morbidity of 10% and mortality of 2% for splenectomy for idiopathic hypersplenism was described by Traetow et al.[10]

The response rates and morbidity and mortality of splenectomy for secondary hypersplenism varies, depending on the underlying disease.

Felty's Syndrome

In 1924 Felty described chronic arthritis, splenomegaly, and neutropenia as a clinical syndrome, and in 1932 the first splenectomy was done for this syndrome. Felty's syndrome is seen in only one of 300 patients with rheumatoid arthritis.

Diagnosis

Symptoms include acute and chronic recurrent infections and nonhealing leg ulcers. Infections usually occur in the skin, although pneumonia and lung abscesses are seen (Table 6). Physical examination shows splenomeg-

TABLE 5.
Causes of Hyperspleninsm

- I. Inflammatory
  - A. Felty's syndrome
  - B. Systemic lupus erythematosus
  - C. Sarcoid
- II. Neoplastic
  - A. Myeloproliferative disorders
  - B. Leukemia
  - C. Lymphoma
  - D. Metastatic tumor
- III. Infectious
  - A. Acute and subacute
    1. Viral (infectious mononucleosis and hepatitis)
    2. Bacterial endocarditis
    3. Sepsis
  - B. Chronic
    1. Tuberculosis
    2. Parasites (malaria, shistosomiasis, echinococcus)
    3. Fungus
- IV. Infiltrative
  - A. Storage disease (Gaucher's, Neimann-Pick)
  - B. Amyloidosis
- V. Congestive splenomegaly
  - A. Cirrhosis
  - B. Splenic and portal vein thrombosis
  - C. Congestive heart failure

aly. Polymorphonuclear leukocytes are generally less than 2,000 cells/sq mm. Neutropenia is believed to be caused by immune system stimulation leading to hyperplasia of the germinal centers and aggregates of plasma cells in the sinusoids.

Treatment

Response to splenectomy is generally good, with Laszlo et al.[40] reporting resolution of leukopenia in 88% of patients and resolution of recurrent infections in 77%. Coon[41] reported a good response rate with respect to increasing white blood cell count and anemia. He also described 60% resolution of leg ulcers. Schwartz et al.[6] reported an 83% response rate. Attempts to predict response to splenectomy have not been successful. Morbidity is generally low, despite the debilitated status of the patients. Table 7 shows the morbidity and mortality reported in three series. Complications are generally minor, with the most severe being subphrenic abscess.

TABLE 6.
Infections Associated With Felty's Syndrome

Infection	Laszlo et al.[40]	Coon[41]
Leg ulcers	22%	25%
Pneumonia	11%	25%
Skin infections	11%	20%
Intraoral/pharyngitis	19%	10%
UTI	7%	. . .

TABLE 7.
Morbidity and Mortality Associated With Splenectomy for Felty's Syndrome

Author	Year	No. of Patients	Morbidity (%)	Mortality (%)
Schwartz et al.[6]	1984	16	3 (19)	0
Lazslo et al.[40]	1978	27	2 (7)	0
Coon[41]	1985	24	1 (4)	0

Systemic Lupus Erythematosus

Splenectomy for systemic lupus erythematosus (SLE) does not treat the underlying disease, but helps in the management of the patient. Systemic lupus erythematosus is a multisystem disorder with a host of serologic and hematologic abnormalities. Normocytic and normochromic anemia is common and is the anemia of chronic disease. Although the direct Coombs' test result may be positive, there is no evidence of hemolysis. Leukopenia is often present, in particular, lymphocytopenia. Mild thrombocytopenia also occurs. Bleeding occasionally occurs with low platelet counts. Bone marrow is usually hyperplastic or normal.

Treatment

Treatment of SLE is symptomatic and directed toward the immune-mediated and inflammatory nature of the disease. Salicylates and nonsteroidal antiinflammatory drugs are the mainstay of therapy. Corticosteroids are reserved for failures of salicylates and other antiinflammatory drugs. Leukopenia, anemia, and thrombocytopenia refractory to steroids are often responsive to splenectomy. Results are good, but few cases exist to adequately evaluate the proper indication for splenectomy in SLE and the response rate.

Chronic Myeloproliferative Disorders

This group of abnormalities is generally thought to be interrelated, originating from a common stem cell. Four disorders believed to be interrelated and possibly to share a common final pathway are (1) polycythemia vera (PV), (2) essential thrombocythemia (ET), (3) myeloid metaplasia with myelofibrosis (MM), and (4) chronic myelogenous leukemia (CML).

Polycythemia vera is an autonomous clonal expansion of erythropoiesis with varying increases in leukocytes and megakaryocytes. Symptoms are secondary to the increased hematocrit and blood volume, which cause increased blood viscosity and thrombosis. A palpable spleen is noted in 75% of patients, and half have hepatomegaly. Essential thrombocytopenia is a rare disease of adults with an increase in megakaryocytes resulting in increase of platelets in the peripheral circulation. Other cell lines such as granulocytes and erythrocytes may be involved. Clinical problems are secondary to hemorrhage and thrombosis, and there is an increased risk of hemorrhage and thrombosis in both polycythemia vera and essential thrombocytopenia. Splenectomy is not beneficial and therefore is not currently recommended.

Chronic myelogenous leukemia will be discussed later in this chapter with other malignancies, leukemias and lymphomas. It is believed that PV, ET, MM, and CML are overlapping entities that may all be evolving in the final common pathway—acute myelogenous leukemia (AML).

Myeloid metaplasia with myelofibrosis is a disorder characterized by fibrosis of the bone marrow and extramedullary hematopoiesis. Extramedullary hematopoiesis occurs in the spleen, liver, lymph nodes, and uncommonly in other organs. It is seen in the middle-aged and the elderly and is more common in white persons, but has no sexual or familial predilection. The etiology is unknown, but myelofibrosis has been induced in animals with radiation. It can also be seen in diseases that involve the bone marrow, such as tuberculosis, syphilis, or cancer.

Patients may be asymptomatic, but often have malaise, fatigue, weight loss, anorexia, or symptoms related to organomegaly. One must search for a history of radiation or toxin exposure, as well as other diseases that can involve the bone marrow. Physical examination will show hepatosplenomegaly with the splenic enlargement that is often quite dramatic. Organomegaly is secondary to hematopoiesis. The disease is characterized by progressive pancytopenia and splenomegaly. Complications causing death include bleeding, infection, and anemia. Five percent of patients develop acute leukemia.

Laboratory findings show abnormal red cell morphology with nucleated red cells and reticulocytosis. The alkaline phosphatase level is usually elevated. Interestingly, radiographic evidence of arteriosclerosis is present in half the patients. Hyperuricemia is frequent, and therefore patients should be monitored for gout and renal lithiasis. Diagnosis is made by bone marrow biopsy, since aspirates are usually not satisfactory. Bone marrow biopsy shows fibrosis with foci of hematopoietic cells.

Treatment is usually symptomatic and directed toward the symptoms of secondary hypersplenism and splenomegaly. Transfusions are required for anemia. Corticosteroids, androgens, chemotherapy, and splenic irradiation are used to prevent symptoms of massive splenomegaly and secondary hypersplenism. Splenic irradiation has a minimal initial response of short duration. Allopurinol should be used in patients with hyperuricemia.

As fibrosis progresses, so does hepatosplenomegaly. As the spleen enlarges, the hypersplenic activity exceeds the hematopoietic function. At this point, splenic destruction of formed elements is greater than production and splenectomy is indicated.[42] In 1978, Cabot et al.[43] described the use of preoperative ferrokinetic and chromium survival studies as well as ^{111}In marrow scintigraphy to determine marrow function and degree of splenic sequestration. This was not used as a screening tool to select potential surgical candidates, but to assess possible postoperative prognosis. Wilson et al.[44] found kinetic studies were not effective in prognosis in patients with myeloproliferative disorders.

Although splenectomy does not prolong survival and has considerable risk, there is still a role for splenectomy in the treatment of myeloproliferative disorders. Indications for splenectomy are related to hypersplenism and symptomatic splenomegaly. Hypersplenism exceeding extramedullary hematopoiesis results in anemia, granulocytopenia, and thrombocytopenia. There is an increasing demand for red cell and platelet transfusion. Splenic infarcts are common and are quite painful. In addition, massive splenomegaly causing gastric compression and early satiety are also indications for splenectomy. In some cases, portal hypertension associated with splenomegaly is evidenced by varices and ascites. Disappearance of esophageal varices after splenectomy in patients with myelofibrosis has been documented.[45] Schwartz[45] documented a decrease in portal pressures after splenectomy in patients with ascites and varices in myelofibrosis. Table 8 shows indications for splenectomy.

Results have been similar to those with other hematologic disorders. Schwartz[45] reported 100% palliation of symptomatic splenomegaly with the average splenic weight of 2,250 gm (normal, 75 to 150 gm). Improvement in anemia, thrombocytopenia, and leukopenia occurs in 86%. Coon et al.[46] reported a response rate of approximately 75% but excluded postoperative deaths. Cabot et al.[43] reported a response rate of 95% in symptomatic splenomegaly.

TABLE 8.
Indications for Splenectomy in Myeloproliferative Disorders

	Coon et al.[47]	Cabot et al.[43]	Schwartz[46]
Total patients	34	19	24
Hypersplenism	20 (60%)	8 (40%)	16 (67%)
Symptomatic splenomegaly	11 (30%)	9 (50%)	8 (33%)
Rupture	1 (4%)	. . .	. . .
Others	2 (6%)	2 (10%)	. . .

TABLE 9.
Morbidity and Mortality of Splenectomy for Massive Splenomegaly

	Goldstone[48]*	Schwartz[45]	Cabot[43]	Coon[46]	Musser et al.[16]
Average Spleen size	2,814 gm	3,150 gm	1,700 gm	2,000 gm	1,776 gm
Average age	50 yrs	NA	60.3 yr	40–76 yr	55 yr
Morbidity	56%†	NA	75%	35%	47%
Mortality	14.7%	10%	5%	12%	18%

*87% were for myeloproliferative disorders.
†Half of morbidity was secondary to hemorrhage.

Morbidity and mortality are high. Hickling[47] in 1937 reported a mortality rate of 60% for patients undergoing splenectomy for myelofibrosis. Although morbidity and mortality rates have improved, they are the highest of any group of hematologic diseases for which splenectomy is indicated except chronic myelogenous leukemia. Table 9 shows morbidity and mortality reported in the recent literature.

These data represent several small studies of 15 to 34 patients. In a separate article reviewing splenectomies for massive splenomegaly, 87% of which were for myelofibrosis, Goldstone[48] reported a similar morbidity and mortality. The complication most often seen is hemorrhage, requiring either transfusion or reoperation. Atelectasis, pleural effusion, and pneumonia are the most frequent pulmonary complications. Thrombosis and sepsis occur but are less frequent. The elevated morbidity and mortality are multifactorial. Patients in all the series are elderly, and have advanced disease. While splenectomy is dangerous, survival without splenectomy ranges from six weeks to four years.

Splenectomy should still play a role in myelofibrosis, but the age of the patient and stage of the disease increase the risk of the procedure. Survival is not altered by splenectomy, but very good palliation is obtained.

Splenectomy for Leukemia

Chronic Myelogenous Leukemia

This form of leukemia is believed by some to be a continuum of the myeloproliferative disorder, polycythemia vera, essential thrombocythemia, and myeloid metaplasia. This is a clonal malignancy characterized by excessive proliferation of neutrophil stem cells. There is an associated chromosome abnormality called the Philadelphia chromosome (chromosome translocation 22 9), which is thought to be responsible for loss of control of leukocyte production. Ninety percent of patients with chronic myelogenous leukemia will have the Philadelphia chromosome. Patients who are Philadelphia chromosome-negative have an atypical course and poorer prognosis. Incidence of CML increases with age, with the median at 30 to 40 years, but 5% of childhood leukemias are CML. Males are affected more often (3:2).

Etiology is unknown, but risk factors include radiation exposure, drugs such as benzene, aklylating chemotherapy agents, phenylbutazone, viruses, and genetic factors (i.e., Philadelphia chromosome).

Chronic myelogenous leukemia is a biphasic disease: chronic and acute. The chronic phase is characterized by fatigue, pallor, weakness, and symptoms of hypersplenism and splenomegaly. Abdominal pain infrequently occurs secondary to splenic infarcts. Eighty percent of patients with CML progress to the acute phase.

The acute phase is characterized by high fever, increasing splenomegaly, and resistance to chemotherapy. There is a generalized increase in malaise and muscle and bone pain. Leukemic mass increases at a remarkable rate. Complications are infection and bleeding. Prognosis is very poor, with survival usually less than six months after onset.

Treatment

Chronic myelogenous leukemia may be well controlled for years with busulfan, but patients may develop thrombocytopenia from busulfan toxicity or sensitivity. A multicenter clinical trial evaluating early splenectomy during the chronic phase of the diseases was reported by Wolf et al.[8] These trials suggested that early splenectomy may reduce morbidity during the acute phase by eliminating pain from splenic infarcts, improved oral intake as gastric compression is reduced by the removal of a massive spleen, and by decreasing transfusion requirements. Response to chemotherapy was unaffected by splenectomy.

The most frequent indications for splenectomy are symptomatic splenomegaly or infarcts and large transfusion requirements secondary to hypersplenism.[12, 49, 50] Other indications include splenic rupture or removal of a large splenic focus of leukemic cells prior to bone marrow transplant.[9] The indication for splenectomy in acute disease is limited and heroic, since prognosis is poor.

Results show good relief of symptomatic splenomegaly and a variable response to hypersplenism. Multicenter mortality rates of 0.7% were described by Wolf et al.,[49] with low postoperative morbidity in 145 patients. This differs from the 33% mortality rate and 56% morbidity rate described by Musser et al.[16] in nine patients. Postoperative morbidity in Wolf's series[49] showed major nonfatal infection in 9% with a 4% incidence of thromboembolic complications.

The role of splenectomy in CML is very limited, and its use should be reserved for selected patients. Although it has been shown in some centers to have acceptable morbidity and mortality, its role is strictly palliative, with no increase in survival nor improvement in response to chemotherapy. Others claim little enthusiasm for splenectomy in CML except where it is performed as a prerequisite to bone marrow transplant.[9]

Chronic Lymphocytic Leukemia

Chronic lymphocytic leukemia (CLL) is a neoplasm of mature B cells. It accounts for one fifth to one third of all leukemias. It has a 2:1 male predominance, and rarely occurs in children. It is a disease of the elderly, with the average age in one series 66 years.[50]

Onset is insidious, with painless lymphadenopathy a common presenting symptom. Occasionally, the disease is detected in asymptomatic patients in routine blood examinations. Infrequent symptoms are weakness, fatigue, weight loss, and anorexia. Progression of disease leads to massive lymphadenopathy and splenomegaly. Anemia and thrombocytopenia appear secondary to bone marrow infiltration of leukemic cells, or Coombs'-positive hemolytic anemia. Bleeding and infection are life-threatening complications. Infection is secondary to granulocytopenia and generalized immunodeficiency. Approximately 20% of patients develop secondary malignancies.

Therapy is aimed at controlling complications of the disease. Chemotherapeutic agents such as chlorambucil and vincristine are often used in conjunction with steroids, irradiation, and splenectomy. Depending on the stage, the course may last from months to years, with slow progression of lymphadenopathy, splenomegaly, anemia, and thrombocytopenia. Splenectomy is primarily done to decrease transfusion requirements induced by hypersplenism and to relieve symptomatic splenomegaly. Anemia may be Coombs'-positive, secondary to tumor invasion of bone marrow or sequestration in a massive spleen. After splenectomy, improvement of hematologic disorders occurs in about 80% of patients, but Mentzer et al.[50] noted relapse in patients with antierythrocyte antibodies, i.e., Coombs'-positive anemia. Operative mortality is low.[16, 50]

Hairy Cell Leukemia

Hairy cell leukemia (HCL) first described in 1958 by Bouroncle et al.[51] at The Ohio State University is a monoclonal, lymphoproliferative disorder of mature B cells. This rare disease represents less than 5% of all leukemias. Men comprise more than 75% of all patients. The average age is approximately 55 years, and the disorder is rare in those less than 30 years old. Approximately half the patients have symptoms of weakness and fatigue. Infection and splenomegaly were the initial symptoms in 17% and 14%, respectively, in one study.[53] Bleeding diatheses and an incidental finding each account for about 10%.

Physical findings are nonspecific, but splenomegaly is almost universally present to some degree, with half the patients having a spleen palpable below the umbilicus.[53] Hepatomegaly and lymophadenopathy are less frequent, but often seen.

Diagnosis

The diagnosis must be confirmed by finding the pathognomonic mononuclear hairy cell in the peripheral blood or bone marrow. Ninety percent of patients have the hairy cell in the peripheral blood. The cell derives its name from the morphologic characteristics of its cytoplasmic projections. Various laboratory techniques for visualizing the hairy cell can be used, including supravital staining, phase-contrast microscopy, and electron microscopy. Cytochemical studies such as the tartrate-resistant acid phosphatase reaction are extremely helpful in establishing the proper diagnosis.

The clinical course is usually protracted. Infection is the most common complication, as well as the primary cause of death. Sepsis and pneumonia accounted for 65% of deaths in one study,[53] and infections range from bacterial (most common) to fungal and parasitic. Bleeding complications are the second most common cause of death, and over the course of the illness necessitate numerous transfusions. Less frequently, splenic rupture will complicate the disease, causing death in 3% of patients in a series of 82 patients at the Ohio State University Hospitals.[53]

Treatment

For several years the treatment of choice of HCL was splenectomy, improving the hypersplenic symptoms of anemia and cytopenia, as well as relieving symptomatic splenomegaly (Table 10). Less frequent indications included removal of a large tumor burden and splenic rupture due to massive splenomegaly. Several retrospective studies showed patients undergoing splenectomy for HCL had a longer survival.[9, 52, 53] One retrospective

TABLE 10.
Patients With Hairy Cell Leukemia Undergoing Splenectomy

	Coon[18]	Musser[16]	Brockard[56]	Jansen[55]	Total
# Patients	17	16	37	391	444
% Males	65	94	68	77	77
Morbidity	3 (14%)	3 (19%)	3 (8%)	. . .	. . .
Mortality	1 (6%)	1 (6%)	1 (3%)	2%	. . .

multicenter analysis of almost 400 patients suggested that splenectomy did not improve survival in patients with small spleens (less than 4 cm below the costal margin) and absence of severe neutropenia, anemia, or thrombocytopenia.[53] Hypersplenic complications of HCL have been improved in 70 to 80% of patients undergoing splenectomy.[9, 16]

While splenectomy remains the mainstay of therapy at some institutions, new therapies with low-dose deoxycoformycin (DCF) and alpha-interferon have had excellent results. Bouroncle and associates at The Ohio State University Hospitals, using low-dose deoxycoformycin (4 mg/sq m every two weeks) have achieved complete remission in 92% of patients.[56] Good results have also been achieved with alpha-interferon.[57] Complete remission has been achieved in patients who had splenectomy as well as those who had not. In view of this, splenectomy will eventually play a very limited role in HCL. Presently at The Ohio State University, Bouroncle and her colleagues are no longer recommending splenectomy for their patients with HCL.

In patients undergoing splenectomy, mortality ranges from 2 to 6% in recent studies.[9, 16, 52, 53] Morbidity has also been low, ranging from 8 to 20%.[16, 52] Although these data are encouraging from a surgical standpoint, chemotherapy has supplanted surgery as the treatment of choice. Splenectomy will now be relegated to a very minor role in patients who have failed to respond to deoxycoformycin, alpha-interferon, or other chemotherapeutic agents.

Lymphoma

Hodgkin's Lymphoma

In recent years with advances in radiation and chemotherapy, excellent response rates and five-year survival have been achieved for Hodgkin's disease. Therapy varies according to stage, but overlapping of therapies should be avoided due to potential side effects.

Hodgkin's disease, initially described in the early 1800s by John Hodgkin, is a malignancy of lymphoid tissue characterized by the Reed-Steinberg cell (R-S cell), a multinucleated giant cell. Hodgkin's disease differs from non–Hodgkin's lymphoma in its epidemiology. Hodgkin's has bimodal peak incidence periods in relation to age. It reaches a peak in the 20s to 30 years of age and then declines. Later in life (after 50), risk increases again. Overall, it is more common in men, but the nodular sclerosing type has a higher incidence in women. Etiology is unknown, but certain trends have been identified. Geographic and familial clustering have been seen, and some evidence points to the possibility of viral origin.

Symptoms of Hodgkin's disease are usually peripheral lymphadenopathy with the cervical or supraclavicular area involved in up to 80% of patients. Axillary lymphadenopathy is next frequent, and inguinal nodes least often involved. Lymph nodes are usually firm and mobile in contrast to the hard, fixed adenopathy of metastatic carcinoma. Central adenopathy involving the mediastinum and hilum of the lung is also common. Patients may have cough, dysphagia, or chest pain. The superior vena cava syndrome is rare. Splenomegaly is uncommon as an initial finding. About 66% of patients have either stage I or II disease limited to one side of the diaphragm. This contrasts with NHL, where 70% of patients have stage III or IV. Also described as "almost pathognomonic" is alcohol intolerance.[59] The ingestion of alcohol results in a peculiar pain in areas involved with disease, such as lymph nodes or spleen. Athough uncommon, this may be useful in following disease in remission.[59]

The presence or absence of night sweats, fever, and weight loss of 10% or more over the previous six months are very important. These symptoms are called "B" symptoms and are associated with a poorer prognosis. They also change the mode of therapy in stage III disease. The fever, called Pel-Ebstein fever, is a high, spiking fever followed by days with normal temperature. Other nonspecific symptoms include malaise, fatigue, and anorexia.

The staging and classification of Hodgkin's disease are very important for both prognosis and therapy. Table 11 shows the importance of staging. Stage I disease is confined to one regional lymph node are; stage II disease is confined to two or more contiguous regions of lymph nodes on the same side of the diaphragm. Stage III disease occurs on both sides of the diaphragm, but is confined to lymph nodes and spleen. Stage IV disease is diffuse and disseminated, involving organs such as liver, bone marrow, and lungs. Each stage is also described as A—absence of fever, weight loss, and night sweats, or B—presence of these symptoms. Recently, these stages also include a subscript E for the presence of extranodal, localized disease and subscript S for splenic involvement only.

TABLE 11.
Hodgkin's Lymphoma: Stage-Related Treatment and Survival

Stage	I	II	III	IV
At presentation (%)	10	50	30	10
Treatment	Radiation	A. Radiation B. Radiation Chemotherapy	A. Radiation B. Radiation Chemotherapy	Chemotherapy
5-yr survival	90%	A. 90% B. 60–80%	A. 80% B. 50%	50%

The Rye classification was initially described in 1965 as a modification of the older Lukes-Butler histologic classification:

Lymphocyte predominant
Nodular sclerosis
Mixed cellularity
Lymphocyte depleted

Lymphocyte predominant and nodular sclerosis subgroups are usually seen in younger patients and have a more favorable prognosis, in contrast to lymphocyte-depleted and mixed cellularity types, which occur in older patients and are more ominous. As stated, Hodgkin's is more common in men overall, but in the nodular sclerosis subgroup, women predominate.

Initially, the first step is to obtain a histologic diagnosis. This is quite easily done from cervical, supraclavicular, axillary, or other peripheral nodes. Mediastinal adenopathy is biopsied via mediastinoscopy or thoracotomy if necessary. Once a histologic diagnosis of Hodgkin's has been made, the clinical stage is assessed.

Clinical staging begins with history and physical examination. Presence or absence of "B" symptoms, splenomegaly, and lymphadenopathy, are easily determined. Hematologic values are assessed. Elevated liver enzymes may indicate hepatic involvement, and an elevated alkaline phosphatase may represent bone metastasis. Chest x-ray will confirm or disprove mediastinal hilar adenopathy. Liver-spleen scan may be used to evaluate organomegaly. Retroperitoneal lymph nodes are evaluated by computed tomography (CT) and bipedal lymphangiogram. Computed tomographic scan is used to assess the bulk of disease if any, while lymphangiography is more specific for tumor involvement in lymph nodes. Scanning with CT cannot detect microscopic disease, but had an overall accuracy of 83% in one retrospective study.[61]

Lymphangiography is an excellent tool for the evaluation of retroperitoneal nodes, which are involved 40% of the time in Hodgkin's disease.[61]

Several studies have shown the test to be accurate 90% of the time; false positives and false negatives are rare.[60, 62] A positive lymphangiogram is good evidence of intraabdominal disease. In the presence of normal studies, the spleen is involved in 20 to 30% of cases. Patients with large mediastinal masses should not undergo lymphangiography because of increased risk of pneumonitis from lipid microemboli.[61] Phlebitis is another complication. Lymphangiography may produce residual nodal opacity for as long as two years, making follow-up evaluation possible.

Bone marrow and percutaneous liver biopsy should also be used to assess for stage IV disease. Patients with a positive bone marrow or liver biopsy do not need staging laparotomy. Chemotherapy is the therapy of choice. Liver involvement rarely occurs in the absence of splenic disease.[61]

Further staging is done by laparotomy. Therapy is based on the stage and has been found to change with laparotomy in over 40% of patients.[61] Prognosis also varies with stage, so accurate staging is paramount. Staging laparotomy is unnecessary in stage IIIB and IV disease, since there will be no change in treatment or prognosis. However, in these cases splenectomy may be occasionally performed to decrease tumor load and to treat hypersplenism. Splenectomy will also obviate any need for splenic irradiation and decrease risk of nephritis and pneumonitis.

Staging laparotomy includes liver biopsy, abdominal exploration, splenectomy with excision of splenic hilar lymph nodes, and retroperitoneal and abdominal lymph node sampling. The procedure is usually performed through a midline incision. The liver is evaluated first for gross involvement. A wedge biopsy is then taken from both lobes, as well as needle biopsy. If the liver is involved with tumor, stage IV disease is confirmed. Splenectomy then follows, with excision of splenic hilar nodes. Surgical clips are placed to mark the splenic pedicle and splenic hilar nodes. Lymph node biopsies are next to be performed. Sampling occurs from the celiac axis and porta hepatis if nodes are available. Paraaortic, iliac, and mesenteric lymph node biopsies are also performed, with surgical clip placement at each site as a marker for possible radiation therapy. Any positive or suspicious nodes on lymphangiography should be excised. This can be confirmed with x-rays in the operating room. Iliac crest biopsy is performed last if needed. This completes the staging procedure.

Oophoropexy may be desirable in women who want children. Oophoropexy removes the ovaries and tubes from the inverted Y portal of abdominal radiation. The lateral attachments to the ovaries are incised, allowing movement of the ovaries and tubes to the midline. The ovaries are marked with clips so they can be excluded from the radiation portal.

Auxiliary operations should be avoided, since they add increased risk to the procedure. A recent study evaluating the use of appendectomy with staging laparotomy showed an increase in wound infections from 1% to 5%.[63] Appendectomy makes a clean operation into a clean-contaminated one and should be avoided in staging laparotomy.

Splenectomy for Hodgkin's not related to staging has an important role.

Secondary hypersplenism, removal of tumor burden, and relief from symptomatic splenomegaly are all indications for splenectomy. In one series, 90% of patients with Hodgkin's had correction of hematologic abnormalities with no operative deaths in 60 patients.[64] It has been suggested that a decrease in the tumor burden and site of production of malignant cells may influence the effects of therapy.

Clinical staging was changed in 43% of cases in one large series of 825 staging laparotomies. The stage was increased 36% of the time, and decreased 7% of the time. This is dramatic evidence of the need for staging laparotomy in Hodgkin's disease.

Morbidity and mortality are low in staging laparotomy. Morbidity is usually less than 10% and mortality less than 1%. Wound infection accounted for one quarter of all complications in one large series.[61] Iliac crest infections constituted 10% of complications. Other complications include pulmonary effusions, pneumonia, sepsis, small-bowel obstruction, subphrenic abscess, and pulmonary embolus.

Mortality remained quite low, with several series showing less than 1% (Table 12).

Non-Hodgkin's Lymphoma

Although similarities exist between Hodgkin's disease and non-Hodgkin's lymphoma (NHL), there are several factors that make the latter a distinct and separate disease, especially to the surgeon. Age, stage of disease at presentation, and the wide variety of histologic findings and route of spread make each patient with NHL a very distinct individual compared with those with Hodgkin's disease.

Although there is no predilection for either sex, the patients with lymphoma are generally older; the average age of 50 years is almost double the average age in Hodgkin's disease. Peripheral lymphadenopathy is similar in distribution, although less frequent. Central adenopathy occurs less often in NHL. Extranodal sites accounted for the initial complaint in about

TABLE 12.
Morbidity and Mortality of Staging Laparotomy: Recent Literature Review

	Taylor et al.[61]	Mitchell et al.[64]	Traetow et al.[10]
No. of Patients	825	140	203
Morbidity	9.5%	10%	4%
Mortality	0.1%	0	0

one fourth of patients. Extranodal disease can include Waldyer's ring, which presents as mass or pain. Gastrointestinal manifestations can be present initially, with hemorrhage or obstruction. Eighty percent of patients with NHL have stage III and IV disease at the time of diagnosis, in contrast to Hodgkin's disease, where the stage at initial presentation is I or II in 60% of patients. Half of the patients with NHL have intraabdominal dissemination at presentation. The presence of "B" symptoms (fever, night sweats, and 10% weight loss) is more frequent initially in NHL. More commonly than Hodgkin's, NHL will involve distal regional nodes, while contiguous nodes are uninvolved.

The clinical course and natural history of NHL varies with stage and histologic type. In NHL, both stage and histologic status are important in prognosis. Most NHL are monoclonal B-cell tumors. Histologic classification uses the Rappaport system, which uses three basic criteria to determine favorable vs. unfavorable histologic findings:

1. Nodular (favorable) versus diffuse (unfavorable).
2. Lymphocytic (favorable) vs. histiocytic (unfavorable).
3. Well-differentiated (favorable) vs. poorly differentiated (unfavorable).

Clinical staging is done, once the histologic diagnosis is made (Table 13). History and physical examination will elicit the absence or presence of "B" symptoms, organomegaly, or multiple areas of lymphadenopathy. Further clinical staging is performed in a manner similar to that used in Hodgkin's disease.

Laparotomy for staging is the exception rather than the rule. Eighty percent of patients have stage III or IV disease, and splenectomy will not alter prognosis or treatment protocol. Chemotherapy and radiation therapy are the treatments of choice. Patients with NHL are elderly and usually have advanced disease.

TABLE 13.
Clinical Staging of Non-Hodgkin's Lymphoma

Chest roentgenogram to evaluate the mediastinum and hilar areas.
Computerized tomography of the chest and abdomen to help adenopathy and bulk of disease.
Bone marrow biopsy to check for advanced disease.
Lymphangiography to evaluate retroperitoneal lymph nodes as well as initial nodal and extranodal sites.
Gallium 67 scans to confirm or deny previous studies.
Liver biopsy if previous studies do not show disseminated disease.
Staging laparotomy to prove stage I disease.

In NHL, splenectomy is indicated for secondary hypersplenism as well as symptomatic splenomegaly and painful splenic infarcts. Pancytopenia responds to splenectomy quite well, with one series reporting 86% improvement in hematologic abnormalities.[64] The authors reported no mortality and minimal morbidity. Although splenectomy is infrequent in NHL, if it is performed for a specific, individualized indication it has a definite role in management.

Summary

Splenectomy has a major role in the treatment of hematologic diseases. Although it is rarely curative, splenectomy removes the site of the destruction or sequestration of erythrocytes, leukocytes, and platelets. Destruction occurs in such diseases as hemolytic anemia and ITP, whereas sequestration occurs as an idiopathic disease or secondary to a host of other diseases described above. Splenectomy is also indicated for symptomatic splenomegaly associated with leukemia, lymphoma, or myeloproliferative disorders. It is palliative, increasing the comfort of the patient by removing a massive spleen. Splenectomy also serves as a staging tool in lymphoma, Hodgkin's disease, and NHL, although it is much more beneficial in Hodgkin's disease, owing simply to stage at presentation. Splenectomy can be performed safely with minimal risk in most patients, but certain diseases carry increased risks of fatality and complications. Such diseases include leukemia, lymphoma, and myeloproliferative disorders, but even in these, splenectomy may be indicated in a select group of patients. The decision to perform splenectomy should therefore be made individually in these cases. Because it can be palliative in some cases, splenectomy can play a role in patient management, even though it may not alter survival.

References

1. Sherman R: Perspectives in management of trauma to the spleen. *J Trauma* 1980; 201:1.
2. Morganstern L: The surgical inviolability of the spleen: Historical evolution of a concept, in *Wellcome Institute of the History of Medicine.* London, 1974, pp 62–68.
3. Sabiston D, et al.: *Textbook of Surgery,* ed 13. Philadelphia, WB Saunders Co, 1986.
4. Lawrie GM: Surgical treatment of hereditary spherocytosis. *Surg Gynecol Obstet* 1974; 139:208–210.
5. Leonard AS, Giebink GS, Baesl TJ, et al: The overwhelming postsplenectomy sepsis problem. *World J Surg* 1980; 4:423.
6. Schwartz SI, Adams JT, Bauman AW: *Splenectomy for Hematologic Disorders.* Chicago, Year Book Medical Publishers Inc, 1971.
7. Evans RS, Duane RT: Acquired hemolytic anemia. *Blood* 1949; 4:1196–1213.

8. Bryant T: Case of excision of the spleen from an enlargement of the organ attended with leucocythemia. *Guy's Hosp Rep* 1966; 12:444–455.
9. Coon WW: The limited role of splenectomy in patients with leukemia. *Surg Gynecol Obstet* 1985; 160:291–294.
10. Traetow WD, Fabri PJ, Carey LC: Changing indications for splenectomy. *Arch Surg* 1980; 115:447–451.
11. Wintrobe MM, Hanrahan EM Jr, Thomas CB: Purpura hemorrhagica with special reference to course and treatment. *JAMA* 1937; 109:1170–1176.
12. Doan CA, Bouroncle BA, Wiseman B: Idiopathic and secondary thrombocytopenic purpura: Clinical study and evaluation of 381 cases over a period of 28 years. *Ann Intern Med* 1960; 53:861–876.
13. Barker K, Martin FFR: Splenectomy in congenital microspherocytosis. *Br J Surg* 1969; 56:561.
14. Krueger HC, Burgert E Jr: Hereditary spherocytosis in one hundred children. *Mayo Clin Proc* 1966; 41:821.
15. Diamond LK, et al: The hazard of overwhelming infection postsplenectomy. *J Pediatr* 1965; 67:1022.
16. Musser G, Lazar G, Hocking W, et al: Splenectomy for hematologic disease. *Ann Surg* 1984; 200:40–45.
17. Feretis CB, et al: Prophylactic cholecystectomy during splenectomy for beta thalassemia homozygous in Greece. *Surg Gynecol Obstet* 1985; 160:9–12.
18. Coon WW: Splenectomy in the treatment of hemolytic anemia. *Arch Surg* 1985; 120:625–628.
19. Allgood JW, Chaplin H: Idiopathic acquired hemolytic anemia. *Am J Med* 1967; 43:254–273.
20. Evans RS, Duane RT: Acquired hemolytic anemia. *Blood* 1949; 4:1196–1213.
21. Schwartz S, Hoepp L, Sachs S: Splenectomy for thrombocytopenia. *Surgery* 1980; 88:497–506.
22. Akwari DE, et al: Splenectomy for primary and recurrent immune thrombocytopenic purpura. *Ann Surg* 1987; 206:529–539.
23. Difino SM, et al: Adult idiopathic thrombocytopenic purpura. *Am J Med* 1980; 69:430–442.
24. Harrington WJ, Minnich V, Hollingsworth JW, et al: Demonstration of a thrombocytopenic factor in the blood of patients with thrombocytopenic purpura. *J Lab Clin Med* 1951; 38:1–10.
25. McMillan R: Chronic ITP. *N Engl J Med* 1981; 304:1135–1147.
26. Leeuwen EF, et al: Idiopathic thrombocytopenic purpura in children: Detection of platelet autoantibodies by immunofluorescence. *Scand J Haematol* 1981; 26:285–291.
27. Karpatkin S: Autoimmune thrombocytopenic purpura. *Blood* 1980; 56:329–423.
28. Kaynelson P: Verschwinden der hamarrhagischer diasthese bei einem talle von essentieller thrombopenie nach milzerstirpation splenogene thrombolytische purpura. *Wien Klin Wochenschr* 1916; 29:1451–1454.
29. Coon WN: Splenectomy for ITP. *Surg Gynecol Obstet* 1987; 164:225–229.
30. Spence AW: The results of splenectomy for purpura hemorrhagica. *Br J Surg* 1928; 15:466–499.
31. Yam LT, Crosby WH: Spontaneous rupture of the spleen in leukemic reticuloendotheliosis. *Am J Surg* 1979; 137:270–273.

32. Coon WW: Splenectomy for idiopathic thrombocytopenic purpura. *Surg Gynecol Obstet* 1987; 164:225–229.
33. Adams JG, Nichols AG: *Principles of Pathology*. Philadelphia, Lea & Febiger, 1909, vol 2, p 222.
34. Burns TR, Saleen A: Idiopathic thrombocytopenic purpura. *Am J Med* 1983; 75:1001–1007.
35. Picozzi VJ, Roeske WR, Creger WP: Fate of therapy failures in adult ITP. *Am J Med* 1980; 69:690–694.
36. Myers TJ, Wakem CJ, Ball ED, et al: Thrombotic thrombocytopenic purpura: Combined treatment with plasmapheresis and antiplatelet agents. *Ann Intern Med* 1980; 92:149–155.
37. Schneider PA, Rayner AA, Linker CA, et al: The role of splenectomy in multimodality treatment of thrombotic thrombocytopenic purpura. *Ann Surg* 1985; 202:318–321.
38. Amoros EL, Ultmann JE: Thrombotic thrombocytopenic purpura: Report of 6 cases and review of the literature. *Medicine* 1966; 45:139–159.
39. Rutkow IM: Thrombotic thrombocytopenic purpura and splenectomy: A current appraisal. *Ann Surg* 1978; 188:701–705.
40. Laszlo J, Jones R, Silberman HR, et al: Splenectomy for Felty's syndrome. *Arch Intern Med* 1978; 138:597–602.
41. Coon WW: Felty's syndrome: When is splenectomy indicated? *Am J Surg* 1985; 149:272–275.
42. Fabri PJ, Carey LC: Splenectomy in leukemia, lymphoma, and mixed profiferative disorders. *Surg Rounds* June 1984, pp 82–89.
43. Cabot EB, Brennen MF, Rosenthal DS, et al: Splenectomy in myeloid metaplasia. *Ann Surg* 1978; 187:24–30.
44. Wilson RE, Rosenthal DS, Moloney WC, et al: Splenectomy for myeloproliferative disorders. *World J Surg* 1985; 9:431–436.
45. Schwartz SI: Myeloproliferative disorders. *Ann Surg* 1975; 182:464–471.
46. Coon WW, Liepman M: Splenectomy for agnogonic myeloid metaplasia. *Surg Gynecol Obstet* 1982; 154:561–563.
47. Hickling RA: Chronic non-leukemic myelosis. *Q J Med* 1937, p 253.
48. Goldstone J: Splenectomy for massive splenomegaly. *Am J Surg* 1978; 135:385–388.
49. Wolf DJ, Silver RT, Coleman M: Splenectomy in chronic myeloid leukemia. *Ann Intern Med* 1978; 89(pt 1):684–689.
50. Mentzer SJ, Osteer RT, Staines HF, et al: Splenic enlargement and hyperfunction as indications for splenectomy in chronic leukemia. *Ann Surg* 1987; 205:13A.
51. Bouroncle BA, Wiseman BK, Doan CA: Leukemic reticuloendotheliosis. *Blood* 1958; 13:609.
52. Anderson KC, Boyd AW, Fisher DC, et al: Hairy cell leukemia: A tumor of pre-plasma cells. *Blood* 1985; 65:620–629.
53. Bouroncle BA: Leukemic reticuloendotheliosis. *Blood* 1979; 53:412–435.
54. Bouroncle BA, Grever MR, Kraut EH: Treatment of hairy cell leukemia: The OSU experience with deoxycoformycin. *Leukemia* 1987; 1:350–354.
55. Jansen J, Hermans J: Splenectomy in hairy cell leukemia. *Cancer* 1981; 47:2066–2076.
56. Brochard M, Sigauy F, Flandrin G, et al: Splenectomy performed upon thirty-seven patients with hairy cell leukemia. *Surg Gynecol Obstet* 1987; 165:305–308.

57. Quesada JR, Reuben J, Manning JT, et al: Alpha interferon for induction of remission in hairy cell leukemia. *N Engl J Med* 1984; 310:15–18.
58. Kaplan HS: *Hodgkin's Disease.* Cambridge, Mass, Harvard University Press, 1972, p 452.
59. Jones SE: Importance of staging in Hodgkin's disease. *Semin Oncol* 1980; 7:126–135.
60. William SF, Golomb HM: Perspective on staging approaches in the malignant lymphomas. *Surg Gynecol Obstet* 1986; 163:193–201.
61. Taylor MA, Kaplan AS, Nelson TS: Staging laparotomy with splenectomy and Hodgkin's disease: The Stanford experience. *World J Surg* 1985; 9:449–460.
62. Castellino RA, Blank N: Roentgenologic aspects of Hodgkin's disease. *Natl Cancer Inst Mono* 1973; 36:271–276.
63. Morris DM, et al: Effect of incidental appendectomy on the development of wound infection in patients undergoing staging laparotomy for Hodgkin's disease. *Am J Surg* 1982; 153:226–229.
64. Mitchell A, Morris PJ: Splenectomy for malignant lymphomas. *World J Surg* 1985; 9:444–481.

Occult Gastrointestinal Bleeding: Newer Techniques of Diagnosis and Therapy

Ashby C. Moncure, M.D.

Associate Clinical Professor of Surgery, Harvard Medical School; Visiting Surgeon, Massachusetts General Hospital, Boston, Massachusetts

Ronald G. Tompkins, M.D., S.D.

Assistant Professor of Surgery, Harvard Medical School; Assistant in Surgery, Massachusetts General Hospital, Boston, Massachusetts

Christos A. Athanasoulis, M.D., M.P.H.

Professor of Radiology, Harvard Medical School; Head, Section of Vascular Radiology, Massachusetts General Hospital, Boston, Massachusetts

Claude E. Welch, M.D.

Clinical Professor of Surgery, Emeritus, Harvard Medical School; Senior Surgeon, Massachusetts General Hospital, Ambulatory Care Center, Boston, Massachusetts

"Occult" gastrointestinal bleeding in the past has referred to chronic blood loss from the gastrointestinal (GI) tract manifested by anemia and a positive test for blood in the stool.[1]

Other investigators have used the term "obscure" GI tract bleeding; it includes those cases that still have not been diagnosed after upper and lower GI tract endoscopy and standard radiologic studies. Thirty-seven such cases originating in the small intestine were seen in the Hammersmith Hospital (London) in an eight-year period, and reported in 1984. They included eight Meckel's diverticula, seven smooth-muscle tumors, 14 vascular abnormalities, one duodenal diverticulum, one jejunal diverticulum, one duodenal duplication, one angiosarcoma, one solitary jejunal ulcer, an ulcerated lymphoma, one with multiple ischemic ulcers, and one with leukemia.[2]

A glance at the causes of major and minor episodes of GI tract bleeding show that nearly every one can be manifested either by overt, ranging from minor to major, or by occult or obscure blood loss. Some start as occult and end as major hemorrhages (Table 1).

Adv Surg 22:141–178, 1989

0065-3411/89/22-141–178-$04.00

TABLE 1.
Occult Gastrointestinal Bleeding: Causes*

Esophagus, Stomach, Duodenum	**Jejunum, Ileum**	**Colorectum**
(Esophageal varices)	*AV malformations*	*(Angiodysplasia)*
Esophagitis	Angiodysplasia	AV malformations
(Gastritis)	Ulcers	*(Ulcerative colitis)*
(Gastric varices)	*(Anastomotic)*	*(Diverticulosis)*
(Mallory-Weiss tears)	Simple	*Cancer*
(Peptic ulcer)	*(Diverticula)*	*Polyps*
AV malformations	Meckel's	*Hemorrhoids*
Cancer	Acquired	Anal fissure
Polyps	Crohn's disease	Stomal varices
(Leiomyoma, sarcoma)	Varices	Postoperative
	Ischemic ulcer	Postpolypectomy
Brunner's adenoma	Tuberculosis	Anastomotic
Angiodysplasia	Arteritis	(Trauma)
Pancreatic rest	Blind loop	Ulcers
(Trauma)	Angioma	Simple
(Postoperative)	(Leiomyoma)	Stercoral
Retained ulcer	Cancer	Typhoid
Residual gastritis	Sarcoma	Amebic
Anastomotic ulcer	*Polyps*	
	Uremic ulcer	
	Stomal varices	
	Lymphoid hyperplasia	
	(Trauma)	

*Lesions in parentheses are usually manifested by acute severe bleeding, but also may cause chronic blood loss, anemia and positive tests for blood in the stool. The most common lesions are italicized.

The boundaries between these types of hemorrhage are thus ill-defined and artificial. We propose that it is better to revert to the original meaning of the word "occult," namely something that is hidden or mysterious. By this definition all bleeding is considered to be occult until the exact cause and site are determined.

In this review all types of GI tract hemorrhage must receive attention. Major emphasis is placed on the most difficult cases in which either the source or cause is elusive. Inasmuch as available methods of diagnosis and therapy, as well as degrees of expertise, vary in different geographical locations, one other problem associated with the old definition of occult is obviated, i.e., what was occult in one locality or era is not occult in another.

Despite all modern methods of diagnosis, in many cases either the cause or the location of the bleeding remains unanswered. The exact percentage has decreased in recent years but still is a matter of speculation. From 1952 to 1968 at the Johns Hopkins Hospital 203 patients had a laparotomy because of GI tract bleeding; a source was not found in 141, or approximately 70%.[1] This figure was almost the same as that reported by Stone in 1944.[3] In contrast, between 1977 and 1981 at the Charing Cross Hospital, diagnoses were made in all but 17, or 6%, of 286 recorded cases of GI tract bleeding.[4] At the Hammersmith Hospital, where a very difficult group of referred patients was treated, all but 16% of 131 patients had a diagnosis made.[5]

Failure of diagnosis and therapy may be ascribed to several factors. The major reason is that the entire jejunum and ileum are not available for endoscopy except at the time of laparotomy. In other cases the source may have been obvious but it was missed. The involved viscus may be identified but the exact source or cause is not clear. A second bleeding area due to the same or other disease may appear very soon or later at another area in the digestive tract. The operation performed may increase chances of later bleeding from another source, as, for example, an anastomotic ulcer may develop after some operations for bleeding peptic ulcer. Endoscopy or selective angiography may have been done at an inappropriate time when the bleeding site was not visible.

In summary, the most satisfactory treatment of hemorrhage involves control of the immediate problem, and, insofar as possible, prevention of further bleeding. Unfortunately, long-term studies of these cases are rare; some available data will be cited in the text.

In this chapter no attempt has been made to make a comprehensive survey of all reported cases. The references cited are representative of numerous reports that have appeared both in this country and abroad.

Diagnostic Methods

In this section, the various methods of diagnosis of the source and cause of bleeding are considered briefly.

History

Assuming that all bleeding is occult until a probable site and cause are discovered, the first step is to obtain an adequate history. It usually furnishes a presumptive guide insofar as diagnosis is concerned. The age of the patient, the type and amount of bleeding, and the location in which the individual is seen are factors that influence the diagnosis of the cause and site of the bleeding.

The history aids in the categorization of bleeding as either upper or lower depending upon the source. Vomiting of blood signifies it comes either from esophagus, stomach, or duodenum, or, very rarely, from the upper jejunum. A history of tarry stools also indicates bleeding from the upper part of the GI tract. Lower GI tract lesions may cause either maroon or bright red stools. However, if there is severe, brisk bleeding from an upper source such as a peptic ulcer, red blood also can be passed by rectum.

In addition to suggestions concerning the source of bleeding, the history also provides valuable information concerning the amount of blood loss. Thus a history of collapse and fainting means blood loss has been sudden and severe. On the other hand, the possibility must be recognized that everything that is red is not blood. Color-blind persons cannot identify red, so that they may not know they are passing blood.

Lack of space prohibits discussion of many important guides to diagnosis provided by the history. A few points deserve emphasis. A history of drugs (aspirin, ibuprofen, prednisone, warfarin), surgery, or illness is important. A previous history of surgery for peptic ulcer suggests further bleeding may come from an anastomotic ulcer. In an elderly patient, heart disease, renal disease, or dialysis correlate with angiodysplasia as a cause of bleeding. However, the diagnosis that seems most likely from the history may turn out to be wrong. Esophageal varices may be present but the bleeding arises from a gastric ulcer. Bleeding that apparently arises from a duodenal ulcer may come from gastritis.

Physical Examination

If the hemorrhage is acute, the amount of bleeding can be measured roughly by the degree of shock. A low blood pressure (BP), rapid pulse, sweating, and prostration, combined with a history of fainting or coma suggest that at least a third of available blood volume has been lost. On the other hand, if the bleeding has been slow, the patient's condition may appear to have stabilized and is relatively asymptomatic, even though the hemoglobin level is low.

The skin should be examined for angiomas; if present they suggest the possibility of GI tract vascular malformations. Pigmented lesions on the lips or mucous membranes occur frequently with the Peutz-Jegher syndrome. A palpable liver and/or spleen or spider angiomas raise the possibility of esophageal varices. Petechiae or subcutaneous hemorrhages on various parts of the body accompany blood dyscrasias or excessive amounts of anticoagulants. Rectal examination may reveal a fissure or tumor. External hemorrhoids are visible, but internal hemorrhoids, unless they are prolapsed, are not visible unless anoscopy is done.

In the most difficult cases the physical examination can be entirely normal, and it is impossible to know at the outset whether or not the patient is bleeding or the site from which the blood comes. Whenever a source of bleeding is unknown, and in every case of possible upper GI tract bleeding, the most important evidence is provided by the passage of a nasogastric tube and gastric lavage. The presence of blood or coffee grounds, or of a guaiac-positive aspirate make it almost certain the blood is coming from the upper rather than the lower GI tract.

Laboratory Tests

The important laboratory tests required in patients with GI tract bleeding include examination of the stools and of the gastric aspirate, certain hematology examinations, and blood chemistry determinations.

Examination of the Stool

Hematochezia (passage of gross blood in the stool) means the source of the blood nearly always is in the anorectum or colorectum; however, severe upper GI tract bleeding may lead to bloody stools in rare instances. When blood streaks appear on the outer margin of the stool the source is usually in the rectum or anal area. Melena (black stools) customarily follow an upper GI tract hemorrhage of moderate severity, but also may occur with continued slow bleeding from the proximal colon; it may persist for three to five days after cessation of the hemorrhage. The color of stools is not always due to blood; black stools can follow the ingestion of iron or bismuth, and red stools follow red dyes or such food as beets or tomatoes.

Relatively large amounts of blood can be passed by rectum with apparently normal stools; it has been estimated that at least 50 ml/day, briefly can escape in this way without symptoms. In normal persons, 1 to 2 ml of blood is lost per 100 gm of feces. Therefore, in order to determine pathological loss, any test for blood should not be unduly sensitive. At the present time Hemoccult tests are used most frequently; they usually detect about twice the normal daily blood loss, and false positive reactions are found in only 1% of examinations even if a meat-free diet is not used.

Examination of Gastric Contents

If a patient enters the hospital and is bleeding severely with both vomiting of blood and passing bright-red stools, the bleeding almost surely is coming from the esophagus, stomach, or duodenum. If there has been no vomiting of blood and the patient has had tarry stools, the bleeding also probably comes from stomach, duodenum, or, rarely, the upper jejunum. Under all circumstances it is important to pass a nasogastric tube. Gastric aspirates also should be tested with guaiac to detect occult blood. Coffee-ground aspirate with a positive guaiac test also is confirmatory of upper GI tract bleeding, but if the nasogastric aspirate is negative for blood, the bleeding probably comes from beyond the ligament of Treitz.

Hematology

Abnormalities include depletion of blood, particularly of red blood cells and platelets, abnormal bleeding and clotting times, and elevation of certain substances in the serum, such as blood urea nitrogen (BUN) and blood ammonia. Previously, blood volume determinations were made to determine the amount of blood loss, but at present most decisions are made on the clinical condition of the patients. A low hemoglobin level combined with shock indicates roughly the loss of 30% to 40% of an individual's blood. However, if the blood loss has been slow, the hematocrit level may be low but the patient tolerates the anemia with a normal pulse and BP.

Blood Chemistry

The BUN level rises with an acute hemorrhage from the upper GI tract because of the increased load of nitrogenous products from blood absorption and often because of reduction in liver and kidney function. Massive hemorrhage from bleeding varices secondary to liver cirrhosis produces large amounts of urea and other substances that cannot be metabolized, so ammonia intoxication and coma can follow. A high BUN level also can indicate renal failure, which can be accompanied by GI tract angiodysplasia and superficial ulcers.

The hematocrit is the best guide to the amount of blood loss, but equilibration may take several hours to occur; hence, early readings may be too optimistic insofar as estimates of the amount of blood loss is concerned. Prothrombin and partial thromboplastin times are essential if anticoagulants have been used. Aspirin reduces the ability of platelets to agglutinate; this probably is one reason that many patients with hemorrhage give a history of aspirin ingestion prior to the bleeding episode.

Endoscopy

Fiberoptic endoscopy, introduced by Hirschowicz in 1958, has developed into an extremely important diagnostic and therapeutic tool. In this section preoperative studies will be considered. The type of endoscopy chosen in an individual case will depend upon the suspected site of bleeding. If bleeding appears to be from the upper GI tract or the site of origin is uncertain esophagogastroduodenoscopy is the first choice. If the origin appears to be in the anorectum or colorectum several procedures are available; they include anoscopy, rigid sigmoidoscopy, flexible sigmoidoscopy, and total colonoscopy.

Esophagogastroduodenal Endoscopy

Esophagogastroduodenal endoscopy is an extremely important procedure. However, it is necessary for the observation to be made promptly and at a time when bleeding has slowed to a trickle, and clots have been evacuated from the stomach by a large bore tube.

In practice, some patients enter with torrential bleeding; a nasogastric tube is passed and the stomach is irrigated. If severe bleeding continues endoscopy is not likely to be satisfactory; the choice then lies between selective angiography or immediate operation unless the bleeding is suspected to be due to a ruptured esophageal varix. If the bleeding slows, it is desirable to perform an endoscopy at that time, since the site often will not be visible if examination is delayed until the aspirate clears.

Ruptured esophageal varices demand either immediate sclerotherapy, or, if that is not available, control with a balloon. If a bleeding site is found in the stomach or duodenum, control of bleeding by electrocoagulation or laser may be possible.

There are, however, some limitations to the value of this type of endoscopy. Unless the observation is made at the right time, the source of bleeding may not be found. The upper portion of the fundus of the stomach may be difficult to observe. Too much bleeding may make it impossible to identify the source. Observation of the third and fourth portions of the duodenum may be impossible. It has been estimated that approximately 15% of all endoscopies done for bleeding are unsatisfactory. In a series of 129 endoscopies done for gastric bleeding at the Massachusetts General Hospital, there was active bleeding but the exact source could not be determined in 11 (9%); in five others there was blood in the stomach but no active bleeding; and in six the stomach appeared to be normal. Thus endoscopy failed to identify the exact site in the stomach from which bleeding originated (as determined later by angiography or operation) in 22 patients, or 17% of the total[6] (Table 2).

Endoscopy of the Jejunum and Ileum

Endoscopy of the jejunum and ileum was first reported in 1972. At the present time it is still impossible to examine the whole small bowel in a nonanesthetized patient. In one series the terminal 15 to 40 cm of the ileum was examined in 400 patients in conjunction with colonoscopy.[7] Some Japanese authors and others have reported examinations of the upper jejunum in nonanesthetized individuals. Usually, however, observations of the jejunum and ileum are not satisfactory unless they are combined with surgical exploration, when the surgeon can guide the endoscope through the entire length of the intestine.

Colorectal or Anorectal Bleeding

When bleeding presumably originates from colorectum or anorectum, the choices include the following.

Anoscopy.—Hemorrhoids or fissures are common. The source of bleeding from hemorrhoids often cannot be found but if the hemorrhoids are large, no other lesions are found on sigmoidoscopy, the stool guaiac is negative and the history is typical, the diagnosis is almost certain. A barium enema or colonoscopy prior to hemorrhoidectomy should be done in all but young patients. Any persistent bleeding after hemorrhoidectomy demands further investigation.

Rigid Sigmoidoscopy.—This is the next simple procedure, and is indicated when bleeding apparently comes from the colon or rectum. Polyps

TABLE 2.
Endoscopic Findings: Acute Gastric Bleeding*

Finding		Number
Gastritis		68
Small gastric ulcers		17
Gastritis and varices		8
Gastritis and ulcers		5
Gastrojejunostomy bleeding		4
Mallory-Weiss tear		3
Gastric tumor		2
Active bleeding (?) etiology		11
Gastroesophageal junction	7	
Lesser curvature	4	
No active bleeding, blood in stomach		5
Normal		6
TOTAL		129

*From Eckstein MR, et al: Occult gastrointestinal bleeding: Newer techniques. *Radiology* 1984; 152:644. Used by permission.

or cancers are not uncommon. At times an angioma or arteriovenous malformation bleeds vigorously and can be identified only if it is bleeding actively at the time of the examination. On the other hand, if the examination is done in the interval phase, the bleeding site may not be found.

Flexible Sigmoidoscopy.—This is a simpler procedure than total colonoscopy but may miss many bleeding lesions, since a high proportion of them occur in the right colon.

Total Colonoscopy.—Colonoscopy is a very important diagnostic tool. It is far superior to a barium enema for the diagnosis of polypoid lesions under 1 cm in diameter. It also is particularly valuable when a radiologic examination that had been done because of rectal bleeding identified diverticula but no other lesion; the endoscopist often finds polyps or small cancers that are the true cause of the bleeding.

However, there are definite limitations in the value of colonoscopy. They include inability to examine the colon adequately in the presence of serious hemorrhage, inability to visualize the whole colon in perhaps 10% to 15% of patients due either to colonic obstruction or lack of skill of the endoscopist, and inability to identify the minute lesions of angiodysplasia unless they are bleeding at the time of the examination. Therefore, total colonoscopy is most valuable when the colon can be prepared adequately and the patient is not bleeding severely.

Radionuclide Studies

Technetium (^{99m}Tc-pertechnetate) may be coupled to sulfur colloid or autologous red blood cells (RBCs) to detect bleeding from the GI tract. Technetium-99m–pertechnatate may be used alone to detect ectopic gastric mucosa, which it will identify, when it is present, in Meckel's diverticula. Scans also have been reported to identify bleeding in ulcerative lesions in the small bowel such as can be seen with lymphoid hyperplasia.

Technetium pertechnetate, when coupled with sulfur colloid (SC) or RBCs, may identify bleeding into the GI lumen if the bleeding rate is greater than 0.1 to 0.4 ml/minute. The relative sensitivities and specificities of ^{99m}Tc coupled to each of the two materials (SC and RBCs) has not been well-defined in controlled populations. Properties of the two materials are different and offer various advantages and disadvantages. Technetium-99m–SC has a short half-life because of its rapid clearance by the reticuloendothelial system. A short half-life in the blood pool will allow extravasation at the area of active bleeding and a high target to nontarget ratio of radioactive signal and thus identify small bleeding sites. Because of the short half-life, another advantage is that little pertechnetate is excreted into the gastric mucosa leading to false positive results. Technetium-99m–SC has the disadvantage, because its short half-life in the blood stream may detect active bleeding only during a short time period following injection. Since intestinal bleeding tends to be intermittent, the bleeding phase may be missed. Furthermore, the hemorrhage must be in regions that are not obscured by uptake of the radiolabel by the reticuloendothelial system, particularly liver and spleen.

Technetium-99m labeled red cells have a longer half-life in the bloodstream and therefore may detect intermittent bleeding over a 24-hour period. A disadvantage of this method is that more pertechnetate therefore is excreted into gastric mucosa and may lead to more false positive results. Generally, backgrounds are much higher for the ^{99m}Tc-SC and therefore may obscure small extravasations and result in a lower sensitivity. Nuclear medicine scans such as ^{99m}Tc-RBC or SC scans are useful in confirmation of hemorrhage but have not been accurate in the detailed localization of the source of bleeding within the bowel.[8–15]

Not unexpectedly, there has been a great deal of controversy concerning the clinical value of radionuclide scans in the diagnosis of GI tract hemorrhage. Several conclusions seem warranted. In the first place it is of little value in the detection of lesions that are bleeding at a slow rate and manifested only by guaiac-positive stools and anemia; active bleeding is necessary. Background activity makes any interpretation of upper GI tract hemorrhage very difficult. Technetium-99m–SC can be obtained commercially, can be injected rapidly, and, if the patient is bleeding actively, a reading can be obtained rapidly. Technetium-99m red cells pick up intermittent bleeding over a much longer period of time, perhaps require a bit more bleeding (0.4 ml/minute vs. 0.1 for ^{99m}Tc-SC), and require at least an hour for a reading. Peristalsis may interfere with localization of the bleeding point.

At Massachusetts General Hospital at the present time, if a patient enters with acute active hemorrhage that appears to be from the lower GI tract, blood is immediately drawn and RBCs are tagged with the ^{99m}Tc. Meanwhile the angiography suite is alerted. The tagged RBCs are ready an hour later; they are reinjected and if a bleeding point is identified, the patient is taken immediately to the angiographic suite. If the scan is negative, the patient is admitted to the ward, put on a bleeding watch, and if bleeding recurs, angiography is done.

Radiologic Studies

The radiologist can provide valuable information in many instances.

Plain Abdominal Films

Plain abdominal films are unlikely to provide pertinent data. At times calcification suggestive of an aneurysm can be observed either in the aorta or iliac arteries.

Selective Angiography

Selective angiography is the optimum preoperative method of determining the exact source of major continuing GI tract hemorrhage, since endoscopy will be unsatisfactory if the stomach or colon cannot be cleared sufficiently to permit observation. It is effective as a diagnostic measure regardless of the source of active arterial hemorrhage, provided that the blood loss is 0.5 ml/minute or more. It is also a valuable therapeutic tool.

Several important observations can be made by selective angiography.[16–18]

1. Provided there is continuing active arterial or capillary bleeding of at least 0.5 ml/minute, extravasation of contrast material can be identified. In the Massachusetts General Hospital studies this was possible in 121 of 222 cases (55%) of gastric bleeding, in 27 of 54 cases (50%) of jejunal or ileal hemorrhage, and 72 of 104 cases (69%) of colon hemorrhage.

2. In cases of bleeding from gastritis, one may see extravasation or a blush of the gastric wall indicating marked hyperemia. In 222 cases of gastric bleeding there was extravasation in 121 and blush in 95.[6]

3. A tumor blush, indicative of marked hyperemia, is also seen in other instances. Leiomyomas are particularly apt to be demonstrated in this way.

4. Selective catheterization of small branches of the superior mesenteric artery can localize sites of bleeding in the jejunum and ileum. This has been followed by the intraoperative injection of methylene blue by the angiographer through the catheter to allow the surgeon to identify the exact source of bleeding in the jejunum or ileum.

5. In cases of colonic bleeding, the demonstration of a vascular tuft and an early filling vein in the ileocecal area is diagnostic of angiodysplasia.

6. Varices can be demonstrated in many cases of portal hypertension. Some of them may be in unusual positions.[18] On the other hand, bleeding from the venous system very rarely can be shown because of dilution of contrast medium before it reaches the venous system.

7. Patients with a stoma, either of the colon or small bowel, and portal hypertension may bleed severely from the stoma. Selective arteriography can demonstrate a plexus of vessels about the stoma.

There are certain ways by which angiography can be made more effective. The site of injection is important. For gastric bleeding, the left gastric artery gives better results than the celiac axis. For colonic hemorrhage, the superior mesenteric, the inferior mesenteric, and the celiac arteries should be injected.

The main limitation of selective arteriography is that it is chiefly applicable to severe bleeding when the bleeding is arterial in nature and bleeding is occurring at the time of the catheterization. It follows that there will be some cases in which the bleeding is intermittent or less severe, and the source cannot be determined by this method.

Another problem is that when characteristic findings of angiodysplasia are shown by catheterization of the superior mesenteric artery, the actual source of bleeding actually may be elsewhere in the colon or even from a source as high as the duodenum. This is the reason that in cases of severe colonic bleeding both the superior and inferior mesenteric and celiac arteries must be catheterized; in one of the authors' cases (C.A.A.) angiodysplasia in the cecum was associated with severe bleeding from a diverticulum in the splenic flexure. Furthermore, angiodysplasia has been associated with malignant tumors of both the colon and the ileum. Further diagnostic tests such as endoscopy, barium studies, and/or exploration may be necessary to make a final diagnosis.

Selective arteriography also can be of great value in the therapy of many lesions. Selective vasopressin infusion or embolization may control the bleeding.

Barium-Contrast Studies

It is very important to note that barium studies must be done electively and not in the presence of active bleeding because angiography will be useless if barium is present in the gut.

However, when conditions permit, and the patient seems unlikely to bleed massively in the near future, barium-contrast studies are often very helpful. For example, in a patient with a bleeding gastric ulcer, concomitant extensive duodenal deformity shown on barium studies will help to plan the subsequent anastomosis after gastrectomy. In cases of angiodysplasia, an unexpected tumor may be demonstrated. If the bleeding is due to diverticulosis, a barium enema gives the best conception of the extent of the disease and a clue as to the amount of colon that preferably should be resected. Small-bowel enemas, produced by injection of barium through a tube passed into the upper jejunum, give better delineation of the jejunum and ileum than the usual upper GI tract series with follow-through films of the small intestine.

Ultrasound

This examination can aid to identify aortic or iliac aneurysms, or hepatic angiomas.

Computerized Body Scans

In general these examinations are not helpful. They do provide a method to aid in identification of aortoenteral fistulas secondary to insertion of a prosthetic graft after resection of an aneurysm.

String Tests

Tapes that carry radiopaque markers can be swallowed and the location in the small bowel determined. After a few hours the tape can be withdrawn and tested for blood. Localization of a site of slow but persistent bleeding can be determined at times in this fashion.

Blakemore-Sengstaken Balloon

The Blakemore-Sengstaken balloon has been used in the absence of endoscopy for suspected bleeding from esophageal varices. If bleeding stops after inflation, the diagnosis of varices is almost certain.

Methods Involving Laparotomy

Surgeons who are forced to operate to discover an unknown source of bleeding have an extremely difficult task. The problem arises in two special classes of patients. In the first, acute massive hemorrhage prevents certain preoperative studies, or if they were done, they were unsatisfactory. In the second, bleeding has been characterized by chronic anemia and positive tests for blood in the stools; all the standard preoperative tests have been carried out and were negative.

In general terms, there are four methods that can be used.

1. Exploratory laparotomy alone. An observing eye and palpation, aided by transillumination, are the most effective. Opening a viscus to search for a bleeding point is most likely to be successful in the stomach or duodenum or small intestine. Exact quantitation of the success of laparotomy alone to determine the source of hemorrhage is impossible; however, it has been estimated in cases of chronic bleeding with complete preoperative studies that today it is successful in about 80% of cases.[19] In the absence of what are now regarded as complete studies, the success rate was only about 30% in 1970.[1]

2. Exploratory laparotomy combined with operative endoscopy. This

method is particularly important for lesions of the jejunum and ileum and will be discussed in more detail later; it has also been used for the esophagus, stomach, duodenum, and colon.

3. Exploratory laparotomy plus operative arteriography. This method also is valuable for lesions of the jejunum and ileum and will be considered later.

4. "Blind" resections. In some instances all attempts to determine an exact source of bleeding fail. In such cases the surgeon, who has exhausted all alternatives, as a life-saving procedure, is forced to carry out an extensive blind resection. Obviously such a maneuver is practical only with the stomach or colon but not with the jejunum or ileum. Careful observation by the pathologist still may fail to find the causative lesion, and the only proof that it has been excised will be the cessation of bleeding.

A comparison of the value of various diagnostic methods was made in the Hammersmith Hospital (London) in 1985. Since 87% of their cases had been referred from other hospitals, the group was a particularly difficult one to treat. A diagnosis eventually was made in all but 16% of cases. Diagnoses were made primarily by visceral angiography in 60%, by surgery in 22%, by endoscopy in 10%, by barium studies in 3%, and by endoscopic retrograde pancreatography (ERPC) in 2%.[5]

The most difficult lesions to diagnose include arteriovenous malformations (AVMs), which include hemangiomas of various types, Osler-Weber-Rendu's disease, and cirsoid aneurysms. Angiodysplasia and vasculitis are distinguished by special histologic criteria. Other diseases in which bleeding is common, but determination of the exact site is difficult to determine, include gastritis and diverticulosis (see Table 1).

Methods of Therapy

Techniques of diagnosis and therapy overlap in many instances. For example, the Blakemore-Sengstaken balloon serves as both a diagnostic and therapeutic agent. In general terms, the methods can be classified as follows.

Conservative Methods

Roughly 80% of patients survive a single episode of bleeding. On the other hand, survival after massive bleeding (defined as loss of 5 units or more of blood) is dependent on numerous factors, such as cause, age, physical condition of the patient, and type of treatment. At present, the mortality for emergency operations for massively bleeding peptic ulcer is 22% at the Massachusetts General Hospital due primarily to multiple-organ failure but not to recurrent bleeding.[20]

In cases of severe hemorrhage, blood replacement and correction of clotting factors are the most important factors in addition to vigorous attempts at diagnosis and specific therapy. Additional techniques applicable in upper GI tract hemorrhage include continuous nasogastric aspiration to relieve gastric distention, antacids, mucosal-coating agents, and H2 antagonists. Prostaglandins reduce mucosal blood flow but have had no substantial effect in changing the pattern of bleeding.

Peripheral intravenous injection of vasopressin decreases the BP in the portal system and theoretically should be effective for hemorrhage for stomach, small intestine, or colon. However, side effects that include cardiac arrhythmias and intense peripheral vasoconstriction limit its use.

Endoscopic Methods

Endoscopic techniques include mono- or bipolar electrocoagulation and laser photocoagulation.[21–24] Endoscopic sclerotherapy of esophageal varices is the accepted initial treatment.

Angiographic Methods

Angiographic detection of bleeding arterial lesions can be supplemented either by selective intraarterial injection of vasopressin or of emboli formed of a clot of the patient's blood, Gelfoam, polyvinyl alcohol, or a small coil. Injection of vasopressin directly into the arterial segment supplying the lesion is more effective and less hazardous than peripheral use of the drug. A summary of the results from Massachusetts General Hospital is in Table 3.

Surgical Methods

Surgical methods include excision of the offending lesion, resections of portions of various organs, and ligation of bleeders; additional procedures are considered in the discussion of bleeding from specific viscera.

In summary, various methods of therapy can be used. However, the

TABLE 3.
Selective Angiography

Location	No. of Cases With Active Bleeding	Intraarterial Vasopressin Initial Control	Recurrent Bleeding
Stomach	200	82%	16%
Jejunum, ileum	27	62%	11%
Colon	65	90%	17%
TOTAL	292		

salvage of patients who have not responded to conservative measures, coagulation, laser, or selective arterial infusion of pitressin depends on the surgeon. Surgeons often complain that they receive patients who are depleted and have deteriorated in the interval when other therapeutic measures have been tried.

The application of these methods in bleeding from specific viscera and clinical situations now will be considered.

Esophagus

This mucosa-lined muscular tube without recesses can be evaluated quite accurately by endoscopy. Thus, the cause of major hemorrhage from this organ usually is identified promptly. The esophagus and esophagogastric junction are seldom sources of exsanguinating hemorrhage except in two circumstances—esophageal varices associated with portal hypertension and Mallory-Weiss tears. With hemorrhage from esophageal varices, because bleeding occurs directly into the esophagus, copious hemorrhage is common; the patient often describes blood welling into the mouth, rather than forceful vomiting. Most patients have a history of episodes of upper GI tract hemorrhage and of liver disease, and frequently have the physical signs of liver disease.

If varices are the suspected source, a balloon tamponade tube may be placed as a trial. Cessation of bleeding indicates that the esophagus, rather than a more distal site, is the source of the hemorrhage. Subsequent endoscopy with variceal sclerotherapy may allow acute control of the bleeding. Mallory-Weiss tears are short, linear lacerations at the esophagogastric junction, usually produced by violent vomiting. The bleeding is from small arteries that have been torn, and usually is not controlled by balloon tamponade. The diagnosis is established by endoscopy (retroflexing the flexible gastroscope to visualize the esophagogastric junction), or angiography and controlled by angiographic therapy, endoscopic cauterization, or operation.

More rarely, exsanguinating hemorrhage from the esophagus is seen with erosion by an expanding thoracic aneurysm, or from an acute esophageal ulcer that penetrates into the neighboring aorta. The former is suggested by the presence of the characteristic mediastinal abnormality on the chest radiograph and confirmed by aortography, and the latter by massive arterial hemorrhage encountered at esophagoscopy. Prompt operative intervention is necessary to control the hemorrhage.

Giant hiatal hernias ("paraesophageal") may be complicated by major GI tract hemorrhage. The hemorrhage associated with this condition is usually not from the esophageal mucosa, but rather from gastric mucosal erosion in the portion of the stomach entrapped within the mediastinum. Because strangulation of the blood supply of the mediastinal stomach may occur, prompt operation is necessary to reduce the stomach into the abdominal cavity and repair the hiatal defect.

Trauma, usually either from endoscopic laceration or caustic ingestion, may cause hemorrhage from the injured esophagus. The diagnosis is suggested by the circumstances of the clinical presentation and confirmed by esophagoscopy. In the absence of full-thickness perforation, immediate operative intervention is not usually necessary to control the hemorrhage. The esophagus fortunately is infrequently injured by external trauma.

Chronic blood loss leading to positive tests for blood in the stools and anemia is not common with esophageal lesions. However, such bleeding is characteristic of cancer. This low-grade bleeding is similar to the hemorrhage produced by erosive esophagitis that is secondary to esophageal reflux. These causes may be suggested by barium-contrast studies and confirmed by esophagoscopy.

Finally, occasionally, massive hemoptysis may be confused with hematemesis. The presence of an abnormal chest radiograph and bronchoscopy and esophagoscopy should enable the distinction to be made between the two.

Stomach and Duodenum

Bleeding from the stomach or duodenum is manifested by episodes of tarry stools or vomiting of blood in over 90% of the cases. In less than 10% of cases the loss of blood is manifested solely by anemia and by the detection of blood in the stool; however, many of these patients also have minor episodes of acute bleeding. Even when bleeding is overt, it often is very difficult to establish the exact cause or location of the bleeding. Hence there are several groups of patients that need to be considered.

The chief concern here is with individuals who have only anemia and positive tests for fecal blood, or those who, in addition, have minor episodes of overt bleeding. Cancer, either of the stomach or the duodenum, must be considered to be the most likely cause. Polyps, including villous adenomas of the distal duodenum, Brunner's gland adenomas of the proximal duodenum, gastric polyps, and pancreatic rests are rarer causes. Small peptic ulcers may be too small to be observed by the endoscope. There are two other lesions that are common.

Gastritis

The first is gastritis. The term refers clinically to an abnormally hyperemic mucosa that often is subject to superficial erosions. The abnormality may be generalized throughout the stomach, or be localized chiefly within either the antrum or the fundus. The endoscopic appearance does not necessarily correlate with the pathologist's description. At any rate, bleeding is one of the common symptoms. The bleeding can range from acute and massive to chronic and asymptomatic except for mild anemia. Bleeding is initiated or exacerbated by agents that irritate the gastric mucosa, such as aspirin and ibuprofen, or other medications such as warfarin or prednisone.

The great majority of patients with gastritis have hyperacidity and many also have duodenal ulcers. For them, gastric resection and vagotomy should be curative.

Chronic bleeding can be illustrated by two female patients, both of whom had anemia and positive stools for blood. Both patients were thin; both had evidence of gastritis by endoscopy that extended throughout the stomach, but no bleeding points were seen. Since it seemed undesirable to carry out any such radical procedures as total gastrectomy, both patients were given a string test. Strips of tape, marked with radiopaque discs, were swallowed; they passed into the small intestine. Several hours later they were withdrawn. The only areas positive for blood were located in the fundus of the stomach. Proximal gastrectomy, vagotomy, and pyloroplasty led to relief in both cases.

An unusual diagnostic method was used in another case. A patient who was known to have severe antral gastritis and extensive diverticular disease came into the hospital with a history of several instances of moderately severe rectal bleeding. There was no vomiting and the blood that appeared by rectum was quite red. Gastroduodenoscopy showed antral gastritis but no bleeding point. Doubt about the source of the bleeding was resolved readily when a nasogastric tube was passed and 50 ml of blood furnished by the blood bank was put into the stomach. Within a few minutes the patient passed a bloody stool similar to those he had passed previously. His bleeding stopped after andrectomy and vagotomy.

The second lesion is angiodysplasia. Heretofore it has been considered to be rare, but at present it is recognized much more frequently. In a series of 676 patients who underwent endoscopy at Barnes Hospital, St. Louis, for upper GI tract bleeding, angiodysplasia was diagnosed in 4% of the cases.[25] There was a strong correlation with age (the mean age was 63 years), with renal failure, and with dialysis. Previous studies also had implicated cardiac valve disease. Brief episodes of overt bleeding had been noted in 23 of the 30 patients. The lesions were flat, bright red, and ranged from 2 to 10 mm in size and occurred both in the stomach and duodenum. Typical pathologic findings were reported on excised specimens. They tended to appear in other areas after endoscopic cauterization or, in a few cases, after gastric resection.

Other very extensive localized angiodysplastic lesions of the antrum of the stomach have been described, and, because of their appearance, dubbed "watermelon stomachs."[26]

Angiodysplasia must be distinguished from congenital arteriovenous malformations such as occur in Osler-Weber-Rendu disease; these lesions appear in youth. They also, after destruction by cauterization or excision, tend to develop in other areas of the GI tract.

There are other lesions that also can be manifested by chronic bleeding, but they are rare compared with the great bulk of lesions that tend to bleed overtly and severely.

Patients With Severe Bleeding

In this group, patients have severe bleeding, but diagnosis either of the source or the cause is difficult or impossible. Causes include gastritis, cirsoid aneurysms, multiple superficial mucosal erosions, and tiny peptic ulcers. Endoscopic examination may be unsatisfactory because bleeding is either absent or too brisk. It is in this group that angiographic diagnosis and therapy have been the most successful. In the Massachusetts General Hospital series 222 patients had angiography for gastric bleeding. Contrast material extravasation was seen in 121 and blush of the gastric wall consistent with gastritis in another 95 patients. Only six had negative examination results. One hundred ninety-four were treated with intraarterial vasopressin and 17 of them later had transcatheter embolization because of further bleeding. The bleeding finally was controlled in 79% of the entire group. Seventy-seven percent of angiography failures were operated on and half of the patients operated on died during the same hospital admission.[6] The postoperative deaths usually were due to multiple organ failure; recurrent bleeding was rare.

How well these patients would have fared with endoscopic cauterization or laser therapy is a matter of conjecture. When the 17% of patients in whom a bleeding site could not be established by endoscopy are deducted, only 83% would be available for therapy. Small gastric ulcers were found in an additional 13%; they are not as likely to be cured by endoscopic means as gastric erosions.

There has been a great deal of interest in the use of the Nd:YAG laser in the bleeding of lesions in the stomach. The experience with this modality has not been sufficient in the Massachusetts General Hospital to draw any firm conclusions. Reports generally have been optimistic. However, another recent study has shown no advantage in the treatment of bleeding ulcers over controls.[22] We agree that the efficacy of the method still is sub judice, as indicated by Fromm.[23] The subject has been reviewed recently in *Advances in Surgery*.[24]

Severe cases of bleeding gastritis may require heroic surgery. In the Massachusetts General Hospital in the last 12 years we have relied on high subtotal gastrectomy and vagotomy in the few patients who had required operation for severe bleeding due to gastritis. Only one of these patients had to have a second operation in which the remainder of the stomach was removed; he died postoperatively.

Cirsoid aneurysms (Dieulafoy's lesions) bleed vigorously, apparently through essentially normal mucosa. Unless they are bleeding they are difficult to identify either during endoscopy or at operation. The majority of the lesions occur in the fundus of the stomach. Our preference has been either for local excision of the aneurysm or gastric resection, though simple suture has been advocated by others.[27]

At least one group of surgeons has resorted recently to blind gastrectomies as a last resort in several cases of massive gastric hemorrhage in which both endoscopy and angiography had failed to make a diagnosis. Total gastrectomy was done with recovery in four of six cases.[28]

Stress Bleeding

Another group of patients have stress bleeding. Cases include those patients with severe trauma, burns, or infections, or those who do poorly after surgical operations. This group includes not only patients with typical multiple erosions, but also those with Cushing's ulcers, or Curling's ulcers, and some with exacerbations of preexisting gastric or duodenal ulcers. The surgical mortality following operations for such patients always has been high.

Fortunately, vigorous preventive therapy has led to a great reduction in the number of these patients who develop bleeding. Prevention of gastric distention by nasogastric suction, and maintenance of low acidity in the stomach by instillation of antacids have been more effective than cimetidine prophylaxis.[29] For example, in the patients treated in the Boston Shriner's burn center, where this method has been used routinely in serious cases, there have been no patients with such bleeding in many years. Sucralfate also appears to be a good agent to prevent bleeding. It also has the advantage of maintaining gastric acidity and preventing gastric colonization by gram-negtive bacteria.

Severe Overt Bleeding From Various Causes

The final group of patients includes those who have severe overt bleeding from other causes such as peptic ulcer, cancer, or the Mallory-Weiss syndrome. Usually the diagnosis of the cause is clear. However, some ulcers, just as cirsoid aneurysms, are small and essentially invisible. The mucous membrane may appear entirely normal when viewed through a gastrotomy incision. It is a good plan, if no bleeding point can be found, to rough up the mucosa of the stomach and duodenum with a finger; at times this minimal trauma will cause an elusive vessel to spout from apparently normal mucosa.

Angiographic control of peptic ulcers is difficult. It is reserved for patients who are poor surgical risks; hence it is used only in unusual circumstances. When endoscopic cauterization is done, recurrences preferably are treated by surgery rather than by repeated cauterization.

Twenty years ago, continued bleeding after 5 units of blood in older patients was considered an indication for surgical exploration. Today, because of the ready availability of endoscopists, a trial either of electrocoagulation or laser therapy usually is made before the surgeon sees the patient. Whether or not it is wise to delay surgery and permit surgeons to operate only on failures of other types of therapy is a controversial question. One recent prospective controlled study from Birmingham, England, led to the conclusion that prompt operation was life-saving for patients 60 years of age or over with severe hemorrhage. Patients under that age tolerated attempts at control by electrocoagulation; even if they were unsuccessful, the mortality rate was not increased by the delay.[30]

Jejunum and Ileum

General Survey of Bleeding Lesions

Lesions manifested by chronic anemia and occult blood in the stool include AVMs, angiodysplasia, tumors such as angiomas, polyps, smooth-muscle tumors (leiomyoma is the most common), cancers, sarcomas, lymphomas, diverticula (including Meckel's diverticulum), ulcers (anastomotic, ischemic, simple ulcers in diverticula or blind loops), Crohn's disease, mesenteric varices, arteritis, ileal loop and ileostomy, tuberculous enteritis, and aortoenteric fistulas.

All of these lesions can also be manifested by severe bleeding.[31] In the cases with severe bleeding subjected to selective angiography in the Massachusetts General Hospital, the diagnoses are listed in Table 4.

In toto the most common causes of bleeding from the small bowel are

TABLE 4.
Angiography for Small-Bowel Hemorrhage*

Lesion	No. of Patients
Active bleeding demonstrated—27 cases	
Marginal ulceration	11 (40%)
Ischemic ulceration	3 (12%)
Ileostomy/ileal loop	2 (8%)
Meckel's diverticulum	2 (8%)
Other†	9 (32%)
Total	27
Active bleeding not demonstrated—27 cases	
Mesenteric and small-bowel varices	11 (40%)
Leiomyoma/leiomyosarcoma	6 (24%)
AVM	6 (24%)
Ischemic ulceration	2 (8%)
Arteritis	1 (4%)
Crohn's disease	1 (4%)
Total	27

*Adapted from Tillotson: CL, et al: Small bowel hemorrhage: Angiographic localization and intervention. *Gastrointest Radiol,* in press.

†Includes one each of SMA false aneurysm, jejunal diverticulum, ovarian cancer metastases, incarcerated inguinal hernia, AVM, arteritis, vascular/enteric fistula, tuberculous enteritis, jejunal intussusception. Percentages are rounded.

AVMs, anastomotic ulcers, diverticula (including Meckel's diverticulum) and tumors (particularly leiomyomas, leiomyosarcomas, angiomas, and malignant tumors).

Diagnostic and Therapeutic Methods

Enteroscopy.—Endoscopy is a very effective method to identify GI tract bleeding if the source is in the esophagus, stomach, first or second portions of the duodenum, or the colon. The third and fourth portions of the duodenum, jejunum, and ileum are not routinely accessible to the endoscope under normal conditions. Limited experience indicates that enteroscopy (endoscopic examination of the distal duodenum, jejunum, and ileum) may be possible with improvements in construction of the endoscope. However, before enteroscopy becomes routine, problems that must be overcome include (1) the length of the small bowel, (2) acute angulations of the bowel, (3) adhesions between intestinal segments, and (4) pain that results from distention of the small bowel during the examination.[32] However, either limited or total enteroscopy has been reported nearly a thousand times in the literature.

The Japanese have been particularly active in the development of enteroscopy. Tada et al.[32] described its use in 224 patients in an 11-year period in Kyoto. Meanwhile, as an indication of its comparative rarity, 34,000 upper and 7,000 lower GI tract endoscopies had been done in addition to 6,000 ERPCs.[32]

Tada et al. investigated three types of enteroscopes. They are (1) the push-type, in which a long duodenoscope is inserted perorally and directed into the upper jejunum; (2) the pull-type fiberscope, which is pulled through the intestine by a Teflon "string" that was swallowed two to five days before the examination; and (3), the sonde-type fiberscope, which has a balloon cuff, and is pulled down the intestinal tract by peristalsis.

The push-type scope can examine only the upper jejunum in the unanesthetized patient but usually is well tolerated. The pull-type scope potentially can examine the whole intestine but this examination must be done with the patient under general anesthesia and is time-consuming. In addition, if there is an area of intestinal stenosis or if there is ileus, the string will not pass the entire distance and the procedure cannot be performed. The sonde-type is subject to the same objections. Possibly, if these limitations can be overcome, more routine enteroscopy eventually will be feasible.

Examination of the distal 15 to 40 cm of ileum has been accomplished during routine colonoscopy in 400 cases by Borsch et al.[7] It contributed information of value in nearly 30% of the examinations.

Thus total enteroscopy is not successful in nonanesthetized patients. It requires general anesthesia and should be done at the time of laparotomy.

Radionuclide Scanning.—As mentioned above, ^{99m}Tc-pertechnetate scanning is of value in patients who have Meckel's diverticula containing gastric mucosa. In general, however, because of background activity and intestinal peristalsis, scans done during acute hemorrhage arising from the jejunum and ileum are not helpful.

Selective Angiography of the Small Intestine.—As mentioned above, in half of our cases that were examined at a time of active bleeding extravasation of contrast medium into the bowel was observed (see Table 4). In the other half of the patients, also examined for acute hemorrhage, other causes of bleeding were found. On the other hand, the site or cause of slow persistent bleeding rarely can be identified. The therapeutic value of selective vasopressin injection in cases with massive bleeding is shown in Table 3.

Laparotomy.—The surgeon may take advantage of several maneuvers if laparotomy is necessary and the source or cause of bleeding is not known. They are as follows.

INSPECTION.—Careful inspection of the entire GI tract is necessary. Palpation of the entire small bowel is essential and transillumination is very helpful.

ENTEROTOMY.—Enterotomy is advantageous, especially in young patients. In infants and children the entire small-intestinal mucosa can be everted through a single incision at the level of the junction of the jejunum and ileum. By age 15 the intestine becomes relatively fixed, so a second or third transverse incision may be necessary, and in adults, this maneuver is not successful. It is possible, however, to insert a sterile sigmoidoscope in an enterotomy incision and view a much wider section of the mucosa.

LAPAROTOMY COMBINED WITH INTRAOPERATIVE ENTEROSCOPY.—[15, 32–35] This is an important method and generally is the next step if careful inspection of the intestine has failed to reveal a lesion. A long endoscope is introduced orally after the abdomen has been explored. After the endoscope enters the duodenum, the surgeon and endoscopist work as a team, gently advancing the instrument.

When the duodenal C-loop has been traversed and the tip of the instrument passes the ligament of Treitz, the remainder of the examination is easy. A noncrushing occluding clamp is positioned at the ileocecal valve to prevent air escaping into colon. Gentle manipulation in the "push-pull" action telescopes the small bowel over the instrument and advances the scope while avoiding small intestinal trauma. Any lesions are marked by a suture placed in the serosa; this will reduce the chances of misinterpretation of any small traumatic hematoma. As the scope advances, the endoscopist keeps the lumen in the center of the field. After the scope reaches the terminal ileum, the room lights are dimmed and the scope is withdrawn from the transilluminated and insufflated bowel. This allows a careful examination of the luminal aspect by the endoscopist and examination of the transilluminated bowel by the operating surgeon.

The scope may also be passed transrectally and advanced to the sigmoid colon by the endoscopist; the scope can then be assisted to the cecum by the surgeon, and the small bowel can be examined in a retrograde fashion.

Once lesions all are identified, they may be removed by simple ellipse wedge resection, a limited intestinal resection, or, at times, by endoscopic polypectomy. The intestines are decompressed as the scope is withdrawn.

Approximatley 100 cases have been recorded in the literature in which this method was used. The experience in the Massachusetts General Hospital has been confined to six cases; it has proved to be very effective. The first one of our cases was referred in 1974 to Professor Judah Folkmann at the Boston Childrens' Hospital. This patient was a 10-year old boy with chronic bleeding. He had over 200 polypoid angiomas in the jejunum and ileum ranging from 0.5 to 1.0 cm in diameter. They were identified by a colonoscope introduced in a retrograde fashion from the rectum as high as the ligament of Treitz. The midileum was then opened and the entire intestine intussuscepted in both directions through the incision. All of the lesions were individually excised. The patient did well for nine years, when because of 85 new angiomas a second similar procedure was carried out. Three years later further bleeding led to laser photocoagulation and snare cautery excision of remaining polyps and distal duodenum in 1984 by Drs. Dixon and Gaisford in Salt Lake City. He has remained well since that time (personal communication, Dr. Folkman).

LAPAROTOMY COMBINED WITH SELECTIVE ANGIOGRAPHY.[36, 37]—This method has been used in five cases at the Massachusetts General Hospital. Essentially it consists of identification of a bleeding site by a catheter that was superselectively positioned in the appropriate mesenteric branch prior to the operation. The method involves placement of a No. 6.5-F catheter in the jejunal artery supplying the lesion, and an inner No. 3-F catheter within the larger one. The patient is taken to the operating room and the inner catheter is passed to the margin of the intestine and injected with 1 ml of methylene blue. The stained area is resected. Several other surgeons have used a similar procedure; Crawford has used indigo carmine.[37]

OTHER METHODS.—Other methods to localize bleeding lesions in the jejunum and ileum have been suggested. They include Doppler investigations and estimations of PO_2 levels in venous blood to detect high flow areas or evidence of arteriovenous communications. These methods seem to us to be less practical and accurate than those described above.

Specific Lesions

Diverticula.—Bleeding from a Meckel's diverticulum usually occurs in childhood and adolescence and is manifested by intermittent brisk rectal hemorrhages. Rarely bleeding may be chronic, with anemia and stools positive for blood.[38] Technetium-99m–pertechnetate scans are positive if gastric mucosa is present in the diverticulum. Occasionally, the diverticulum can be seen on barium examination of the small bowel. Resection of the diverticulum and adjacent small bowel, which is usually the site of the peptic ulceration, is indicated.

Diverticula in adults may be single near the ligament of Treitz, but usually are multiple and occur chiefly in the upper jejunum. When hemorrhage arises from one of them it usually is due to an ulcer, and is likely to be severe, but in exceptional cases may be chronic rather than acute.[39, 40] A resection for single or localized multiple diverticula is advisable. Preliminary angiography is advisable in all cases of severe bleeding; if it positively localizes the site of bleeding and very extensive diverticulosis is found, localized segmental resection is possible.

Tumors.—The most common benign tumors of the small intestine are primarily adenomas (adenomatous polyps, villous adenomas, Brunner's gland adenomas). Leiomyomas, lipomas, fibromas, angiomas, pancreatic rests, and hamartomas such as the Peutz-Jegher polyps are other benign lesions. The most common malignant tumors are adenocarcinomas, carcinoids, lymphosarcomas, and leiomyosarcomas. All of them may bleed but except for leiomyomas the bleeding tends to be chronic and low grade. Leiomyomas frequently bleed massively. Many of them can be diagnosed by their peculiar appearance on selective angiography.

Vascular Malformations.—Arteriovenous malformations are quite common in the small bowel. Angiodysplasia appears to have a different cause, since it occurs in the elderly, in contrast to AVMs, which occur in the young. Both of them can lead either to chronic blood loss, anemia, and positive tests for blood in the stools, or to intermittent episodes of brisk bleeding. Intraoperative enteroscopy is the best method of diagnosis. The lesions usually are multiple. New lesions develop in other areas of the bowel in some instances at a later date.

In one of our cases, a 65-year-old woman presented with a second episode of massive upper GI tract bleeding resulting in shock. The bleeding was identified by the endoscopist as coming from an AVM in the distal duodneum near the ligament of Treitz. With aid of the endoscopist at the time of surgery the lesion was identified easily; no other area of AVMs were found in the remainder of the bowel.

Mesenteric Varices.—In the presence of portal hypertension, varices may form within the abdominal cavity. They are particularly common in the omentum. At times a varix may lead to ulceration of the intestine and bleeding. In six cases treated at the Massachusetts General Hospital all of them developed at the site of previous intestinal adhesions. Bleeding from this lesion usually is brisk, but may be intermittent over a long period.[41] At times the bleeding is chronic. The varices nearly always are secondary to cirrhosis of the liver, though occasionally there are other causes. In 1982, 97 case reports were collected from the world literature.[18]

Pancreatitis may lead to thrombosis of the splenic and superior mesenteric veins; varices result. They may involve the small intestine. In one reported case, bleeding was intermittent but severe. After several operations, all of which failed to stop the bleeding, a shunt from a large ileocolic vein to the inferior vena cava was effective.[42]

Ulcers.—Anastomotic ulcers following operations for peptic ulcer disease, such as gastroenterostomy and gastric resection with a Billroth II anastomosis, especially if a vagotomy is not added, may lead to anastomotic ulcers. A retained antrum at the time of gastric resection also is a potent ulcerogenic operation. The most common sign of an anastomotic ulcer is bleeding. Diagnosis by barium-contrast studies usually is impossible, and even the endoscopist may find it difficult to see the ulcer. If the bleeding is minimal, angiography is useless, but such ulcers often bleed massively and angiography is very helpful.

Other ulcers may occur in diverticula, proximal to adhesions, and in blind loops. Ulcers may develop in uremic patients or in those on hemodialysis. Typhoid ulcers can occur massively; despite wide involvement of the ileum in this disease, bleeding points in one reported case were in the cecum.[43]

Crohn's Disease.—Small intestinal ulcerations may lead to hemorrhage in this disease. However, all bleeding usually is minimal, in contrast to that of ulcerative colitis, which often is massive.

Intussusception.—In children, diagnosis is made by a history of abdominal cramps followed by rectal bleeding and at times a palpable right lower quadrant mass. A barium enema is frequently both diagnostic and therapeutic. In adults intussusception usually is due to a tumor of the right colon; the signs are those of intestinal obstruction, and bleeding is not common.

Strangulating Intestinal Obstruction.—Diagnostic signs of severe abdominal pain, vomiting, and obstipation may occasionally also include vomiting of blood and bright blood by rectum. All symptoms are acute and the treatment is that of the intestinal obstruction.

Trauma.—Trauma may lead to bleeding either from a penetrating wound or from blunt trauma. In most instances the diagnosis is obvious from examination or abdominal tap. Retroperitoneal ruptures of the duodenum lead initially to few abdominal signs. Computed tomographic scans, or extravasation of contrast material given by mouth may aid in diagnosis of questionable cases.

Colon, Rectum, Anal Canal

The common causes of bleeding from the lower bowel are listed in Table 1. The diagnosis and treatment of the great majority of these lesions are standardized and furnish little controversy. In this section the more difficult problems encountered in clinical practice will be considered.

The source of colorectal bleeding often is very difficult to determine. The exact origin of hemorrhoidal bleeding may be invisible a few minutes later. The lesions of angiodysplasia are so minute that they may be missed by endoscopy and by the surgeon; even the pathologist has trouble finding them unless special injection techniques are used. Very few specimens of the colon resected for diverticular bleeding actually demonstrate the site of origin of the hemorrhage.

Clinical patterns of bleeding give a clue concerning the source and cause of the bleeding. Several types can be identified as follows:

1. The patient has microcytic anemia suggesting blood loss and the

stools are positive for occult blood. The prime sources in the colon are cancer of the right colon and angiodysplasia. However, all of the lesions discussed above from the esophagus to the colon may be responsible.

2. Bleeding in an adult is intermittent and bright red, varying from streaking on the toilet paper to larger amounts. Hemorrhoids are the likely diagnosis, but further studies are necessary to rule out cancer or polyps.

3. Bright red blood or streaking is seen in every bowel movement. The diagnosis in an adult is probably cancer or polypoid disease.

4. The bleeding is severe or massive. If there is any possibility that it might arise from the upper GI tract, a nasogastric tube is inserted. If the aspirate is positive for blood, endoscopy of the stomach and duodenum is necessary. Meanwhile, a sample of blood is drawn, and tagged with ^{99m}Tc. If the gastric aspirate is negative, the angiography staff is alerted. If the radionuclide scan is positive when it is available about an hour later, the patient is taken to the angiography suite. However, if bleeding is severe, angiography is done without waiting for results of the scan.

The angiogram usually will demonstrate either a bleeding point with extravasation or a vascular tuft and early filling vein in the right lower quadrant typical of angiodysplasia. If there is extravasation, selective infusion of the artery with vasopressin is done; control of bleeding can be expected in 90% of patients. The catheter is left in place in case there should be recurrent bleeding within 48 hours. Recurrent bleeding may at times be controlled with a second injection of vasopressin, but usually a segmental colectomy is necessary.[17]

It is apparent that we place great confidence in angiography for diagnosis and control of massive colonic bleeding. Meanwhile total colonoscopy is reserved until a time when the colon is either clear of blood or there is minimal bleeding. Many surgeons have combined intraoperative irrigation of the colon (through the scope or a catheter placed in the cecum) with intraoperative colonoscopy.[44, 45] We have been somewhat dubious about the value of this method because of the great difficulty in finding the lesions either of angiodysplasia or the actual bleeding diverticulum.

In the course of the last few years a great deal has been learned about certain types of bleeding from the large bowel. Bleeding from angiodysplasia and from diverticulosis has received the most attention. Some of the most pertinent information will be listed concerning these lesions as well as others in which specific treatment is possible.

Angiodysplasia

This disease, identified in 1960 by Margulis and named by Galdabini in 1974, occurs in older patients and apparently is developmental and not congenital as occurs with other AVMs. In our experience, it has occurred nearly exclusively in the right colon. The lesions typically are 1 to 5 mm in diameter; unless they are bleeding they are almost impossible to identify either by the endoscopist or pathologist. Injection techniques have shown their microscopic pathology. The lesions may be single or multiple; as many as five have been identified in a single specimen. The average age of our patients is about 70; many have had preceding heart disease, such as aortic stenosis.

The cardinal angiographic signs, a vascular tuft and early filling of a right lower quadrant vein, do not mean that an angiodysplastic lesion is the cause of bleeding. Angiography of the inferior mesenteric artery must be done at the same time because either diverticula of the left colon or cancer may be the cause. Signs of intraluminal bleeding such as true extravasation do not occur commonly with angiodysplasia.

Endoscopic electrocoagulation has been successful in the treatment of some of these lesions. However, unless there is active bleeding, they frequently cannot be found. Angiographic control is not likely to be used because of the rarity with which active bleeding is demonstrated. Segmental colectomy is considered to be the procedure of choice. In a follow-up study of 31 of our patients, two had rebled within an average period of 18 months after right colectomy.[46] Boley reported three recurrent bleeding episodes after 24 operations.[47]

Diverticulosis

One of the surprising discoveries that was made early in the use of angiography was that diverticular bleeding was found in the majority of cases to originate from diverticula of the colon proximal to the splenic flexure, although diverticula are far more common in the left colon than in the right. The reason has never been discovered. Angiography demonstrates a bleeding point in 75% of cases, provided it is done at a time when the bleeding is at a rate of over 0.5 ml/minute. It is estimated that if all angiographies were done when bleeding actually was occurring at this rate that positive findings would be obtained in over 95% of cases of diverticular bleeding.

Although segmental resection is considered to be adequate in the cases in which a single source of diverticular bleeding is demonstrated, most authorities agree that subtotal colectomy is wiser if diverticula are scattered throughout the colon.

Postoperative Bleeding

Hemorrhage is not uncommon after endoscopic polypectomy. Fortunately, it responds well to selective arteriographic vasopressin injection. In these cases the major mesenteric vessels are still intact. Following more radical resections and anastomoses in which the major vessels or their major tributaries have been interrupted, vasopressin still has been effective in stilling anastomotic bleeding. It also has been used for bleeding after colostomy closure.

Major bleeding from the colon is a very serious problem if selective angiography is not available. We have had no experience with intraoperative washing of the colon, and either intraoperative endoscopy or segmental clamping in an attempt to localize the bleeding point. Assuming that rigid sigmoidoscopy had shown no lesion and the laparotomy shows no lesion other than a colon filled with blood, subtotal colectomy is a reasonable choice. Thus Drapanas had a mortality of only 11% when he pursued this more radical method in 1972.[48] More recently, in the same institution, angiography was used; 14 patients had subtotal and 21 had segmental colectomy. The overall postoperative mortality in the 35 patients still was 11%, but postoperative morbidity had been reduced from 37% to 11%.[49]

The main arguments against routine subtotal colectomy are (1) that the postoperative mortality usually is less after segmental than subtotal colectomy, and (2) that in some elderly patients subtotal colectomy may lead to serious postoperative diarrhea that can be avoided by segmental resection. On the other hand, under these circumstances, the occurrence of later bleeding after subtotal colectomy in our cases was reduced to zero, while it remained approximately 6% after segmental colectomy. This series was small but suggested later development of similar lesions in the remaining bowel after segmental colectomy.

At the present time, balancing these arguments, most surgeons believe that segmental colectomy is wise in the presence of angiodysplasia. For diverticular bleeding when the bleeding site has been shown by angiography, segmental colectomy is preferred, unless diverticula are found throughout the large bowel, when the proper operation is subtotal colectomy. Subtotal colectomy also is preferred if the site of origin of the bleeding cannot be determined. In all cases, careful examination of the entire intestinal tract at the time of laparotomy is essential. If any other lesions potentially could be the source of hemorrhage, they should be removed.[50]

Liver and Bile Ducts; Hemobilia

Hemobilia is a form of GI tract bleeding that results from fistula formation between the hepatic artery and the bile duct system and is therefore an arteriobiliary fistula. This GI bleed may present as massive hematemesis, melena, or hematochezia. According to Sandblom, the bleeding into the bile ducts in 75% of the cases is from the liver or gallbladder, in 22% directly into the extrahepatic biliary tree, and in 3% from the pancreas. The diagnosis is suggested by the following three factors: (1) a history of trauma, (2) right upper quadrant pain, and (3) GI bleeding.[51]

Trauma is the etiology in approximately 50% of cases; the etiology in the remaining cases is inflammation, gallstones, or tumors. The fistula may be the result of simultaneously produced lacerations of the hepatic artery and a biliary radical that produces the initial fistula. The fistula also may develop later as a result of erosion of the bile duct and artery by an expanding liver cavity or by a gallstone. Lastly, the delayed appearance of a fistula may be the result of expansion of a false aneurysm of the hepatic artery that has produced pressure necrosis of a biliary radical.

If the diagnosis is considered strongly the most accurate and direct diagnostic procedure is a celiac or hepatic angiogram. The angiogram may identify either extravasation of contrast into the biliary tree or a collection of contrast material within an aneurysm sac or hepatic cavity. Endoscopy and ERCP also are essential; bleeding from the ampulla of Vater can be seen. Cholangiography can demonstrate clots or tumors. Other studies that may be helpful include ultrasound, computed tomography (CT), magnetic resonance imaging, and barium studies.

The treatment of hemobilia depends on the etiology and location of the fistula.[52] The most common type, due to trauma, usually develops because of an intrahepatic injury. Rarely, conservative management is successful in children, as has been reported from the Massachusetts General Hospital; this can be appropriate if the bleeding is not life-threatening and serial monitoring by angiography is possible.[53]

Intrahepatic aneurysms and arterial fistulas usually may be treated adequately by angiographic embolization. If operation is necessary three general options are available: (1) formal resection of the involved portion of the liver if the lesion is localized to one lobe or segment; (2) opening the liver cavity, suture ligation of the involved artery and bile duct, and drainage of the cavity; or (3) ligation of either the common hepatic, right or left, or proper hepatic artery, depending upon which method causes the bleeding to stop.

The choice of treatment for extrahepatic aneurysms is more difficult. An operation can be very dangerous; on the other hand, angiographic embolization can lead to liver infarction in some instances. The options must be weighed carefully; much depends on the comparative skills of the surgeon and the angiographer.

If the aneurysm is in the common hepatic artery, a patent gastroduodenal artery makes either arteriographic embolization or surgical operation safer than if the proper hepatic artery is involved. Surgically, an aneurysm of the common hepatic artery can be ligated proximally and distally because collateral flow through the gastroduodenal artery will provide arterial perfusion of the liver. If collateral blood flow is not expected to be sufficient, bypass grafting of the common hepatic artery is recommended.

Aneurysms or fistulas involving the proper hepatic artery are even more problematic; although ligation or embolization probably are safe because of compensatory increase in portal venous flow, this cannot be assured. Optimal treatment includes either excision or exclusion of the aneurysms and arterial reconstruction.

For the other causes of hemobilia, surgical treatment should resolve the problem. Cholecystectomy will cure the disease if gallstones are the cause. In the rare case of hemobilia resulting from arterial erosion from a pancreatic pseudocyst, the cyst may be opened or resected, the artery ligated, and the cyst decompressed either by internal or external drainage.

Pancreas

The most common instance of major GI hemorrhage from diseases of the pancreas is that of diffuse gastric mucosal hemorrhage ("stress gastritis"), which is seen with pancreatic necrosis from acute pancreatitis or undrained pancreatic abscess. The diagnosis is suggested by the occurrence of upper GI hemorrhage in the setting of acute pancreatitis and confirmed by gastroscopy, and CT scan of the abdomen with contrast. The gastric mucosal hemorrhage is best treated with selective intraarterial vasopressin and the pancreas with operative debridement and drainage.

Other less common pancreatic causes of GI hemorrhage include erosion of an infected pancreatic necrotic mass into a neighboring viscus (usually the stomach), erosion of a primary pancreatic tumor into a neighboring viscus with arterial bleeding, and, occasionally, hemorrhage from arterial erosions from tumor or pancreatitis into the pancreatic ductal system and thence into the duodenum. Necrosis of the transverse mesocolon from pancreatitis may produce ischemia of the transverse colon with hemorrhage. Computed tomographic scans of the abdomen with contrast and mesenteric angiography should allow the diagnosis to be made and may allow angiographic control of the bleeding.

Chronic relapsing pancreatitis or advanced pancreatic malignant disease may produce occlusion of branches of the portal venous system with the formation of varices and hemorrhage. Computed tomographic scan of the abdomen with contrast and mesenteric angiography (venous phase) suggest this diagnosis.

Both penetrating and blunt trauma may produce hemorrhage from the pancreas that is more frequent into the retroperitoneum and free abdominal cavity than into the GI tract. The circumstances of the clinical presentation make the diagnosis, which in a stable patient may be pursued with CT scan and angiography.

Vascular System Causes of Gastrointestinal Hemorrhage

Acute mesenteric ischemia, from embolic occlusion or thrombosis of the superior mesenteric artery, from cardiac dysfunction and a low flow mesenteric arterial state, or from spontaneous mesenteric thrombosis, initially produces ischemic injury to the more vulnerable bowel mucosa. This leads to variable mucosal sloughing and consequent GI bleeding. The overriding symptom in this clinical entity is that of abdominal pain, usually out of proportion to the abdominal physical findings in the absence of transmural bowel infarction. The finding of low-grade GI bleeding is a further variable to lead the clinician to consider the diagnosis. The hemorrhage itself is not usually a major consideration in the management of acute mesenteric ischemia.

The most common long-term complication of the placement of vascular grafts in the abdominal aorta is erosion of the overlying bowel (usually duodenum) with the production of a graft-enteric fistula and consequent GI hemorrhage. The site of difficulty is usually at the proximal aortic anastomosis, but may be at the distal anastomosis. Occasionally, the graft itself may erode into the bowel and hemorrhage occurs through the interstices of the graft. The diagnosis should be considered in any patient with GI bleeding and previous surgery on the aorta or iliac arteries. Somewhat surprisingly, hemorrhage from such fistulas is not necessarily profuse nor continuous, but ultimately if not appropriately treated will invariably lead to the demise of the patient.

Upper GI endoscopy carried into the fourth part of the duodenum will usually allow the diagnosis to be made; however, intraluminal thrombus may preclude diagnostic certainty. Biplane aortography may show irregularity of the involved anastomosis, but thrombus may prevent clear delineation of the anatomic defect and if active extravasation of contrast into the bowel lumen is not seen, the diagnosis will remain uncertain. A CT scan with contrast may strongly suggest this diagnosis if the fat plane between the overlying duodenum and aortic graft at the level of the proximal anastomosis is not seen. Occasionally, it may be necessary to operate on the patient to determine the source of the hemorrhage. The appropriate management of this condition involves removal of the graft, oversewing of the aorta above the proximal anastomosis, and extraanatomic reconstruction with axillo femoral and femoro-femoral grafting to ensure adequate arterial perfusion of the lower extremities and pelvis. Appropriate use of antibiotics and drainage of the retroperitoneum also are essential.[54, 55]

Pseudoaneurysms, usually produced by operative or violent trauma, and true aneurysms of splanchnic arteries may erode into a neighboring hollow viscus, leading to massive GI hemorrhage. Frequently, if hemorrhage is unrelenting, the abdomen is explored. If the patient is stable, arteriography reveals the diagnosis and allows planning of the operation, which involves gaining proximal and distal control of the vessel affected and the selection of the appropriate reconstructive alternative, if it is needed. Rarely, an abdominal aortic aneurysm may erode into the duodenum so that GI bleeding is the first symptom.[54]

Traumatic arteriovenous fistulas involving the splanchnic vessels may lead to portal hypertension at a later date, with resultant GI bleeding from thin-walled submucosal varices. An audible abdominal bruit and a previous history of trauma should lead to abdominal angiography. This will demonstrate both the early venous filling from the involved artery and varices of the portal venous circulation, which can be seen on the venous phase of the angiogram. The treatment is directed to interruption of the arteriovenous communication with repair of the artery.

Lower GI bleeding from the colonic mucosa may result from sudden deprivation of its blood supply. This may occur in two circumstances, either following occlusion of the inferior mesenteric artery, usually during aortic operations, or occasionally as a spontaneous event in older patients with arterial disease. In the former circumstance, the clinical situation should suggest the diagnosis, which is confirmed by colonscopy, and after which operative resection of the ischemic colon is usually the safest approach. Spontaneous ischemic colitis may be a manifestation of both occlusive mesenteric arterial disease or nonocclusive disease, with ischemia most marked in the watershed between the superior and inferior mesenteric circulation.

Lower GI bleeding usually is accompanied by colicky lower abdominal pain and diarrhea, and the patient may be febrile and have abdominal tenderness. Again, colonoscopy is useful to suggest the diagnosis and angiography may confirm it. Barium-contrast examination of the colon may show edema of the ischemic colonic mucosa (''thumbprinting''). Those cases with intestinal gangrene will require emergency resection and those with mild symptoms and signs may be followed closely. Occasionally, a colonic stricture is a late manifestation of a localized colonic ischemia.

Postoperative Gastrointestinal Hemorrhage

Hemostasis, essential to success in all surgical endeavors, may fail because of inadequacy of mechanical control of severed blood vessels, or because any of the natural occurring mechanisms for maintaining hemostasis are not effective. In general, if the preoperative assessment of the patient based on the history, physical examination, and commonly used screening tests (prothrombin time, partial thromboplastin time, platelet count, and bleeding time) fail to uncover an abnormality, and during the conduct of the operation difficulty in obtaining hemostasis is not encountered, the surgeon must reasonably suspect that an early GI hemorrhage after a GI operation is related to mechanical failure of hemostasis. The appropriate management in such circumstances is directed toward maintenance of circulating intravascular volume, reassessment of the patient's ability to make and form thrombus, and clearing of thrombus from the intestine to avoid distention of the bowel at the area of anastomosis. In these patients receiving multiple transfusions, empiric use of fresh frozen plasma and platelet transfusions may overcome the thrombocytopenia and/or factor deficiency (especially V and VII) that occurs with the transfusion of large quantities of older bank blood.

Postoperative anastomotic bleeding may be confirmed by angiogram and controlled with infusion of vasopressin or transcatheter embolization, but the surgeon must weigh carefully the advantages of this approach with that of prompt reoperation to directly control the bleeding in a timely and definitive fashion.

Hemorrhage following endoscopic polypectomy may be effectively controlled with selective infusion of vasopressin into the bleeding artery. Hemorrhage from a retained peptic ulcer is managed on an individual basis, weighing the likelihood of success from vasopressin infusion or angiographic transcatheter embolization against that of direct suture ligation or resection.

Finally, in a patient with continuing hemorrhage after mechanical control of major bleeding points, consultation with a hematologist may be helpful in defining and managing an identifiable coagulopathy.

Gastrointestinal Hemorrhage From Bleeding Diatheses

Gastrointestinal hemorrhage may be a manifestation of a failure of the natural occurring mechanisms for maintaining hemostasis that may be categorized as platelet disorders, vessel wall abnormalities, and disorders of coagulation, congenital and acquired.

Platelets have an important role in initiating hemostasis; hence, inadequate platelets, in number or function, may lead to hemorrhage. An excessive number of platelets, usually associated with thrombosis, may also be associated with bleeding that frequently occurs from the mucous membrane of the GI tract. Qualitative platelet disorders rarely initiate spontaneous bleeding in contradistinction to quantitative disorders. Qualitative platelet disorders are quite common, frequently being caused by drugs affecting platelet adhesion, release, or aggregation, such as aspirin. The transfusion of 4 to 6 units of platelet concentrates will normally restore hemostasis in patients with platelet disorders.

When a vessel is injured, the smooth muscle of the vessel contracts, controlling hemorrhage. A number of congenital and acquired disorders of this mechanism have been recognized, including in the former instance hereditary hemorrhagic telangectasia, and in the latter, purpura and drug induced disorders.

Disorders of coagulation—coagulopathies—may be caused by congenital or acquired abnormal production, consumption, or losses of coagulation factors. The activation of factor X leads to the production of thrombin from prothrombin and the subsequent conversion of fibrinogen to fibrin, the final pathway to coagulation. This may occur through the intrinsic or extrinsic pathways of coagulation. Activation of the intrinsic system begins with the activation of factor XII when it comes into contact with foreign substances, and the extrinsic system by the release of tissue thromboplastin from injured tissues. The partial thromboplastin time monitors function of the intrinsic system; the prothrombin, the external system.

Occasionally, the history, physical examination, or screening test may alert the clinician to the strong possibility that an abnormality in the mechanisms of hemostasis is the major factor in the production of the GI tract hemorrhage. As the hematological diagnosis is being refined by additional investigation, the surgeon must also keep in mind that, in practical terms, GI tract hemorrhage is usually produced by a mucosal lesion of the GI tract. The presence of the congenital or acquired bleeding diathesis may bring to light the presence of this lesion and/or exacerbate a hemorrhage.

All patients bleeding from the GI tract should be investigated from the standpoint of an abnormality of platelets or coagulation ability, but also must be managed from the standpoint of the nature of the lesion causing the hemorrhage. Appropriate hematologic consultation may assist greatly in the management of such patients. Certainly those patients using drugs that interfere with platelet function or the production of coagulations factors should initially be managed by reversal of these drugs. They include aspirin, warfarin, and ibuprofen, among others. As an optimal hemostatic state is approached or reached, and GI hemorrhage continues, the diagnostic studies should be conducted according to the principles described earlier. If operative management is necessary, the surgeon must be guided by the operative findings to determine further action.

Summary

Complex problems occur concerning the diagnosis and treatment of GI bleeding. How often can the exact cause and site of the bleeding be determined? What are the advantages and complications of various forms of treatment? There are no universal answers, applicable to all situations.

Nevertheless, certain assumptions seem to be justified. Diagnosis of the cause of severe bleeding, often suggested by the patient's history, is confirmed most effectively by selective angiography, which should give an answer in over 95% of cases. The causes of slow, persistent bleeding, manifested either by gross blood or by positive tests for blood in the stools, are diagnosed in about the same percentage of cases by endoscopy. It is when the bleeding is intermittent and of minimum or moderate severity that determination of the site of origin is the most difficult; angiography cannot help in the majority of cases, and endoscopy can miss tiny lesions that are not bleeding at the time of examination. However, laparotomy, especially when it is combined with intraoperative enteroscopy or angiography, should reduce the number of unsolved diagnoses to under 5% of the total.

Surgery is the primary method of therapy in many cases. Primary control of bleeding also can be obtained in approximately 80% of cases of severe bleeding by endoscopy, by the use of coagulation or laser, or by selective arterial infusion of pitressin. Recurrences must be treated by surgery, except in some instances where selective embolization by the angiographer may result in a cure. The surgeon must attempt to cure the hemorrhage and to prevent recurrence at a later date by such measures as gastric resection and vagotomy for bleeding duodenal ulcers to prevent stomal ulcers, or by subtotal rather than segmental colectomy for widespread colonic diverticulosis.

There will be an irreducible percentage of lesions that continue to develop in other sections of the GI tract after successful primary treatment of the original cause of bleeding; AVMs, angiodysplasia, and vasculitis are examples. Fortunately, such diseases are relatively rare. It is not unreasonable today to expect that the measures discussed herein will cure bleeding in 95% of cases; if death occurs it rarely is due to hemorrhage, but to some type of organ failure.

References

1. Stafford ES, Zuidema GD, Cameron JL: Unusual causes of occult bleeding from the gastrointestinal tract. *Am J Surg* 1970; 119:208–212.
2. Thompson JN, Hemingway AP, McPherson GAD, et al: Obscure gastrointestinal hemorrhage of small-bowel origin. *Br Med J* 1984; 288:163–165.
3. Stone HW: Large melena of obscure origin. *Ann Surg* 1944; 120:582–585.
4. Spiller RC, Parkins RA: Recurrent gastrointestinal bleeding of obscure origin: Report of 17 cases and a guide to logical management. *Br J Surg* 1983; 70:489–493.
5. Salem R, Thompson JN, Hemingway AP, et al: Specialist investigation of obscure gastrointestinal hemorrhage. *Gut* 1985; 28:A1154–A1155.
6. Eckstein MR, Kelemouridis V, Athanasoulis CA, et al: Gastric bleeding: Therapy with intraarterial vasopressin and transcatheter embolization. *Radiology* 1984; 152:643–646.
7. Borsch G, Schmidt G: Endoscopy of the terminal ileum: Diagnostic yield in 400 consecutive examinations. *Dis Colon Rectum* 1985; 28:499–501.
8. Winzelberg GG: The versatility of Tc-99m red cell blood pool imaging and demonstrating bleeding sites, in *Nuclear Medicine Annual.* New York, Raven Press, 1985, chap 3, pp 73–106.
9. Alavi A, Ring EJ: Localization of gastrointestinal bleeding: Superiority of 99m Tc sulfur colloid compound compared with angiography. *Am J Radiol* 1981; 137:741–748.
10. Alavi A: Detection of gastrointestinal bleeding with ^{99m}Tc-sulfur colloid. *Semin Nucl Med* 1982; 12:126–138.
11. Barum S: Angiography and the gastrointestinal bleeder. *Radiology* 1982; 143:569–572.
12. Fredlich JW, Winzelberg GG: Radionuclide detection of gastrointestinal hemorrhage, in Athanasoulis CA, Greene RG, Pfister RC, et al (eds): *Interventional Angiology.* Philadelphia, WB Saunders Co, 1982, chap 9.
13. McKusick KA, Froelich J, Callahan RJ, et al: ^{99m}Tc red blood cells for detection of gastrointestinal bleeding: Experience with 80 patients. *AJR* 1981; 137:1113–1118.
14. Winzelberg GG, McKusick KA: Froelich JW, et al: Detection of gastrointestinal bleeding with ^{99m}Tc-labeled red blood cells. *Semin Nucl Med* 1982; 12:139–146.
15. Yamamoto Y, Sano K, Shigemoto H: Detection of the bleeding source from small intestine: Intraoperative endoscopy and preoperative abdominal scintigraphy by technetium 99m pertechnetate. *Am Surg* 1985; 51:658–660.
16. Athanasoulis CA: Upper gastrointestinal bleeding of arteriocapillary origin, in Athanasoulis CA, Greene RG, Pfister RC, et al (eds): *Interventional Angiology.* Philadelphia, WB Saunders Co, 1982, chap 6, pp 55–89.
17. Athanasoulis CA: Lower gastrointestinal bleeding, in Athanasoulis CA, Greene RG, Pfister RC, et al (eds): *Interventional Angiology.* Philadelphia, WB Saunders Co, 1982, chap 8, pp 115–148.
18. Reis HE, Moschinski D, Borchard F: Isolierte Dunndarmvarikosis ohne pfor-

taderblock als ursache einer massiven oberen gastrointestinalblutung. *Leber Magen Darm* 1982; 12:23–31.
19. Richardson JD, Harriot TJ, Athanasoulis CA, et al: Hepatic and splenic infarctions: Complications of therapeutic transcatheter embolization. *Am J Surg* 1980; 139:272–277.
20. Welch CE, Rodkey GV, Gryska PR: A thousand operations for ulcer disease. *Ann Surg* 1986; 204:454–467.
21. Laine L: Multipolar electrocoagulation in the treatment of active upper gastrointestinal tract hemorrhage: A prospective controlled trial. *N Engl J Med* 1987; 316:1613–1617.
22. Krejs GJ, Little KH, Westergaard H, et al: Laser photocoagulation for the treatment of acute peptic ulcer bleeding: A randomized controlled clinical trial. *N Engl J Med* 1987; 316:1618–1621.
23. Fromm D: Endoscopic coagulation for gastrointestinal bleeding (editorial). *N Engl J Med* 1987; 316:1652–1654.
24. Joffe SN, Schroeder T: Lasers in general surgery. *Adv Surg* 1987; 20:125–154.
25. Clouse RE, Costigan DJ, Mills BA, et al: Angiodysplasia as a cause of upper gastrointestinal bleeding. *Arch Intern Med* 1985; 145:458–461.
26. Jabbari M, Cherry R, Lough JO, et al: Gastric antral vascular ectasia: The watermelon stomach. *Gastroenterology* 1984; 87:1165–1170.
27. Hoffmann J, Beck H, Jensen HE: Dieulafoy's lesion. *Surg Gynecol Obstet* 1984; 159:537–540.
28. Primrose JN, Gledhill T, Quirke P, et al: Blind total gastrectomy for massive bleeding from the stomach. *Br J Surg* 1986; 73:920–922.
29. Hastings PR, Skillman JJ, Bushnell LS, et al: Antacid titration in the prevention of gastrointestinal bleeding: A controlled randomized trial in 100 critically ill patients. *N Engl J Med* 1978; 293:1441–1445.
30. Morris DL, Hawker PC, Brearley S, et al: Optimal timing of operation for bleeding ulcer: Prospective randomized trial. *Br Med J* 1984; 288:1277–1280.
31. Tillotson CL, Geller SC, et al: Small bowel hemorrhage: Angiographic localization and intervention. *Gastrointest Radiol,* in press.
32. Tada M, Kawai K: Small bowel endoscopy. *Scand J Gastroenterol* 1984; 19(suppl 102):39–52.
33. Bowden TA Jr, Hooks VH, Mansberger AR: Intraoperative gastrointestinal endoscopy. *Ann Surg* 1980; 191:680–687.
34. van Coevorden F, Mathus-Vliegen EMH, Brummelkamp WH: Combined endoscopic and surgical treatment in Peutz-Jeghers syndrome. *Surg Gynecol Obstet* 1986; 162:426–428.
35. Lau WY, Fan ST, Chu KW, et al: Intra-operative fiberoptic enteroscopy for bleeding lesions in the small intestine. *Br J Surg* 1986; 73:217–218.
36. Athanasoulis CA, Moncure AC, Greenfield AJ, et al: Intraoperative localization of small bowel bleeding sites with combined use of angiographic methods and methylene blue injection. *Surgery* 1980; 87:77–84.
37. Crawford ES, Roehm JOF Jr, McGavran MH: Jejunoileal arteriovenous malformation: Localization for resection by segmental bowel staining techniques. *Ann Surg* 1980; 191:404–409.
38. Farthing MG, Griffiths NJ, Thomas JM, et al: Occult bleeding from Meckel's diverticulum. *Br J Surg* 1981; 68:176.
39. Civetta JM, Daggett WM: Gastrointestinal bleeding from jejunal diverticula. *Ann Surg* 1967; 166:976–979.

40. Helin I, Flodmark P, Lindhagen T, et al: Occult bleeding from giant small bowel diverticula. *Acta Pediatr Scand* 1983; 72:463–465.
41. Moncure AC, Waltman AC, Vandersalm TJ, et al: Gastrointestinal hemorrhage from adhesion-related mesenteric varices. *Ann Surg* 1976; 183:24–29.
42. Poole GV Jr, Meredith JW: Gastrointestinal hemorrhage from small bowel varices: A rare complication of pancreatitis. *Contemp Surg* 1987; 30:79–83.
43. Reyes E, Hernandez J, Gonzalez A: Typhoid colitis with massive lower gastrointestinal hemorrhage: An unexpected behavior of *Salmonelli typhi. Dis Colon Rectum* 1986; 29:511–514.
44. Batch AJG, Pickard RJ, DeLacey G: Preoperative colonoscopy in massive rectal bleeding. *Br J Surg* 1981; 68:64.
45. Mendoza CB Jr, Watne AL: Value of intraoperative colonoscopy in vascular ectasia of the colon. *Am Surg* 1982; 48:153–156.
46. Welch CE, Athanasoulis CA, Galdabini JJ: Hemorrhage from the large bowel with special reference to angiodysplasia and diverticular disease. *World J Surg* 1978; 2:73–80.
47. Boley SJ: Invited commentary. *World J Surg* 1978; 2:80–81.
48. Drapanas T, Pennington DG, Kappelman M, et al: Emergency subtotal colectomy: Preferred approach to management of massively bleeding diverticular disease. *Ann Surg* 1973; 177:519–526.
49. Browder W, Cerise BJ, Litwin MS: Impact of emergency angiography in massive gastrointestinal bleeding. *Ann Surg* 1986; 204:530–536.
50. Steger AC, Galland RB, Hemingway A, et al: Gastrointestinal hemorrhage from a second source in patients with colonic angiodysplasia. *Br J Surg* 1987; 74:726–727.
51. Sandblom P: *Hemobilia (Biliary Tract Hemorrhage): History, Pathology, Diagnosis, Treatment.* Springfield, Ill, Charles C Thomas Publisher, 1972.
52. Mathisen DJ, Athanasoulis CA, Malt RA: Preservation of arterial flow to the liver: Goal in treatment of extrahepatic and post-traumatic intrahepatic aneurysms of the hepatic artery. *Ann Surg* 1982; 196:400–411.
53. Hendren WH, Warshaw AL, Fleischli DJ, et al: Traumatic hemobilia: Nonoperative management with healing documented by serial angiography. *Ann Surg* 1971; 174:991–993.
54. Yeager RA, Sasaki TM, McConnell DB, et al: Clinical spectrum of patients with infrarenal aortic grafts and gastrointestinal bleeding. *Am J Surg* 1987; 153:459–461.
55. Vetts JT, Culp SC, Smythe TB, et al: Iliac arterial-enteric fistula arising after pelvic irradiation. *Surgery* 1987; 101:643–647.

Hepatic Trauma

George F. Sheldon, M.D.

Professor and Chairman, Department of Surgery, The University of North Carolina at Chapel Hill, Chapel Hill, North Carolina

Robert Rutledge, M.D.

Assistant Professor, Department of Surgery, The University of North Carolina at Chapel Hill, Chapel Hill, North Carolina

The liver is the most common abdominal organ injured after both blunt and penetrating trauma. Hepatic trauma constitutes a broad spectrum of injuries, ranging from minor lacerations with minimal bleeding that require little or no intervention, to massive crush injuries and lacerations of the retrohepatic vena cava that tax the limits of the best surgical teams and are often lethal. The magnitude of the injury and the complexity of the operative procedure required for repair are determined by the extent, anatomic location, and the mechanism of injury (blunt or penetrating). The majority of hepatic wounds are minor; in one study, 79 (59%) of 134 hepatic injuries required only minor operative repair.[1] In other studies up to 88% of hepatic injuries require little or no operative intervention. Given the large percentage of minor hepatic injuries there has been an increasing number of reports describing nonoperative treatment for selected hepatic injuries. Nonoperative management of hepatic injury will be discussed subsequently.

Because exsanguinating hemorrhage is responsible for most of the early deaths from hepatic injury, surgeons must be familiar with the range of alternatives available in managing hepatic trauma. Although the majority of hepatic injuries can be managed with simple operative techniques, major liver injury requires the most advanced surgical skills and resuscitation.[2]

Anatomy of the Liver

Management of major hepatic injuries requires a thorough understanding of hepatic anatomy. The liver is divided into right and left lobes of relatively equal size (Fig 1). A sagittal section through the gallbladder fossa, which extends superiorly to the diaphragm, left of the falciform ligament and posteriorly to the inferior vena, divides the liver into the right and left lobes (Fig 2). The left lobe of the liver is divided by the falciform ligament into medial and lateral segments. The left lobe lateral segment is drained by the left hepatic vein and supplied by the left hepatic artery and left portal vein. The medial segment of the left lobe is drained by the middle

Adv Surg 22:179–194, 1989

0065-3411/89/22-179–194-$04.00

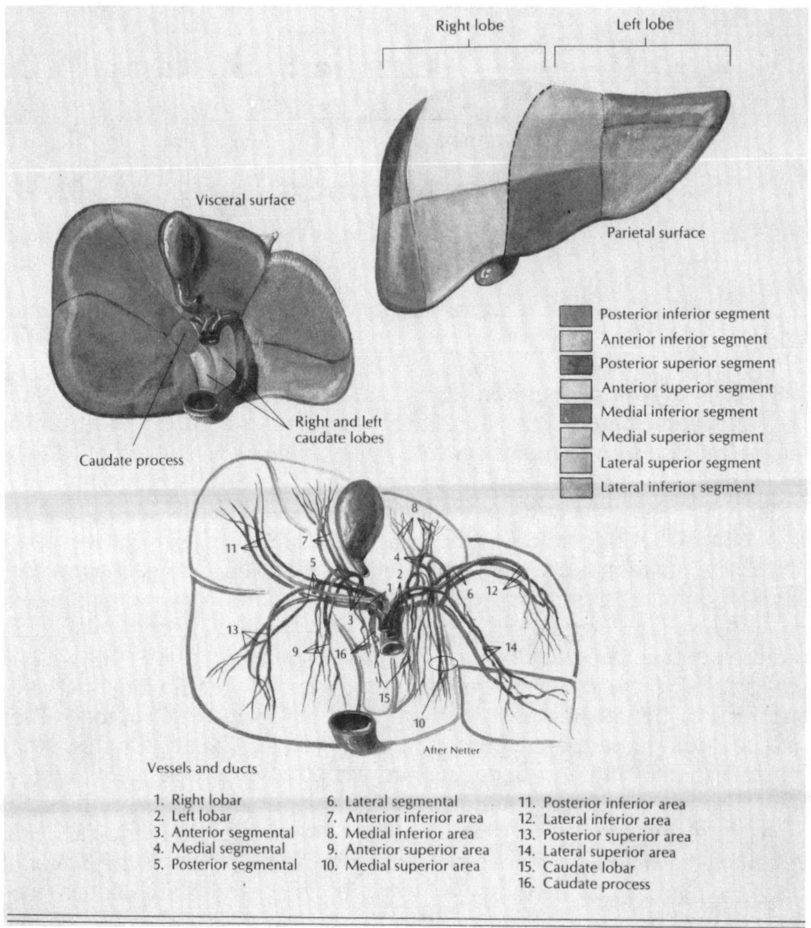

FIG 1.
Anatomy of the liver. (From Lim RC Jr, Crass RA: Liver, in Davis JH, et al (eds): *Clinical Surgery*. St Louis, CV Mosby Co, 1987. Used by permission.)

hepatic vein. The middle hepatic vein may at times join the left hepatic vein prior to entering the vena cava.

The right lobe of the liver is drained by the right hepatic vein and is the largest portion of the liver. It is made up of the liver lateral to the plane through the fossa of the gallbladder. The right and left hepatic arteries usually arise from the common hepatic artery, but the left hepatic artery may arise from the left gastric artery. The superior mesenteric artery may occasionally supply the right or left hepatic artery. The biliary tree generally follows the arterial and venous drainage, but minor anatomical variations of the gallbladder and bile ducts are common.

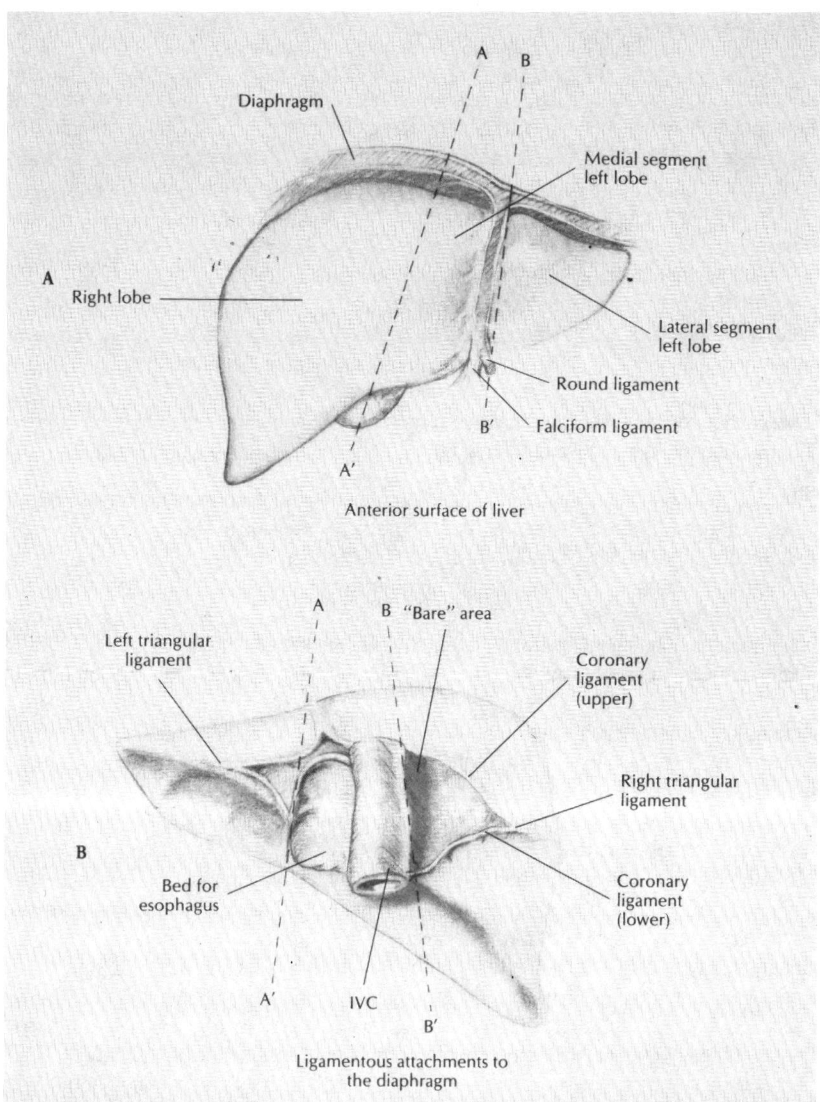

FIG 2.
Anatomy of the liver. (From Lim RC Jr, Crass RA: Liver, in Davis, JH, et al (eds): *Clinical Surgery*. St Louis, CV Mosby Co, 1987. Used by permission.)

Physiology

All forms of injury are associated with alterations in amino acid, glucose, and fatty acid metabolism.[3] After trauma there is an accelerated release of amino acids from muscle and an increase in amino acid uptake for protein synthesis by the liver and other visceral tissues. Trauma increases protein synthesis in the hepatic tissue by 42%. In skeletal muscle, amino acid synthesis is decreased by 50% while protein degradation in muscle is enhanced by about 70%.[4]

Trauma results in a progressive decrease in hepatic phagocytosis. After trauma there is a failure in hepatic Kupffer's cell phagocytosis and an increase in plasma lysosomal enzyme levels proportional to the severity of the injury.

Mechanism of Hepatic Injury

Hepatic injury is usually subdivided into blunt and penetrating types. Blunt trauma is usually secondary to motor vehicle accidents, falls, birth trauma, pregnancy, explosion, or war injuries.[5–7] Penetrating injury is secondary to gunshot wounds, stab wounds, or impalement.

Penetrating injuries are more common in series reported by inner city hospitals, while blunt trauma is more common in other series. In 1,000 patients with hepatic injuries treated at Baylor College of Medicine, Houston, Texas, 86.4% of hepatic injuries were secondary to penetrating wounds.[8] In contrast, 60% of hepatic injuries were secondary to blunt trauma in a series from the University of California at Irvine. In a series from Canada 141 to 145 patients (97%) were treated with liver trauma that was secondary to blunt injury.[1]

Spontaneous rupture of the liver during pregnancy can occur and apparently represents extreme vascular complication of toxemia pregnancy. The mortality rate has been generally attributed to uncontrolled hemorrhage. Hepatic dysfunction may proceed to hepatic necrosis and multiple organ system failure even after successful hemostasis of the liver has been activated. Ligation of the hepatic artery, which has been employed in treatment of liver injury by other causes, may contribute to ischemia and necrosis of the liver in this situation and therefore should be avoided.[9] Patients undergoing routine cardiac surgical procedures can rarely incur liver injury during operation.[10]

Diagnosis of Liver Injury Trauma

The majority of deaths from blunt liver trauma that occur soon after injury are caused by large stellate fractures that involve the posterior lateral aspect of the right lobe of the liver. These injuries can extend into the hepatic veins. In the presence of hypotension, evisceration, or a rigid abdomen, the patient should be operated on immediately. When liver injury is suspected and the patient is stable, peritoneal lavage or computed tomographic (CT) scan followed by prompt laparotomy for definitive treatment gives the best chance for early and successful management of major hepatic injury. In some selected cases blunt hepatic injury is being managed nonoperatively. This new approach will be discussed later in the chapter.

Results of Liver Injury

Liver laceration with exsanguination is the commonest intraabdominal injury resulting in mortality. In 1,000 patients with hepatic injuries reported from Baylor College of Medicine, hepatic injuries were divided into those that were amenable to simple hepatorrhaphy, topical hemostatic agents, or drainage, and those requiring major surgical intervention. Of the 1,000 patients, 881 were satisfactorily treated with minor surgical procedure and only 7.3% died. Extensive hepatorrhaphy, hepatotomy with ligation of bleeding vessels, resection and debridement, resection with selective hepatic artery ligation, or perihepatic packing was required in 119 patients (11.9%); 30 (25%) of these patients died. Uncomplicated recovery occurred in 798 of the 918 patients surviving longer than 48 hours (87%). In the remaining 13% of patients intraabdominal abscess formation was the most common late complication, occurring in 32 of 918 (3.5%). Mortality overall was 10.5% with 78% of all deaths occurring in the perioperative period from shock or hemorrhage.[8]

In 179 patients with hepatic injury from blunt trauma treated at the Maryland Institute for Emergency Medical Services, a mortality rate of 35% was reported.[11] As in the Baylor series, patients with simpler forms of injuries were easily treated with good results. Major injuries involving lobar destruction and vena caval injury were associated with higher mortality and morbidity. Hepatic artery ligation was successful in only seven of 17 cases. Hepatic lobectomy was successful in three of 16 and atrial caval shunting was successful in both patients in whom it was attempted. Twenty-six percent of the deaths after hepatic injury occurred in patients with severe head injury. As in other series, hemorrhage was the most frequent cause of early death (49%) in patients dying of liver injury. Late infection contributed to the death of 27 patients; eight of these 27 infections were related to the hepatic injury.

In 58 patients with hepatic injury treated by The Department of Surgery, University of Goteborg, Sweden, blunt trauma occurred in 30 patients (52%), stab wounds in 26 (45%), and gunshot wounds in 2 (3%). In 45 patients (78%), the injury could be managed by simple methods such as suturing or minimal debridement and suture ligation. Hepatic lobectomy was performed in five patients (9%).[12] Overall mortality rate in this series was 19%. The mortality from the hepatic injury itself was 5%. The mortality rate after blunt trauma was 30%; after stab wounds the mortality was only 4%. The mortality rate was much higher in patients with multiple injuries and after more severe hepatic injuries, as might be expected. The Swedish experience with liver injury, unlike the United States, includes almost no gunshot wounds because of the limits of handgun availability.

A series from San Francisco General Hospital (1976 to 1981) included 143 patients with hepatic injury, 42% due to blunt trauma, 32% due to stab wounds, and 26% from gunshot wounds. This series also demonstrates that most patients with hepatic injury are easily treated, i.e., 72% simple repair. Infection, and pulmonary problems were the most common postoperative complications in this series. The overall morbidity was 38%. Associated injuries occurred in 34% of patients and the overall mortality was low at 9%. Mortality for blunt trauma was 14%, 8% for gunshot wounds, and 2.8% for stab wounds. The majority of deaths (58%) occurred in the perioperative period, with the primary cause being exsanguinating hemorrhage. Multiple organ system failure accounted for most of the late postoperative deaths.[13]

The group from Charity Hospital in New Orleans described 546 patients with hepatic injury. Seventy-six had blunt injury, 306 had gunshot wounds, and 162 had stab wounds. As in other series, stab wounds were associated with the lowest mortality (0.6%), with gunshot wounds (12%) and blunt injuries (28%) associated with higher mortality rates.[14]

Of 233 hepatic injuries reported from the University of Texas Health Sciences Center, San Antonio, the mortality rate was 11%. Death was due to either uncontrollable intraoperative hemorrhage or postoperative complications from mutliple organ system failure.[15]

Techniques of Operative Management

Successful operative management of severe liver injury requires a well prepared and skilled operative team, prompt resuscitation, ready availability of blood products, and an intensive care unit team. Patients are operated on because of physical signs, hemoperitoneum, abnormal hepatic scintigrams, arteriograms, or CT scans. The abdomen is entered through a generous midline incision. If brisk bleeding is immediately encountered, manual compression and packing are applied while transfusion and resuscitation are intensified. Exploration assesses the nature of the injury. The Foramen of Winslow is immediately identified and the structures of the portal triad occluded by finger pressure, vascular clamp, or rubber vascular slings (Pringle maneuver). The subdiaphragmatic area is examined for hepatic vein bleeding. If bleeding is from that area or exposure suboptimal, the midline incision is extended using a midline sternotomy to expose the subdiaphragmatic area and allow access to the heart in the event that atriocaval shunting is required. With exposure improved, the cruciate ligaments can be divided allowing bimanual compression of the right lobe, which is sometimes aided by use of a Penrose drain as a tourniquet. If the left lobe is injured, a similar maneuver can be performed by dividing the triangular ligament.

Most hepatic injuries are satisfactorily managed by manual compression and suture ligation of the bleeding points. More severe injuries are usually managed by hepatotomy and suture ligation. Anatomic resection, packing of the damaged liver, or control of the hepatic venous injury by an atriocaval shunt are infrequently necessary. After the Pringle maneuver is performed, differential occlusion to the hepatic artery and portal vein may reveal a pure arterial source for bleeding deep within the hepatic parenchyma. In this event, the right or left hepatic artery is dissected as close to the bleeding point as possible and ligated.

For major injury to the liver, hepatotomy and ligation of bleeding vessels are the usual and preferred methods of operative management. This technique exposes the laceration widely (hepatotomy), allowing direct visualization and ligation of the bleeding vessels.

Occlusion of the porta hepatis (Pringle maneuver) is a valuable adjunct for management of injuries of this magnitude. Forty-seven of 75 injuries in a series from Bellevue required in-flow occlusion for periods of up to 60 minutes, with a mean occlusion time of 30 minutes. Ischemic time exceeded 20 minutes in 70%, 30 minutes in 40%, and 60 minutes in 7%. While there is periodic concern as to the length of time that the Pringle maneuver can be employed, in practice little demonstrated harm comes from occlusion times that do not exceed 20 minutes. Our practice is to reperfuse and then reocclude the liver at 20-minute intervals.[16]

Once hemorrhage is controlled, the injury can be evaluated completely and specific operative techniques employed. Liver injuries are frequently formidable in appearance. However, morbidity and mortality are the result of hemorrhage, devitalized tissue, or injury to bile ducts.

In a study of 51 patients with major blunt hepatic trauma, 29 (56.8%) survived. Nine patients required insertion of atriocaval shunt because of uncontrollable hemorrhage due to disruption to hepatic veins. Eight of these nine patients sustained injury to the hepatic veins or retrohepatic vena cava. Four of these patients were long-term survivors.[17]

Routine drainage of liver wounds has been studied and prompted a randomized trial of drainage with a Penrose drain vs. no drain in patients having emergency laparotomy for trauma. Patients with definite bile leaks have an absolute indication for placement of a drain and were excluded from this study. Of 167 patients studied, six had obligatory drainage because of an obvious bile leak.[18] Among the remaining 161 there were no significant differences as to demographics, mode of injury, volume of blood lost, volume of blood used for resuscitation, incidence or severity of shock, number or types of associated injuries, or magnitude of liver wound between 78 allocated to drainage and 83 left without a drain. Resultant mortality, duration of hospitalization, incidence of wound and/or intraabdominal infection, and likelihood of subsequent bile fistula were not different. These as well as other data suggest the routine use of drain in hepatic injury is unnecessary and should be used *only* if bile leakage is present. When a drain is required, a closed suction drain, not a Penrose drain, is the drain type of choice.

At one time, routine use of T-tube drainage of the common bile was performed in patients with liver injury. In a prospective randomized double-blind study, Lucas and Wait[19] demonstrated higher complications and lack of usefulness of routine common bile duct drainage. Today, common bile duct drainage is performed only for injuries to the bile duct.

Moore et al. reported a series of 319 hepatic injuries identified at laparotomy. Fifty-three patients (17%) sustained major hepatic trauma necessitating complex operative intervention, including lobectomy in 21, segmentectomy in 6, selective hepatic artery ligation in 3, and temporary packing in 7. The study demonstrated a progressive shift toward nonresectional treatment. Lobectomy for major injuries had a mortality rate of 64%, while alternative procedures such as hepatotomy and ligation, selective hepatic artery ligation, and packing had a lower mortality rate from hemorrhage without an increase in delayed death from sepsis. Hepatotomy to gain access to the retrohepatic vena cava laceration was also employed.[20] Similar management and results have been reported from other institutions.[14]

Packing

Packing of the injured liver is an effective method of temporary hemostasis. Packing as a means of hemostasis beyond the initial emergency operation remains controversial. Liver packing and planned reoperation are being used for the management of hemorrhage from severe hepatic injury without incurring increased morbidity or mortality in patients whose injuries preclude immediate definitive correction.[21] This technique is useful for the experienced trauma surgeon to arrest hemorrhage and gain hemodynamic stability before attempting definitive repair. It may also be usefully employed by surgeons at smaller hospitals prior to transfer of the patient to a major trauma center. This can avoid attempts at major hepatic surgery in small poorly equipped hospitals with inadequate capabilities for resuscitation and management. If packing is left for less than 24 to 48 hours, complications such as intraabdominal abscess formation are uncommon.[22–25]

Hepatic Arterial Ligation

Hepatic artery compression or ligation is useful for management of hepatic trauma. In one series, 178 patients who sustained hepatic injuries were treated with selective hepatic arterial ligation. Only two of 20 early perioperative deaths were secondary to hemorrhage. The overall mortality was 20%. Sepsis was the most frequent postoperative complication after hepatic injury.[25] If ligation of the hepatic artery or its branches is employed, cholecystectomy is required if the right hepatic or common hepatic artery is occluded to prevent complications from ischemia in the gallbladder.

Hepatic Resection for Hepatic Trauma

Anatomic resection for liver injury is seldom necessary. Debridement of devitalized tissue may be necessary and sometimes approaches the magnitude of resection involved in anatomical resections.[26]

Fifty-eight hepatic resections were performed at Vanderbilt University between 1968 and 1978 for severe hepatic trauma. Anatomic lobectomies were done on 32 of the trauma cases; of the 42 patients who survived 17 had complications postoperatively, five patients died of exsanguination and another 11 patients died between days 1 and 42 after operation, and four died within two days of cardiovascular collapse. Despite increasing severity of injury, mortality all of trauma victims had improved from 33% to 28%, with a mortality of 24% in the latter half of the series.[27]

Hemostatic Agents

The efficacy of a variety of hemostatic agents, including gelatin foam, oxidized regenerated cellulose, collagen fleece, and microcrystalline collagen as hemostatic agents has been tested in animals with hepatic injury. Microcrystalline collagen and collagen fleece were found to be more effective in control of hematemesis in animal models of hepatic injury, suggesting that they may be the agent of choice in clinical practice as well.[28]

Nonoperative Treatment of Hepatic Trauma

Nonoperative management is occasionally a reasonable mode of management of a selected groups of patients with hepatic injury.[22]

The Hospital for Sick Children in Toronto has championed nonoperative management of both liver and splenic injuries.[29, 30] Thirty-two children were treated for blunt hepatic trauma. Twenty-three injuries were secondary to motor vehicle accidents, and 23 patients had other associated injuries. The hepatic injury was treated surgically in 18 patients. Urgent surgery for massive bleeding was required in seven; eight underwent laparotomy for continued bleeding after initial stabilization, two underwent laparotomy for marked abdominal tenderness and one for an expanding hematoma. Seven patients died (7/18 or 38%), five from uncontrollable bleeding and two from associated severe head injury; 11 survivors did well. The only postoperative complications were two wound infections. Fourteen patients were managed nonoperatively. Five of these patients required blood transfusion, and the mean volume of transfusion was 30 ml/kg, over one third of the blood volume. The hospital course in all cases was uneventful and there were no late complications. Follow-up liver scan obtained in 11 patients showed resolution of the injury in all patients. They concluded that laparotomy is necessary for hepatic injury when associated with continuous or massive bleeding. They concluded that hemodynamically stable patients can be managed nonoperatively even when blood transfusion requirements are significant.[29]

Rainbow Babies and Childrens Hospital in Cleveland, Ohio, described 12 patients during four years with hepatic trauma. Three underwent emergency ceiliotomy because of severity of their injuries, and nine had significant liver injuries that were managed nonoperatively. Hepatic injury was diagnosed and the severity defined by ultrasound, radionuclide study, or CT scan. The stable patients were initially admitted to the intensive care unit (ICU) and on transfer to the ward maintained on restricted activity. Seven of the nine children received transfusions. Initial liver enzymes were elevated, but they returned to normal within seven days. In the hospital and after discharge, imaging techniques documented healing of the hepatic injuries in every case. Eight children were well at three months to four years postoperatively. Only one of the nine nonoperatively managed patients died and this death was secondary to head injury. To date there have been no complications in this series.[11]

Although nonoperative therapy is accepted frequently for renal and for splenic injuries in children, this treatment is now being considered more often in blunt hepatic injury. Surgical repair of traumatized liver has been the generally accepted standard of care for such injuries in the past. The State University of New York at Buffalo presented a report of 17 children between the ages of 2 and 13 with hepatic trauma who were managed nonoperatively. Patients were selected for nonoperative management based on clinical criteria of hemodynamic stability and CT scan findings. Seventeen patients with hepatic trauma identified by CT all responded to conservative resuscitation. The children remained stable and required only a limited number of transfusions. No immediate surgical intervention was necessary for isolated hepatic injuries, however, one patient required exploration due to an associated renal pedicle avulsion. One child required exploration on the fourth postinjury day because of a suspected infected hemotoma. The remaining 15 injuries resolved without operation. Healing was documented on follow-up CT scans. The mean time required for resolution was four months. One child developed late subhepatic hematoma that resolved without drainage. The progress of healing of hepatic injuries was observed by serial CT scans. The liver injury progressed through stages of coalescence, resorption, and remodeling prior to final healing. This group concluded that by utilizing proper patient selection many blunt liver injuries can be managed nonoperatively.

A nonoperative approach to blunt liver trauma has been reported from the University of Capetown, South Africa. Nineteen of 23 children with blunt hepatic injury were treated nonoperatively. Management consisted of observation in the ICU, repeated physical examination, frequent evaluation of hematocrit level, and specialized x-ray evaluation, in particular ultrasonography with bed rest. Nineteen patients all remained stable, required no surgical intervention, and showed resolution of hepatic injuries with no early or delayed complications. Ultrasonography, although not as reliable as CT scan or liver isotopes scan for identification of hepatic trauma, provides a useful method for follow-up. The presence of an isolated hepatic injury is thought to be an insufficient indication for surgery by this group, and indeed they as well as others have documented that, particularly in the pediatric age group, minor liver injuries and some moderate liver injuries can be managed by observation.[31]

Less favorable reports of nonoperative management of hepatic trauma have appeared from the Children's Hospital National Medical Center, Washington, D.C. They reported a study of patients from March 7, 1978, to July 1983 in which seven children with hepatic injury were managed without surgery. Four patients required greater than 50% total blood volume replacement, while the mean packed blood cell transfusion was 28 ml/kg, over one third of the blood volume of the patient. Eight major complications developed in five patients. Hospitalization averaged 23 days with no deaths. This morbidity rate and length of hospitalization are much greater than those described in earlier reports and suggest that observation of anything beyond the most minor of hepatic injuries may be questionable.[32]

Criteria for nonoperative management of splenic and hepatic injuries have been evolving over the last several years. The accumulated experience to date provides some support that this more selective therapeutic approach may result in lower morbidity and mortality for children sustaining certain types of splenic or hepatic injuries.

Interventional Radiology

With the rise in nonoperative management to hepatic injuries there is also a rise in consideration for interventional radiology. As an adjunctive management technique for patients with liver injury, interventional radiology is defined as catheter placement under radiologic guidance and is a technique that is occasionally useful in hepatic trauma, particularly in the management of hemorrhage, infection with hepatic abscess, and hemobilia. Twenty procedures in 17 patients were reviewed in one series. All patients with hemorrhage from vascular lesions and intraabdominal fluid collections were successfully treated without mortality or substantial morbidity. Interventional radiology should be considered as a major important adjunct to the management of patients with liver injury, particularly those with complications following operation.[33]

Selective hepatic artery embolization is useful in controlling hemorrhage from hepatic injury. In two patients described from the Department of Radiology, George Washington University Medical Center, Washington, D.C., selective arteriography identified the hemorrhaging artery in both cases.[34] Transcatheter embolization successfully stopped hemorrhage acutely, and in both patients no further blood replacement was required. Both patients avoided surgery and both were discharged home. In another article from the University of Alabama Medical Center, the right hepatic artery in a patient with traumatic liver injury was embolized, which stopped an otherwise uncontrollable hemorrhage. Interventional radiology has also been documented to be of assistance after two failed laparotomies in a report from South Africa in which intraarterial embolization with gel foam controlled bleeding from a false aneurysm.

In a review of 15 patients with complications after blunt trauma, x-ray evaluation documented that in seven of 15, what was thought to be relatively minor injury was misdiagnosed and there was a large intrahepatic defect.[35] Newer radiographic techniques frequently can be of value in such cases.

Pyogenic liver abscess is a common complication after a major hepatic injury. Physicians should be aware of this and remain alert for the signs of the development of hepatic abscesses in patients who have had major blunt trauma. Treatment is with a combination of intravenous antibiotics and percutaneous drainage placed under fluoroscopic guidance.

Major hepatic injury with damage to vessels and moderate- to major-sized bile ducts can lead to hemobilia, that is, blood that leaves the vascular space and enters the biliary system. Hemobilia can cause pain and present as gastrointestinal tract bleeding or sepsis. Treatment of hemobilia is approached in a nonsurgical manner, with x-ray diagnosis and intraarterial embolization. Embolization techniques are the method of choice in the management of hepatic trauma with delayed hemorrhage or hemobilia.[36]

Pseudoaneurysm formation is another complication of blunt hepatic trauma. The definitive diagnostic test for this is hepatic angiography. Contrast-enhanced CT scanning can also be used as a preliminary test to differentiate between abscess and other postinjury complications.

Hepatic trauma, either penetrating or blunt, may lead to vascular malformations, usually pseudoaneurysm of hepatic artery and sometimes arteriovenus fistula. The true incidence of such traumatic lesions is unknown,[37] but may be higher than previously realized and also can occasionally regress spontaneously. Treatment of arteriovenous malformations as in hemobilia can be managed by arterial catheterization and embolization, and this should be a standard therapeutic measure for lesions. This is due to low morbidity and good precision in limiting the area of devascularization to that desired, as well as a higher success rate reported with this technique.

Summary

Hepatic trauma is a common form of abdominal injury. Although the majority of hepatic injuries are minor and require little or no treatment, many hepatic injuries are major and lethal if not managed appropriately. Good management of these patients requires a thorough understanding of hepatic anatomy and of the options available for surgical management of hepatic injuries. These options include simple suture, hepatotomy to expose the bleeding vessels and ligation, hepatic artery ligation, packing of hepatic injuries, and, rarely, formal anatomic lobectomy and atriocaval shunting. The trauma surgeon must be familiar with these types of management and be able to apply them in appropriate situations. Nonoperative management is now being reported more commonly and it may be appropriate in a selected group of patients. While the most common cause of death after hepatic injury is from exsanguination occurring early after injury, patients with major hepatic injury remain at risk for a variety of complications after the initial injury. These include hepatic abscess, hemobilia, pseudoaneurysm, and arteriovenous malformations that lead to bleeding. All of these are best treated by CT scan and interventional radiologic techniques. A determined and committed approach to these injured patients can significantly decrease the mortality of these injuries.

References

1. Hanna SS, Maheshwari Y, Harrison AW, et al: Blunt liver trauma at the Sunnybrook Regional Trauma Unit. *Can J Surg* 1985; 28(3):220–223.
2. Elerding SC, Moore EE Jr: Recent experience with trauma of the liver. *Surg Gynecol Obstet* 1980; 150(b):853–855.
3. Broom J, Miller JD: Nutritional and metabolic support following acute hepatic trauma. *Scott Med J* 1986; 31(4):251–252.
4. Hasselgren PO, Jagenburg R, Karlstrom L, et al: Changes of protein metabolism in liver and skeletal muscle following trauma complicated by sepsis. *J Trauma* 1984; 24(3):224–228.
5. Hashmonai M, Schramek A, Kam I, et al: Treatment of liver trauma in the Lebanon War, 1982. *Isr J Med Sci* 1984; 20(4):327–329.
6. Bass EM, Crosier JH: Percutaneous control of post-traumatic hepatic hemorrhage by gelfoam embolization. *J Trauma* 1977; 17(1):61–63.
7. Smulewicz JJ, Tafreshi MM: Hematoma of the liver due to birth trauma. *J Natl Med Assoc* 1975; 67(3):214–215.
8. Feliciano DV, Mattox KL, Jordan GL Jr, et al: Management of 1000 consecutive cases of hepatic trauma (1979–1984). *Ann Surg* 1986; 204(4):438–445.
9. Aziz S, Merrell RC, Collins JA: Spontaneous hepatic hemorrhage during pregnancy. *Am J Surg* 1983; 146(5):680–682.
10. Eugene J, Ott RA, Stemmer EA: Hepatic trauma during cardiac surgery. *J Cardiovasc Surg (Torino)* 1986; 27(1):100–102.
11. Brotman S, Oliver G, Oster-Granite ML, et al: The treatment of 179 blunt trauma-induced liver injuries in a statewide trauma center. *Am Surg* 1984; 50(11):603–608.
12. Hasselgren PO, Almersjo O, Gustavsson B, et al: Trauma to the liver during a ten-year period: With special reference to morbidity and mortality after blunt trauma and stab wounds. *Acta Chir Scand* 1981; 147(6):387–393.

13. Carmona RH, Lim RC Jr, Clark GC: Morbidity and mortality in hepatic trauma: A 5 year study. *Am J Surg* 1982; 144(1):88–94.
14. Levin A, Gover P, Nance FC: Surgical restraint in the management of hepatic injury: A review of Charity Hospital Experience. *J Trauma* 1978; 18(6):399–404.
15. McInnis WD, Richardson JD, Aust JB: Hepatic trauma: Pitfalls in management. *Arch Surg* 1977; 112(2):157–161.
16. Pachter HL, Spencer FC, Hofstetter SR, et al: Experience with the finger fracture technique to achieve intra-hepatic hemostasis in 75 patients with severe injuries of the liver. *Ann Surg* 1983; 197(6):771–778.
17. Rovito PF: Atrial caval shunting in blunt hepatic vascular injury. *Ann Surg* 1987; 205(3):318–321.
18. Mullens RJ, Stone HH, Dunlop WE, et al: Hepatic trauma: Evaluation of routine drainage. *South Med J* 1985; 78(3):259–261.
19. Lucas CE, Wait AJ: Analysis of randomized biliary drainage for liver trauma in 189 patients. *J Trauma* 1972; 12:925–930.
20. Moore FA, Moore EE, Seagraves A: Nonresectional management of major hepatic trauma: An evolving concept. *Am J Surg* 1985; 150(6):725–729.
21. Carmona RH, Peck DZ, Lim RC Jr: The role of packing and planned reoperation in severe hepatic trauma. *J Trauma* 1984; 24(9):779–784.
22. Little JM, Fernandes A, Tait N: Liver trauma. *Aust NZ J Surg* 1986; 56(8):613–619.
23. Krause R, Langenberg CJ, van der Starre PJ: Changes of protein metabolism in liver and skeletal muscle following trauma complicated by sepsis (letter). *J Trauma* 1985; 25(3):276–277.
24. Ivatury RR, Nallathambi M, Gunduz Y, et al: Liver packing of uncontrolled hemorrhage: A reappraisal. *J Trauma* 1986; 26(8):744–753.
25. Flint LM, Mays ET, Aaron WS, et al: Selectivity in the management of hepatic trauma. *Ann Surg* 1977; 185(6):613–618.
26. Balasegaram M, Joishy SK: Hepatic resection: The logical approach to surgical management of major trauma to the liver. *Am J Surg* 1981; 142(5):580–583.
27. Lutzker LG, Chun KJ: Radionuclide imaging in the nonsurgical treatment of liver and spleen trauma. *J Trauma* 1981; 21(5):382–387.
28. Zoucas E, Goransson G, Bengmark S: Comparative evaluation of local hemostatic agents in experimental liver trauma: A study in the rat. *J Surg Res* 1984; 37(2):145–150.
29. Giacomantonio M, Filler RM, Rich RH: Blunt hepatic trauma in children: Experience with operative and nonoperative management. *J Pediatr Surg* 1984; 19(5):519–522.
30. Suson EM, Klotz D Jr, Kottmeier PK: Liver trauma in children. *J Pediatr Surg* 1975; 10(3):411–417.
31. Moore EE: Edgar J. Poth Lecture: Critical decisions in the managment of hepatic trauma. *Am J Surg* 1984; 148(6):712–716.
32. Bass BL, Eichelberger MR, Schisgall R, et al: Hazards of nonoperative therapy of hepatic injury in children. *J Trauma* 1984; 24(11):978–982.
33. Sclafani SJ, Shaftan GW, McAuley J, et al: Interventional radiology in the management of hepatic trauma. *J Trauma* 1984; 24(3):256–262.
34. Rubin BE, Katzen BT: Selective hepatic artery embolization to control massive hepatic hemorrhage after trauma. *AJR* 1977; 129(2):253–256.
35. Lawrence D, Dawson JL: The secondary management of complicated liver injuries. *Ann R Coll Surg Engl* 1982; 64(3):186–190.

36. Shenoy SS, Bergsland, J, Cerra FB: Arterial embolization for traumatic hemobilia with hepatoportal fistula. *Cardiovasc Intervent Radiol* 1981; 4(3):206–208.
37. Schmidt B, Bhatt GM, Abo MN: Management of post-traumatic vascular malformations of the liver by catheter embolization. *Am J Surg* 1980; 140(2):332–335.

Thyroid Carcinoma

Jeffrey B. Kramer, M.D.

Resident, Department of Surgery, Washington University School of Medicine, St. Louis, Missouri

Samuel A. Wells, Jr., M.D.

Professor and Chairman, Department of Surgery, Washington University School of Medicine, St. Louis, Missouri

Despite the abundant literature devoted to thyroid neoplasia, there is still much controversy regarding its management. The extreme variability in the biologic aggressiveness of the various thyroid neoplasms has made the establishment of general therapeutic guidelines difficult. The problems most frequently faced by the surgeon are: (1) What constitutes the appropriate evaluation of a thyroid mass? (2) When is operation indicated? (3) What should be the extent of thyroid resection? (4) How should patients be followed and treated if the malignancy recurs? The reason that proper therapy for thyroid malignancies (especially papillary and follicular neoplasms) is not clear is because there have never been clinical trials designed such that patients are staged, then prospectively randomized to various treatment arms, and ultimately followed to death or disease recurrence. Also, since most thyroid malignancies (excepting anaplastic carcinomas) have a favorable prognosis, even if metastatic disease is present, 20 or 30 years follow-up would be required to show meaningful conclusions.

Incidence and Etiology

Carcinoma of the thyroid gland occurs relatively infrequently and constitutes 1% of all malignancies.[1] In the United States there are approximately 10,000 new cases and 1,000 deaths per year.[2, 3] The incidence of thyroid neoplasia at autopsy, especially small, well-differentiated "occult" carcinomas,[4, 5] reflects the usually indolent clinical course of well-differentiated carcinomas. Thyroid carcinoma occurs in a female to male ratio of 2.5 to 1,[6] although there has recently been an increasing incidence in men.[7] In older patients the gender distribution is more equal.[8] The infrequency of clinically apparent thyroid carcinoma contrasts sharply with the prevalence of thyroid nodules, which are present in 1% to 7% of the general population upon neck examination,[9] and in up to 50% of autopsy cases.[10] The

Adv Surg 22:195–224, 1989

0065-3411/89/22-195–224-$04.00

differentiation of malignant from benign nodules is a major challenge for the clinician.

Several factors have been associated with an enhanced propensity toward the development of thyroid malignancy. The major risk factor is the exposure of the head and neck to external beam irradiation during childhood or adolescence.[11] This association was first reported in 1950 by Duffy and Fitzgerald in nine children.[12] Since that time, retrospective reviews and experimental studies have demonstrated an increased incidence of carcinogenesis in patients receiving 500 to 2,000 rad for a variety of conditions,[11] most commonly thymic hypertrophy, tonsillitis, acne vulgaris, and lymphogenous malignancies. The prevalence of clinical thyroid carcinoma in irradiated individuals has been estimated to be 12%,[13] though in irradiated patients undergoing total thyroidectomy for nodular disease, the pathologic incidence of cancer has been reported to be 36% to 59%.[14] Malignancies that occur in patients following x-ray exposure are almost always well-differentiated papillary carcinomas and are usually multicentric.[11, 14, 15] They also metastasize frequently to cervical lymph nodes (up to 50% at the time of initial presentation), and tend to recur frequently, especially if less than total thyroidectomy has been performed.[11, 16] The relatively aggressive behavior that these neoplasms exhibit justifies careful systematic screening of patients with prior irradiation of the head and neck and, if malignancy is detected, an aggressive surgical approach—i.e., total or near-total thyroidectomy.[11, 14, 15] According to one large series of 5,266 irradiated patients,[17] the median latency of the development of cancer is 20.2 years, while delays of up to 40 years[15] have been reported, indicating that careful long-term follow-up is necessary for these individuals. It appears that neither external radiation over 3,000 rad[11] nor exposure to ^{131}I administered for the treatment of Graves' disease[18] predisposes toward the development of malignancy. In addition, individuals receiving radiation after the age of 18 years seem to have a minimally increased risk for the development of carcinoma subsequently.[9]

Another factor seemingly associated with thyroid neoplasia is dietary intake of iodine.[9] In areas of endemic goiter, where deficiency of iodine intake is common, subjects have had higher than expected incidences of follicular carcinoma, whereas papillary lesions have been found to be more prevalent in regions of relatively high iodine intake. The precise mechanism influencing these occurrences is not known, although it has been postulated that elevation of serum thyroid-stimulating hormone (TSH) levels due to iodine deficiency is a possible factor in the genesis of follicular neoplasms.

Other conditions affecting the thyroid gland have also been considered as predisposing to thyroid malignancy. Occult well-differentiated thyroid carcinomas are found in 0.5 to 8.7% of specimens resected in patients with Graves' disease.[19] At particular risk are patients who have also received low-dose external irradiation during childhood or adolescence, since they have even a higher incidence of concurrent malignancy.[18] Toxic multinodular goiter has also been associated with an increased incidence of thyroid carcinoma, occurring in up to 3% of cases.[18] This has led to the hypothesis that either TSH or HTSI (human thyroid-stimulating immunoglobulin) may in some fashion promote the development of thyroid malignancy, since increased plasma concentrations of these substances have been noted in patients with nodular goiter and Graves' disease, respectively. Hashimoto's thyroiditis[20, 21] is another condition that has been linked to the development of both well-differentiated and poorly differentiated thyroid carcinoma. The incidence of thyroid malignancy in patients with Hashimoto's thyroiditis has varied from 5 to 22.5%[20, 21] in different series. It has been speculated that the tumor might arise from the regenerating epithelium, which occurs with Hashimoto's disease. Conversely, it has also been suggested that the dense inflammatory response is instead secondary to the malignant process.

Thyroid malignancy seems to have a better prognosis when associated with Hashimoto's thyroiditis than without it,[21] thus indicating that an immune response to the tumor may indeed take place and retard growth of the neoplasm. In addition, patients with Hashimoto's thyroiditis who also have a past history of radiation exposure do not have a higher risk of carcinoma than do those without such exposure, although the incidence of bilaterality may be somewhat greater in the former group.[20]

Finally, two other associations implicate hormonal responsiveness as being of importance in the recurrence and subsequent behavior of these neoplasms. Rosen and Walfish[22] reported a 43% incidence of carcinoma in 30 pregnant patients evaluated for thyroid nodules, and they suggested that variations in estrogen or placental hormones may be responsible for the growth of these tumors. Also, Cady and associates[8, 23] have shown that the prognosis of well-differentiated carcinoma is largely dependent on age, especially in women. Women 50 years of age and younger have a much better prognosis compared with older patients; Cady and coworkers postulated that alterations in plasma estrogen levels may be responsible for this difference. The fact that a difference in prognosis related to age also occurs in the male argues against the importance of this factor, however. Further definition of this phenomenon awaits the identification of the specific promoting factors involved in enhancing growth of this malignancy.

Pathologic Classification

Tumors of the thyroid gland may be either benign or malignant and, based on histology, fall into the classifications listed in Table 1. In addition, tumors can be clinically staged by the extent of disease[24, 25]: stage I—cancers confined to the thyroid gland, stage II—cancer involving regional nodes, stage III—cancer invading adjacent structures, and stage IV—distant metastases present.

TABLE 1.
Pathologic Classification of Thyroid Tumors

- Benign tumors
  - Follicular adenoma
  - Cyst
  - Teratoma
  - Hürthle cell tumor
  - Autoimmune thyroiditis
  - Colloid nodule
- Malignant tumors
  - Well-differentiated
    - Papillary carcinoma
    - Follicular carcinoma
    - Hürthle cell carcinoma
  - Poorly differentiated
    - Medullary carcinoma
    - Anaplastic carcinoma
  - Miscellaneous
    - Lymphoma
    - Teratoma
    - Squamous cell carcinoma
    - Fibrosarcoma
    - Metastatic carcinoma

The most common benign tumor of the thyroid is a follicular adenoma.[1, 26] The features of an adenoma include fibrous encapsulation, uniform histologic architecture, and compression of surrounding thyroid tissue. This is in contradistinction to multinodular goiters in which the nodules are not true neoplasms but rather consist pathologically of areas of thyroid hyperplasia intermixed with large dilated colloid-filled follicles with an absence of complete encapsulation. Follicular adenomas are collections of acinar cells that may or may not produce colloid and that are associated with a variable amount of interacinar stoma. These lesions may be premalignant and are difficult to differentiate from follicular carcinoma by needle biopsy.

Teratomas of the thyroid gland occur rarely and may be benign or malignant.[1, 27] These lesions represent vestigial remnants of embryonal tissue and contain a variety of cell types. Primary thyroid malignancies are generally divided into papillary, follicular, medullary, and anaplastic types. Rarely the thyroid gland is the site of other malignancies: squamous cell carcinoma, fibrosarcoma, and metastatic carcinoma. Primary lymphoma of the thyroid gland also occurs rarely.[25, 28, 29]

Clinical Presentation

Thyroid carcinoma, regardless of the histologic type, usually presents as a solitary asymptomatic neck mass. Occasionally, however, patients may complain of hoarseness, dysphagia, and dypsnea in association with a rapidly expanding, often painful, neck mass. Such symptoms result from the malignancy's invasion of adjacent structures in the neck and most often develop in association with anaplastic carcinoma. The presence of enlarged cervical nodes also suggests the presence of regional metastatic disease and may occur in the absence of palpable thyroid abnormalities.

Solitary thyroid nodules present a diagnostic challenge[9, 30, 31] and their management depends on the clinician's suspicion of malignancy based on history, physical examination, and results of various studies. The aim of the clinician is to identify patients at high risk for malignancy so that they may be treated surgically. Those patients in the "low-risk" group should be managed nonoperatively, but require careful follow-up. Several historical factors are critical in defining these groups, most important of which are age, sex, history of previous neck irradiation, family history of thyroid disease, and the presence of coexistent thyroid disorders. Although the incidence of malignancy within thyroid nodules increases with age, younger patients with solitary nodules have a high incidence of malignancy—from 45 to 75% in patients less than 15 years of age.[1] The appearance of new nodules in elderly patients also signifies a higher risk of malignancy, cited as approximately 45% in individuals over 65 years of age.[32] The peak ages of the onset of thyroid carcinoma are: papillary 25 to 35 years, follicular 40 to 55 years, medullary 45 years (sporadic form), and anaplastic more than 60 years.[1] Although females much more commonly present with thyroid nodules, the incidence of malignancy within the nodules is greater in males, making young males with such lesions at particularly high risk for cancer. A family history of thyroid malignancy is important, especially with medullary thyroid carcinoma, which may occur in three familial patterns, as will be described subsequently.

Various aspects of the physical examination also may raise suspicion that the nodule is malignant: the solitary nodule that is "cold" on radionuclide scan is more likely to be malignant than is a multinodular thyroid gland. Malignant nodules are usually firm and nontender, and the more aggressive malignancies may present with vocal cord paralysis, dysphagia, dyspnea, or lateral neck adenopathy. The examining physician should carefully question the patient about symptoms suggestive of malignancy, and on physical examination should search for signs of regional lymph node spread. Although the history and physical examination may indicate the need for operative intervention, several noninvasive and minimally invasive diagnostic tests should be considered first.

Diagnostic Evaluation

Thyroid Scan

The routine use of thyroid scintigraphy as the first step in screening patients with thyroid nodules has been criticized on a cost-effective basis[33, 34] and many authors believe that it should not be performed until the results of fine-needle aspiration (FNA) cytology are known. Either ^{123}I or ^{99m}Tc radioisotopes are used since both give much less radiation exposure than ^{131}I (2.8 rad exposure vs. 100 to 200 rad).[9] A malignant thyroid nodule presents as a cold or hypofunctional area, since malignant cells concentrate less isotope than the surrounding parenchyma. Malignant nodules are virtually never hot nor do they concentrate radionuclide as does normal tissue. Scanning of patients at high risk for the development of thyroid carcinoma seems justified—such as in patients with a history of childhood irradiation to the head and neck or those with a family history of medullary thyroid carcinoma. Radionuclide scintigraphy has also proven very important in the postoperative management of patients with differentiated thyroid cancers, specifically in screening for residual thyroid tissue in the neck or for metastatic disease.

Ultrasound

Ultrasonography has a very limited role in evaluation of thyroid nodules. Cystic lesions comprise 10 to 20% of solitary nodules,[1, 35] and most are benign. Ultrasonography has been shown to be 95 to 100% accurate[36] in distinguishing solid from cystic lesions. In two specific populations, pregnant women and pediatric patients, echography might be particularly helpful in avoiding the radiation exposure from radioisotope scanning. At present, fine needle aspiration with cytologic examination of the fluid has replaced ultrasonography as a routine diagnostic technique. A residual thyroid mass following aspiration or recurrence of an aspirated nodule are indications for surgical intervention.

Needle Biopsy and Aspiration

In the 1940s when surgery was recommended for nearly all solitary thyroid nodules, the incidence of carcinoma in the resected specimens was approximately 4.5%,[37] indicating the liberal use of thyroidectomy. Subsequently, techniques have been developed for obtaining thyroid tissue samples for cytologic analysis. With the development of techniques such as FNA and coarse-needle biopsy (CNB), the clinician can plan therapy with the confidence of having a tissue diagnosis.[38] Therefore, the performance of thyroidectomy has become much more selective, and in some series, the incidence of malignancy in resected nodules has risen to 60 to 70%.[38] Coarse-needle biopsy, described in 1930 by Martin and Ellis,[39] was pioneered at the Cleveland Clinic by Crile and associates. The technique[40, 41] involves the percutaneous insertion of a large-bore (Tru-cut or Vim Silverman) needle into the thyroid gland after administration of local anesthesia. In large series using this technique, 90% to 94% of biopsy specimens have been sufficient for pathologic diagnosis. Biopsies are very rarely false positive,[40] but the incidence of false negativity has been reported as high as 25%.[38] The major limitations of the procedure include (1) only lesions 2 cm or more in diameter are amenable to biopsy, (2) adequate sampling is greatly dependent on the expertise of the clinician, and (3) significant complications can occur, such as implantation of tumor along the biopsy tract (only one case reported in over 2,000 biopsies performed at the Cleveland Clinic),[42] hemorrhage requiring urgent exploration of the neck, and recurrent laryngeal nerve injury. Nevertheless, several proponents of the technique stress the importance of combining CNB with FNA, to provide greater sensitivity.[43]

Fine-needle aspiration biopsy cytology has been used in Sweden on over 20,000 patients since 1952[44] and constitutes a major advance in the evaluation of thyroid nodules. Performance of the aspiration is safe and relatively simple; using a 22- or 23-gauge needle with a specially-developed syringe holder,[44, 45] cells are aspirated from the nodule without the necessity for local anesthesia. A May-Grunwald-Giemsa stain[44, 45] is made and the specimen is evaluated microscopically. Several benign and malignant conditions can be differentiated from one another; however, experience with the technique, in both the performance of FNA and interpretation of the cytologic specimen, results in a higher diagnostic accuracy. Three of the four common thyroid malignancies (papillary carcinoma, medullary carcinoma, and anaplastic carcinoma) can be identified with high reliability by FNA cytology, although the differentiation of benign from malignant follicular lesions is difficult if not impossible by this technique, mandating surgical excision of these lesions. Several recent series[46–49] have reported excellent results using this technique, including a prospective trial by Boey and associates[43] examining 600 patients undergoing FNA, 482 of which were negative for malignancy. After a mean follow-up of 30.9 months, the false negative rate for FNA was only 2.1% and none of the subsequently discovered carcinomas proved to be advanced lesions. There was no false positive specimen in this group. When combined with CNB, which was performed in patients with solid nodules still palpable after FNA, the false-negative incidence fell to 1%.[43] Generally, the former technique has been proven equal to or superior to the latter, and because of its simplicity, ease of performance, and patient acceptance, it has become more widely utilized. Also, it can be performed repeatedly in cases in which the sample is inadequate or the diagnosis problematic.

A recently reported application of FNA, suggested by Backdahl and associates,[44] involves analysis of cytologic specimens for the nuclear DNA content of cells. These investigators have observed that malignant cells of low biologic aggressiveness exhibit either diploidy or tetraploidy, whereas highly malignant cells exhibit aneuploidy and are biologically aggressive. To date, this technique has not been useful in differentiating benign from malignant follicular neoplasms; however, it seems likely that information gained from the technique will have prognostic significance.

In evaluating patients with solitary thyroid nodules, the algorithm illustrated in Figure 1 is commonly followed by our group. Following a thorough history and physical examination, FNA should be performed. If a diagnosis of papillary or medullary carcinoma is made, then thyroidectomy is indicated. The treatment of patients with anaplastic carcinoma depends primarily on the cell type and partly on the philosophy of the clinician (see below). If a follicular neoplasm is diagnosed on FNA, then thyroid scintigraphy is indicated. If the lesion is "cold," it should be excised; however, if it is "hot" or "warm," the patient may be followed conservatively. In patients with cystic nodules, the lesion should be excised if the cytology proves malignant or if fluid reaccumulates. In the event of equivocal or nondiagnostic FNA results, either a trial of TSH suppression or re-biopsy is indicated, followed by thyroidectomy if there is no resolution at six months. Of course, this plan should be tempered by various patient-specific factors such as overall operative risk, suspicious signs of malignancy on physical examination, and the presence of risk factors for carcinoma, such as previous head and neck irradiation, positive family history for medullary thyroid carcinoma (MTC), or age less than 25 or greater than 60 years. Adherence to this algorithm should minimize the performance of unnecessary surgical procedures with a very minimal risk of delaying appropriate treatment in patients with early malignancy.

Thyroid Suppression

One approach to the management of patients presenting with either single or multiple thyroid nodules has been TSH suppression by the administration of L-thyroxine. Nodules should shrink when suppressed in this manner; however, the experience of some surgeons fails to support this. Thompson and associates[1] claim that less than 2% of solitary, noncystic nodules regress or disappear with thyroid suppression. If this modality is chosen, patients should undergo frequent (every six months) examinations to monitor changes in the size of the nodule. If complete regression of a solitary or dominant nodule does not occur, neck exploration is mandatory to rule out carcinoma.

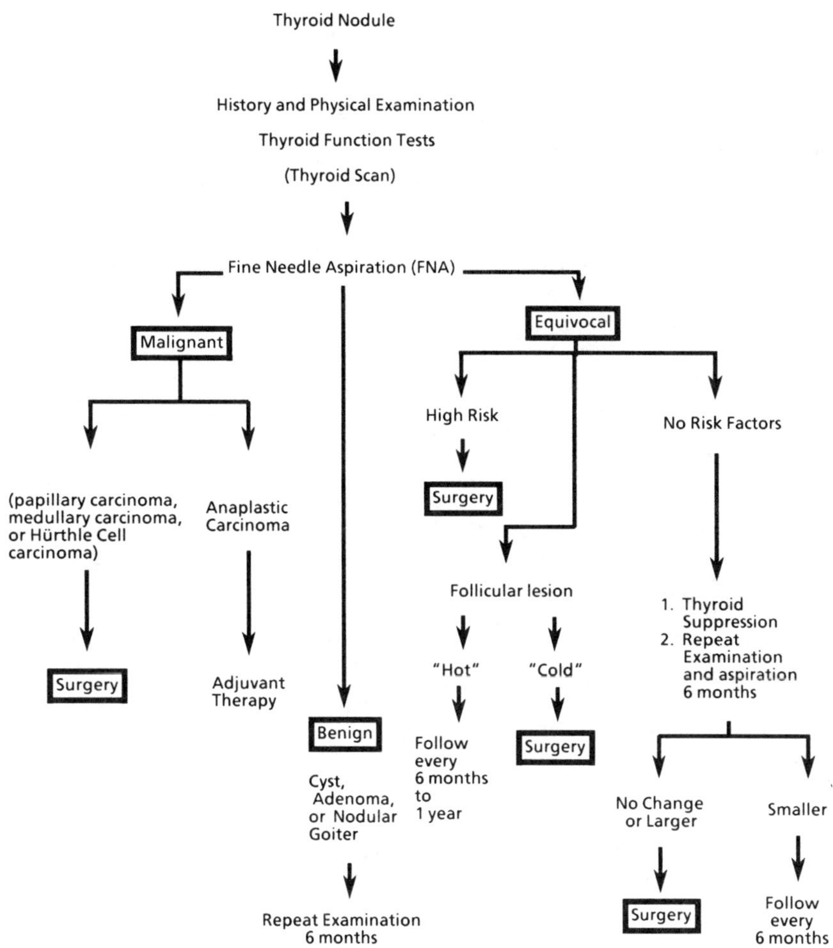

FIG 1.
Algorithm for evaluating patients with solitary thyroid nodules.

Management of Thyroid Carcinoma

Papillary Carcinoma

Papillary carcinoma represents the most prevalent type of thyroid carcinoma, constituting approximately 60% of thyroid malignancies. It is a tumor of some biologic variability, though in most instances it is not extremely aggressive. The net mortality over several decades is less than 10%,[50] and patients with diffuse metastases may live for years following appropriate adjuvant therapy. Although the peak incidence of papillary carcinoma occurs in early adulthood, it is frequently seen in the pediatric age group as well as in the elderly. Also, there is a female preponderance.

Histologically, papillary tumors are made up of branching, tree-like collections of stroma and epithelial cells and are almost always associated with follicular elements, colloid-filled follicles.[26] The papillary cells have been described as containing characteristic "ground glass" appearing nuclei.[1] In addition, psammoma bodies, or collections of necrotic, calcified clumped cells, are frequently seen in papillary lesions. Tumors that contain features of both papillary and follicular neoplasms generally behave as papillary carcinomas clinically, even if histologically they appear predominantly follicular. The only histologic feature of significance is the presence of so-called "tall cells" within the tumor, which allegedly portends a much more aggressive clinical course.[1]

Prognosis

Several factors have been mentioned as important prognostic indicators in papillary carcinoma. One factor of importance is the extent and size of the tumor; generally they may be divided into occult, intrathyroidal, and extrathyroidal lesions. Woolner and associates,[51] in a review of 509 cases of papillary thyroid carcinoma seen at the Mayo Clinic from 1926–1955, noted that 29% were occult, 53% were intrathyroidal, and 11% were extrathyroidal (7% were inoperable and biopsied only). Occult carcinomas (those less than 1.5 cm in diameter) are usually found incidentally. Several autopsy series have demonstrated a high prevalence of occult cancers in routine thyroid specimens. For instance, Sampson[5] reported a rate of 5.7% in Olmstead County, Minnesota, while a 13% prevalence of "minimal thyroid cancer" (< 1 cm diameter) was noted in 100 consecutive routine autopsies performed at the University of Michigan.[4] There also appears to be a differential geographic distribution of these occult lesions, the highest rate being reported in Japan (28%).[5] There are not similar differences in the prevalence of clinically evident cancers. This has led to the postulate that carcinogenic agents and factors that *promote* tumor growth may be quite distinct and vary in their prevalence. Neither are occult lesions necessarily confined to the thyroid gland. In a Mayo Clinic review[52] of 137 patients, lesions were bilateral in 7% and metastatic to the cervical lymph nodes at the time of presentation in 40%. Intrathyroidal lesions were those larger than 1.5 cm, but still contained within the thyroid capsule, whereas extrathyroidal lesions had broken out of the thyroid capsule and invaded surrounding structures such as the trachea, esophagus, and soft tissues of the neck. Patients with occult and intrathyroidal papillary carcinoma had survival rates that paralleled life insurance survival curves, whereas patients with extrathyroidal lesions had an especially poor prognosis.

Another clinical feature that seems to alter prognosis in patients with papillary carcinoma is the age at diagnosis. Children and young adults have an excellent prognosis despite the fact that at least 40% have nodal metastases at the time of diagnosis.[1] Cady and associates[8, 23, 53] found that mortality rates were much higher in both men and women over 50 years of age. In the Lahey Clinic series,[53] the mortality increased from 2% (1/42) in patients under 20 years of age, to 34% (70/205) in patients greater than 50 years of age. This one factor seems to supersede all others in importance, including the histological tumor pattern and the extent of local disease. The presence of distant metastases, most commonly to bone or lungs, denotes an unfavorable prognosis, although age, to some extent, may mitigate this factor. Other factors clearly seem *not* to impact on survival. There appears to be no difference in survival, extent of local invasiveness, or metastatic potential based on gender,[50] although this has been debated.[1] As opposed to the majority of malignancies, the presence of regional lymph nodal metastases has no effect on survival,[1] although the rate of recurrence following initial therapy may be higher in patients with cervical metastases.

Treatment

The primary treatment for papillary carcinoma is surgical excision. The extent of resection, indications for regional lymph node dissection, and the postoperative follow-up of patients are the most controversial aspects of management. Because of the slow growth of these well-differentiated neoplasms and the overall good prognosis, recurrences can occur several years after thyroidectomy, thus follow-up for periods of 20 years or greater are critical for comparative evaluation of treatment modalities. Consequently, recommendations for therapy of well-differentiated neoplasms are based on retrospective studies of large numbers of patients treated in an uncontrolled manner.

The recommended treatment of papillary carcinoma has ranged historically from resection of thyroid nodules to total thyroidectomy. Currently, most surgeons favor either total or near-total thyroidectomy or lobectomy with or without partial resection of the contralateral uninvolved lobe. If regional lymph nodes are involved, a modified neck dissection may be indicated. The various treatment options are discussed as follows:

Total Thyroidectomy

This procedure involves removal of the entire thyroid gland with identification and preservation of the recurrent laryngeal nerves and parathyroid glands. Many proponents of the operation recommend its use in all papillary carcinomas 1 cm or larger (excluding minimal cancers) since, by their estimation, it is a safe procedure and affords the best chance for cure.[1, 30, 51, 54–59] The rationale for this extensive procedure is based on the following reasons.

1. Papillary carcinoma has been reported as being multifocal in 30 to 88% of thyroidectomy specimens, depending on the completeness with which the specimen has been examined.[56] Also, bilaterality is common,[55] and residual foci of papillary carcinoma may be left in the remaining thyroid tissue. Although most of the residual malignant foci are "minimal" cancers, approximately 5 to 10% will subsequently become clinically evident and require completion thyroidectomy.

2. The local recurrence rate following less than total thyroidectomy is greater in several retrospective series than that observed following total thyroidectomy.[56, 57] For example, Mazzaferri[56] reviewed 576 patients after operation for papillary carcinoma and found recurrence rates of 10.9% and 19.2% for total and subtotal thyroidectomies, respectively. As pointed out by Attie,[57] these recurrences may include lesions involving the trachea, esophagus, recurrent laryngeal nerve, and sternocleidomastoid muscle, making secondary removal technically difficult.

3. Reoperations for recurrent disease carry a higher risk of intraoperative complications,[55] such as recurrent laryngeal nerve injury and damage to the vascular supply of the parathyroid glands. Also, the eventual mortality attending patients who develop recurrent disease has been high.

4. Total thyroid excision facilitates the use of ^{131}I thyroid scan for the detection of recurrent disease. In addition, ^{131}I radiotherapy has been used for treatment of metastatic disease and this is optimal if all thyroid tissue has been surgically ablated prior to treatment.

5. Transformation of papillary to anaplastic carcinoma is thought to occur on occasion[60] and elimination of any residual papillary foci would prevent this.

6. Total thyroidectomy is a safe operation in the hands of experienced surgeons. In 430 patients with papillary carcinoma reported from the University of Michigan,[61] treated by total thyroidectomy, the incidence of recurrent laryngeal nerve injury was 0.45% and of permanent hypoparathyroidism 2.7%. Jacobs[58] reported no recurrent laryngeal nerve injuries and a 0.8% incidence of permanent hypoparathyroidism in 213 patients undergoing total thyroidectomy. Several other large series[54, 55, 57, 62] and our results at Washington University Medical Center (unpublished data) have generally supported this concept.

Total thyroidectomy is also indicated in patients undergoing surgery for a thyroid nodule that has developed after exposure of the gland to external beam radiotherapy.[11, 15] This is necessary because in approximately 50% of cases malignancies, if present, are not located in the palpable nodule and may even reside in the contralateral lobe. Results following total thyroidectomy for papillary carcinoma are generally good, with mortality approximating 0.6% after ten to 20 years of follow-up.[1] There are no clear data, however, documenting that this therapy is superior to lesser procedures.

Partial Thyroidectomy

In contradistinction to those advocating total thyroidectomy for all papillary carcinomas, other surgeons believe that total excision is rarely necessary. Specifically, their arguments are:

1. Even though papillary neoplasms do exhibit bilaterality and tend to be multifocal, the vast majority of synchronous lesions are clinically insignificant. Tollefsen[63] reported a series of 45 patients who underwent total thyroidectomy for papillary thyroid carcinoma, and 38% had occult carcinoma in the contralateral lobe. Another 216 patients with papillary carcinoma had excision of the involved lobe only, and carcinoma appeared in the contralateral lobe in 4.6% of these patients after five to 35 years follow-up. Thus, even though occult foci of papillary thyroid carcinoma probably remain in the gland after thyroid lobectomy, only a small percentage of patients ever develop clinically significant disease.

2. The incidence of nodal metastases at the time of thyroid lobectomy or total thyroidectomy is high, approximately 90% in one series,[64] and metastatic disease may not be apparent on examination. Therefore, removal of the entire thyroid gland in these cases will not eliminate the tumor completely.

3. Total thyroidectomy has significant morbidity when compared with lesser procedures, depending on the skill and experience of the surgeon.[65–67] One recent series[65] reported a tenfold higher incidence of complications with total compared to partial thyroidectomy. Twenty-one percent of patients developed hypoparathyroidism, which was permanent in 14%, and the incidence of unilateral recurrent laryngeal nerve damage was 3.4%. Schroder and associates[66] reported a 23.5% incidence of complications following total thyroidectomy compared with only 1.9% after partial thyroidectomy, even though permanent hypocalcemia occurred in only three of 56 patients and no permanent recurrent laryngeal nerve injuries were reported.

4. The frequency of anaplastic transformation by low-grade tumors has perhaps been overstated. Cohn and associates[68] have reviewed this issue and point out that the annual incidence of anaplastic transformation in patients with papillary cancer as estimated by the reported prevalence of anaplastic lesions in several series was only .006% (1 in 17,000 patients annually). Furthermore, the mean age of these patients is 66 years and none has been under 45 years of age.[68] Therefore, the risk in the majority of patients with thyroid cancer, especially those under the age of 50 years, is negligible.

Those who advocate less than total thyroid excision generally perform either a total lobectomy with isthmusectomy on the involved side or unilateral total lobectomy with subtotal excision on the contralateral side, the so-called "near-total thyroidectomy." The latter procedure involves dissecting away and leaving behind a small remnant (1 to 2 gm) of the posterior gland and capsule in order to preserve the adjacent parathyroid glands and recurrent laryngeal nerve. Still, other surgeons feel that lobectomy is safer than near-total thyroidectomy and should be performed in cases not involving both lobes.[63, 65, 66, 69, 70]

Three other issues have also been discussed extensively and are somewhat less controversial. First, the appropriate treatment for occult lesions, i.e., intrathyroidal tumors less than 1.5 cm in diameter, need not include total thyroidectomy. Of the 137 patients treated at the Mayo Clinic[52] from 1926 to 1955 by partial thyroidectomy and followed up for a mean of 25.3 years, no cancer-related deaths occurred, including the previously mentioned 55 individuals with lymph node involvement. Recurrence of the disease did require reoperation in 13 cases, however, all recurrences were localized to the neck and were easily resectable.

Another consideration is the role of neck dissection in patients presenting with or without obvious nodal metastases. In patients with palpably enlarged lateral cervical nodes, most surgeons believe that their removal either by simple excision or modified radical neck dissection is indicated. Even though survival in patients with cervical metastases seems not to differ from those without such disease, the local recurrence rate is considerably higher in the former group.[56] Since this might necessitate further operation or treatment, neck dissection is justified in these cases. Noguchi and Murakami[64] have commented that patients over 40 years of age may have a worsened prognosis when metastatic disease is present, and prophylactic modified radical neck dissection is indicated for primary thyroid tumors greater than 1.5 cm in diameter. Their data also indicate that the surgeon's ability to detect nodal metastases at the operating table, and thereby to decide about the need for radical neck dissection, is poor. Rosen and Maitland[71] have suggested that sampling of nodes lateral to the internal jugular vein should be performed through the standard thyroidectomy incision, and the decision regarding neck dissection made after histologic analysis of those nodes. In patients with normal physical examinations preoperatively, they report a 36% incidence of regional node involvement at the time of total thyroidectomy and modified neck dissection.[71]

Finally, the controversial role of radical resection for papillary lesions involving adjacent structure has been addressed in recent reports.[72–74] On occasion, local tumor control may involve resection of adjacent viscera, including the esophagus, larynx, and trachea. In a recent report from the Massachusetts General Hospital, Grillo and Zannini[74] described 12 patients with airway invasion by papillary cancer who underwent resectional therapy, six of whom were alive and disease-free at follow-up (one month to nine years). They concluded that since local invasion is the most common cause of death from well-differentiated cancer, and is a significant source of morbidity, aggressive resection is warranted. Though their primary goal has been palliation, treatment by removal of gross disease and subsequent adjuvant therapy offers a promise of cure as well.

Postoperative Management

The detection and treatment of recurrence following thyroidectomy are important in preserving the excellent prognosis seen in patients with papillary thyroid carcinoma. There are several adjuvant therapeutic options that should be considered in the postoperative period.

There are substantial data in experimental animals that TSH stimulates the growth of thyroid neoplasms.[75] Unfortunately, the data in humans are less convincing and at best anecdotal. Crile[76] emphasized in 1957 that TSH suppression by administration of thyroid hormone might afford palliation in patients with metastatic neoplasms. This concept has been supported recently by Clark[77] and Mazzaferri,[56] who demonstrated improved survival in patients receiving L-thyroxine suppression. This finding has been contradicted, however, by Cady and associates,[78] who reviewed 671 patients following partial resection for papillary carcinoma. Comparing patients treated and those not treated with thyroid suppression, there was no difference in survival. These investigators concluded, however, that TSH suppression might still play a palliative role in the treatment of metastatic disease by prolonging the disease-free interval or actually shrinking clinically evident metastases.[78] Given the current trend favoring near-total or total thyroidectomy for well-differentiated carcinoma and the innocuous nature of thyroid hormone supplementation, the use of synthroid suppression is universally accepted.

Screening of patients postoperatively for the presence of metastatic disease is of considerable importance, since prompt treatment of metastases can lead to enhanced survival. In addition to careful examination of the neck and periodic chest x-ray, thyroid scintigraphy and the serum concentration of thyroglobulin are often determined. Use of these modalities is facilitated by total or near-total thyroid excision. It is usually recommended that the first postoperative thyroid scan be performed six weeks following thyroidectomy, when no thyroid hormone supplementation has been administered and serum TSH levels are maximal.[79] Since appropriate TSH elevations may be delayed following thyroidectomy, particularly in older patients, measurement of TSH levels prior to scanning may, on occasion, be indicated.[1] Following near-total or even total thyroidectomy, small amounts of normal tissue will remain in the neck and may interfere with the sensitivity of the thyroid scan. The normal in situ thyroid tissue has a much greater avidity for radioiodine (compared with papillary carcinoma), and thus it must be ablated by a therapeutic dose of radioactive iodine before one can fully ascertain the extent of metastatic disease. Whether radioiodine ablation should routinely be performed in the absence of suspected metastatic disease is controversial.[80]

Most often, a 2 mCi dose of ^{131}I is used for the initial scan. Depending on the initial scan results and on the preferences of the individual surgeon and radiotherapist, the patient may then receive an ablative dose of ^{131}I.

For instance, if the scan shows uptake only in the thyroid bed, Freitas,[79] in a recent review, recommends ablation of the remnant with 75 to 100 mCi of ^{131}I and another scan is performed in three to seven days to search for metastatic disease obscured on the original scan. Beierwaltes[81] recommends that a scintiscan be performed within three months following thyroidectomy and the subsequent ablations vary between 100 to 175 mCi depending on involvement of cervical nodes and distant sites.[81] Rescanning is then performed in one year. One potential advantage of obtaining the postablative scan is that a negative scan portends a favorable prognosis and may reduce the necessity for frequent whole-body ^{131}I scans.[82]

Levels of circulating thyroglobulin (Tg) have also been demonstrated to be valuable in postoperative follow-up of patients with thyroid carcinoma. Thyroglobulin can be evaluated in a variety of thyroid disorders such as Graves' disease, thyroiditis, and nodular goiter,[83, 84] perhaps arguing against its use in preoperative screening; however, several recent studies have documented its utility in detecting recurrent or metastatic disease. LoGerfo[85] performed radioimmunoanalysis of Tg levels in the serum of 30 patients following total thyroid resection for well-differentiated carcinoma and found that all 20 patients who were recurrence-free at ten years had minimal levels (< 15 ng/ml). On the other hand, of ten patients with recurrent disease, all had levels exceeding 90 ng/ml, much greater than levels determined in 46 normal controls (range, 10 to 60 ng/ml). Similarly, several other investigations have compared the sensitivity of Tg assay with radioiodine scanning,[83, 84, 86, 87] and found the former technique to be more sensitive. For instance, Ashcraft and van Herle,[83] in a study of 53 patients, reported that no metastases were present in postoperative patients with serum Tg levels less than 1 ng/ml, whereas six of nine patients with Tg levels exceeding 10 ng/ml and with normal total body scans, later proved to harbor metastatic disease. If one uses the thyroglobulin assay there is a reduced requirement for screening total body scans, and thus less radiation exposure. Since even small amounts of normal residual thyroid tissue can produce a significant quantity of Tg, complete extirpation of the gland, followed by radioactive iodine (RAI) ablation, is mandatory.

The precise role of radioactive iodine in the prevention of metastatic disease remains very controversial. Some authors have proposed routine administration of ^{131}I postoperatively as a prophylactic measure, citing improved survival and decreased local recurrence rates when this plan is instituted. In a retrospective review, Mazaferri and Young[56] reported the lowest death and recurrence rates in a group of patients who had received both RAI and thyroid hormone suppression. Even though this philosophy is not generally accepted,[79] there may be subgroups of patients, such as those with extensive capsular invasion or with a history of head and neck irradiation, who might benefit from the prophylactic use of adjuvant ablative therapy. The administration of large doses (> 900 mCi) of radioactive iodine has been associated with significant complications, including bone marrow suppression, pulmonary fibrosis, and even leukemia, thus making its use, especially in young, low-risk patients, problematic. Radiotherapy with ^{131}I seems most beneficial for ablating the thyroid remnant following thyroidectomy, in facilitating immediate and subsequent screening, and in the treatment of metastatic carcinoma detected on scintigraphic studies. Another form of adjuvant therapy that may play some role is external beam irradiation, as reviewed recently by Tubiana and associates.[88] These authors point to the efficacy of external beam radiation in treating local disease not controlled by surgery and claim that it is superior to radioactive iodine. They state that with an adequate therapeutic dose of radiation (> 50 Gy), local control is achieved in 90% of cases. If the extent of tumor excision is questionable, radiotherapy is a reasonable alternative form of adjuvant therapy.

Follicular Carcinoma

The other variant of well-differentiated thyroid cancer, follicular carcinoma, accounts for 20% of thyroid malignancies. Despite the fact that histologic elements of papillary and follicular carcinomas are very commonly but variably mixed within a single tumor, most authors recognize follicular neoplasms as a distinct pathologic and clinical entity. Follicular carcinoma is characterized histologically by sheets of anaplastic cells and, in the more differentiated form, by colloid-filled follicles lined by anaplastic cells. These cancers may be extremely difficult to distinguish both from follicular adenomas and from follicular variants of papillary carcinoma,[89] thereby leading to their significant misclassification in the literature. The aggressiveness and hence the prognosis of patients with follicular carcinoma rest to a great extent on the degree of vascular invasion demonstrated by the tumor. "Encapsulated follicular carcinoma" is a well-differentiated form that shows only minimal invasion of the blood vessels or the thyroid capsule.[90] These lesions, which have been called "microinvasive" or "minimally invasive," are rarely multicentric and infrequently metastasize. They carry, in general, a favorable prognosis. On the other hand, angioinvasive follicular carcinomas, and those that extensively invade the thyroid capsule, are often widely metastatic at the time of presentation and tend to be associated with the enhanced mortality reported for these neoplasms.

The clinical presentation of follicular carcinoma is most often similar to that for papillary carcinoma—a nodule or lump in the neck. As reported in one series,[91] as many as 50% of patients present with a long-standing multinodular goiter that has recently changed in size or shape. These neoplasms tend to occur in areas of iodine deficiency and endemic goiter, thus accounting for their diminishing prevalence in the United States.[1, 91] These tumors may also occur in patients who have previously been exposed to low-dose external beam irradiation to the head and neck. Follicular carcinoma, compared with papillary carcinoma, occurs in older patients and rarely develops in the first two decades of life. Several investigators have pointed out that age is the predominant prognostic factor in follicular, as well as papillary carcinoma. Studies reported by Cady,[8, 23] and Donohue[92] conclude that when controlled for age, papillary and follicular lesions have similar biologic behavior, with older patients having much more invasive, clinically aggressive lesions. Similarly, in Crile's series of 84 patients treated at the Cleveland Clinic,[93] the apparent "cure" rate of patients less than 40 years of age at the time of diagnosis was 86% compared with 26% for patients older than 60 years of age. The relationship of age to prognosis, as in the case with papillary carcinoma, is not understood, but is perhaps influenced by hormonal factors or, alternatively, depressed immunocompetence in the older age group.

The pattern of spread of follicular carcinoma is distinct from that observed with papillary neoplasms; follicular tumors tend to metastasize hematogenously to the lung and bone, and occasionally to brain or soft tissue. Often metastases will present early in the course of the disease, even in the presence of very small primary lesions, and occasionally symptomatic metastases may be the first indicator of disease. Unlike papillary carcinoma, distant metastases due to invasive follicular carcinoma carry an extremely grave prognosis. Cervical lymph node metastases are fairly unusual in pure follicular lesions—reported as 5% by Woolner,[94] 15% by Cady,[53] and 5% by Thompson.[1] This has prompted Harness and associates[91] to comment that isolated nodal metastases are invariably due to papillary cancer when pathologic reevaluation has been undertaken. Not uncommonly follicular lesions can involve lymph nodes by direct spread from the thyroid itself.

Treatment

Surgical therapy for follicular neoplasms, as for papillary carcinoma, also varies considerably among surgeons. Crile[93] and Tollefsen[95] point to the low incidence of multicentricity and suggest that total lobectomy with isthmusectomy is adequate treatment for follicular lesions grossly confined to one lobe in the absence of any evidence of metastatic disease. The extent of operation performed does not, from their experience, correlate with the patient's eventual outcome and thus the less morbid procedure is preferable in their judgment. Both groups, however, agree that more extensive resections are necessary when the tumor is locally invasive or when metastatic disease is evident. Schmidt and Wang,[90] in a review of 19 cases of encapsulated follicular carcinoma, recommend that lobectomy be performed for encapsulated lesions less than 3.5 cm in diameter, since no patient with tumors less than 3 cm in diameter developed metastases in their series, whereas 60% of patients with tumors 3.5 cm diameter or greater had evidence of metastatic disease.

In patients who have metastases at the time of diagnosis or those who present with locally aggressive lesions in the neck, near-total or total thyroidectomy is indicated to facilitate the use of adjuvant ^{131}I treatment. In addition, many authors feel that complete resection should be performed routinely for follicular carcinoma, given its propensity to metastasize widely.[91] The presence of metastatic disease has been reported to be high in several series: nine (11%) of 69 patients reported by Tollefsen,[95] 28 (35%) of 84 in Crile's series,[93] and seven (3.3%) of 214 patients reported by Mazaferri[50] presented with evidence of metastatic disease, while a significant number developed metastases subsequent to thyroidectomy. In addition, the incidence of local recurrence is significant despite the extent of the initial surgical therapy, again mandating the use of adjuvant ^{131}I. Local recurrence is frequently a lethal sequela; for instance, in Crile's series,[93] 14 of 84 patients developed recurrence, of which only two were disease-free at ten years. The role of neck dissection in follicular carcinoma is confined to those situations in which nodes are clinically involved, and prophylactic dissections have not been recommended.

Metastatic disease from follicular neoplasms is commonly treated by administration of ^{131}I. Two groups have noted that the combination of total thyroidectomy and ^{131}I is effective in reducing the mortality from follicular cancer. Young and associates[96] reported a recurrence rate of 4.7% in 42 patients treated by total thyroidectomy, ^{131}I ablation, and synthroid suppression, a lower rate than observed for other modalities. Beierwaltes and associates[97] found 36% survival in 25 patients with widely metastatic follicular carcinoma followed after surgery and treated with ^{131}I, and recommended this form of therapy for metastatic disease. Crile and associates,[93] however, found no improvement in prognosis with administration of ^{131}I to patients with metastatic disease. External beam irradiation has also been used to treat recurrent disease; however, it has had only limited effectiveness.[93]

Hürthle Cell Tumors

Once considered a variant of follicular carcinoma, Hürthle cell neoplasms are thought to represent an entity distinct from other forms of well-differentiated thyroid cancers. This neoplasm, alternately termed Ashkenazy cell tumor, oxyphil tumor, oncocytoma, and eosinophilic cell tumor, is characterized histologically by the presence of large, polyhedral cells with abundant eosinophilic cytoplasm and a large number of cytoplasmic mitochondria. These neoplasms may present as well-encapsulated, tan tumors with orderly cell patterns, or they may present with characteristics of invasive carcinoma. The latter exhibit cytologic anaplasia, frequent mitoses, and either vascular or capsular invasion. Several series[98–105] describing Hürthle cell tumors have been published recently, and the incidence of malignancy ranges from 5% to 55%. In general, Hürthle cell carcinomas are thought to be more aggressive than follicular or papillary carcinomas. They are often multicentric, frequently metastasize to lymph nodes and, via the bloodstream, to distant sites, and they have a high local recurrence rate after initial resection.

The biological behavior of "benign" Hürthle cell tumors, and therefore the extent of resection recommended for adequate treatment of these lesions, has sparked some controversy. Gundry and colleagues at the University of Michigan[100] have presented evidence in 62 patients that Hürthle cells tumors that appear "benign" histologically often behave in an aggressive manner clinically. While the overall mortality of Hürthle cell neoplasms was approximately 25% in this series, 12% of 26 patients with pathologically "benign" tumors died of their disease. Of seven patients in this group undergoing late completion thyroidectomy for "benign" disease (1 to 3 years after initial operation), five (71%) had pathologic evidence of contralateral disease.[100] Furthermore, these investigators found that the size of the lesion did not necessarily influence its biologic behavior[100]; even tumors less than 2 cm carried a 25% incidence of malignancy and had a 25% recurrence rate after thyroidectomy. Because of these findings, total thyroidectomy has been recommended by this group as the treatment of choice for all Hürthle cell lesions. Their retrospective review of patients having had total thyroidectomy or lesser procedures revealed recurrence rates of 21% and 59%, respectively. In patients with no metastases apparent at the time of presentation, recurrence rates were 8% and 21%, respectively. The unpredictable nature of "benign" lesions occasionally recurring eight to ten years following the primary surgery mandates, in their view, an aggressive surgical approach in all cases.

Several recently published series seem to contradict the findings of Thompson and associates in several important respects. First, the percentage of malignant Hürthle cell neoplasms is less—10 to 25%—in most series. Second, most authors believe that the histologic appearance *does* predict biologic behavior. And third, total lobectomy is commonly offered as adequate treatment for noninvasive Hürthle cell neoplasms. In a recent review by Arganini and associates,[105] in 84 patients followed up for a mean of 8.4 years, 74% of lesions were benign, only one of which (2.5%) later developed metastatic disease. Only 13% of lesions were frankly malignant in this series. In a review of the recent literature[105] these authors found that only four (1.5%) of 257 "benign"-appearing Hürthle cell tumors metastasized following thyroidectomy. This concept was supported by the series published by Bondeson and associates,[99] Gosain and Clarke,[106] and Caplan and associates,[101] none of whom reported recurrence or mortality consequent to histologically "benign" Hürthle cell tumors treated by partial thyroidectomy. In each of these series, lobectomy (with isthmusectomy), was recommended as the initial surgical treatment for Hürthle cell neoplasms followed either by total or near-total thyroidectomy for lesions that subsequently proved carcinomatous. Needle biopsy is generally not useful in determining the malignant potential of these tumors preoperatively. In addition to thyroidectomy, Arganini and associates[105] and Rosen and associates[104] recommend lateral node sampling and subsequent neck dissection for lesions metastatic to cervical nodes, similar to the approach commonly used for aggressive papillary carcinomas.

The reasons for discrepancy between the various studies probably relates to a number of factors: (1) The Michigan group reported on a series drawn largely from referral cases, which may represent a distorted population, unlike what one would see in a community setting. (2) The length of follow-up may be too short in some series of benign neoplasms. (3) Pathologic classification and criteria may differ between investigators. There could also conceivably be geographical differences accounting for the disparate results, though this seems much less likely.

The prognosis for metastatic Hürthle cell cancer is generally dismal; in the Michigan series,[100] 79% of patients with metastatic disease at the time of operation died of recurrent disease. Hürthle cell lesions do not, as a rule, concentrate ^{131}I, and these investigators noted only one response (in 14 patients with metastatic disease) to ^{131}I, external radiation, or chemotherapy. On the other hand, Arganini and associates[105] recommended the use of ^{131}I postoperatively in patients with malignant Hürthle cell tumors and in patients with previous head and neck irradiation with benign Hürthle cell tumors. They argue that ablation of the thyroid remnant with 30 mCi ^{131}I destroys contiguous residual tumor in the thyroid gland, facilitates later total-body scanning, and allows for the use of thyroglobulin as a tumor marker in follow-up. Bondeson and associates[99] have also reported anecdotal successes with adjuvant radioactive iodine.

Medullary Thyroid Carcinoma

A recent review by our group[107] has detailed the clinical and pathophysiologic features of medullary thyroid carcinoma (MTC), an aggressive neoplasm of the parafollicular or C-cells of the thyroid gland. These tumors, which constitute approximately 10% of thyroid neoplasms, are unique from several vantages. Medullary carcinoma cells have a prolific biosynthetic capacity in the production of tumor markers—especially calcitonin (a 32 amino acid protein polypeptide) and carcinoembryonic antigen (CEA)—allowing for early diagnosis and subsequent follow-up after thyroidectomy. Furthermore, MTC is frequently associated with the hereditary endocrinopathies, multiple endocrine neoplasia (MEN) types IIa and IIb. Medullary carcinoma may present in one of four ways[107]:

1. Multiple endocrine neoplasia type IIa, an autosomal dominant disorder characterized by the concurrence of MTC, pheochromocytoma, and hyperparathyroidism.
2. MEN-type IIb, the association of MTC, pheochromocytoma, multiple mucosal neuromas, and ganglioneuromatosis.
3. Familial non-MEN MTC, which presents without the involvement of other neuroendocrine organs.
4. Sporadic MTC.

The familial MTC syndromes are characterized by an autosomal dominant pattern of inheritance, complete penetrance and expression of the MTC, and, in the cases of MEN-IIa and MEN-IIb, variable expression of the other components of the syndrome. Furthermore, with familial MTC, the tumors are always bilateral, as opposed to the sporadic form, in which the tumor is unilateral. The MTC grossly is white to grey-tan in color and firm and, microscopically, is composed of spindle cells that stain positively for amyloid.

Medullary thyroid carcinoma commonly presents clinically as a palpable nodule with or without regional or distant metastases. Virtually always the basal serum calcitonin level is elevated in patients with clinically evident disease. Kindred members at risk for developing one of the familial forms of MTC may be studied by measuring serum calcitonin levels both basally and following the intravenous administration of calcium and pentagastrin. Specifically, serum samples for the calcitonin assay should be drawn basally and at 1, 2, 3, 5, and 10 minutes following the injection of calcium gluconate (2 mg/kg/1 min), immediately followed by administration of pentagastrin (0.05 μg/kg/5 seconds). Patients with undetectable basal calcitonin levels that increase to greater than 300 pg/ml are suspect for the presence of MTC and should be either retested in six months or subjected to provocative testing with blood samples collected from the inferior thyroid veins, which are subsequently analyzed for calcitonin. In a recent study,[108] 92 patients with MTC were evaluated and the preoperative stimulated calcitonin level was correlated with the amount of regional lymph node spread at the time of thyroidectomy, the presence of residual MTC postoperatively (as indicated by elevated plasma calcitonin levels following provocation in the postoperative period), the presence of distant metastases, and death.[108] The data are shown in Table 2. Clearly, there is a direct relationship between the stimulated preoperative plasma calcitonin level and stage of disease. The cure rate is higher in patients with early disease who have minimally elevated levels compared with patients with clinically evident disease whose plasma calcitonin levels are markedly increased.

Once the diagnosis of MTC has been made, total thyroidectomy is recommended. Meticulous dissection of central zone lymph nodes—those present from the hyoid bone superiorly, to the innominate vessels inferiorly, and to the internal jugular veins laterally—is essential in all cases because of the high rate (50% in a recent review by Russell)[109] of metastases in this region. In addition, jugular node sampling is also performed, and if positive nodes are revealed, modified neck dissection is recommended.

Prior to surgery, appropriate studies should be performed to screen for the presence of pheochromocytomas, which, if present, are removed first. The presence of hyperparathyroidism should be determined by measuring the serum concentrations of calcium and parathyroid hormone (PTH). In patients with MEN-IIa, removal of all enlarged parathyroid glands is advised, and in the event of four gland enlargement, parathyroid autotransplantation is recommended.[110]

Adjuvant therapy for MTC has been largely unsuccessful. Tumor regression and prolonged survival have been noted anecdotally in some patients receiving external beam irradiation. However, both ^{131}I and various chemotherapeutic regimens have not been effective in recent reports.[111, 112]

TABLE 2.
Plasma Calcitonin (CT) and Prognosis*†

Group‡	Preoperative CT pg/ml	Regional Lymph Node Metastases No. (%)	Postoperative CT No. (%) > 300 pg/ml	Distant Metastases No. (%)	Death No. (%)
1 (N = 25)	250–1,000	1 (4)	1 (4)	0 (0)	0 (0)
2 (N = 36)	1,000–5,000	3 (8.3)	6 (16.7)	0 (0)	0 (0)
3 (N = 8)	5,000–10,000	2 (25)	1 (12.5)	0 (0)	0 (0)
4 (N = 23)	> 10,000	13 (57)	14 (61)	4 (17)	2 (8.7)

*From Wells SA, et al: The importance of early diagnosis in patients with hereditary medullary thyroid carcinoma. *Ann Surg* 1982; 19:505–511. Used by permission.

†Ninety-two patients with hereditary MTC were divided into four groups based on their preoperative CT levels after stimulation with calcium gluconate and pentagastrin. Stimulated CT levels correlate with the presence of nodal metastases as well as with mortality.

‡Group 1 or group 2 vs. group 4; $P < .001$.

Careful follow-up of patients by serial measurements of stimulated plasma calcitonin levels may reveal the appearance of recurrent disease amenable to surgical resection. Elevated calcitonin levels occasionally are noted postthyroidectomy in patients without physical or radiologic evidence of recurrence, indicating that small foci of medullary carcinoma may lie dormant for several years and be virtually impossible to eradicate. These patients should be followed closely.

Anaplastic Carcinoma

The most virulent thyroid neoplasm, anaplastic carcinoma, accounts for less than 5% of thyroid malignancies. It generally presents in elderly individuals, the peak incidence being about 65 years of age. Patients with long-standing nodular thyroid disease often present with recent enlargement of the thyroid which rapidly expands to involve adjacent structures. Hoarseness, dysphagia, and dyspnea are not uncommon modes of presentation, indicating far-advanced local disease. These tumors have been subgrouped into those of "follicular cell" origin, i.e., spindle and giant cell carcinomas, and those of "nonparenchymal" origin, i.e., small cell and squamous cell carcinomas.[60] The small cell tumors behave much like lymphomas clinically, in that they are often radiosensitive, and are considered as such by many authors.[60]

An enlarged thyroid gland suspected of harboring anaplastic carcinoma is best evaluated initially by FNA, although occasionally an open incisional biopsy is necessary. Surgical resection or debulking is rarely indicated, since vital structures are frequently invaded, though tracheostomy for airway control may at some time in the course of the disease become mandatory. Therapy for these lesions optimally includes combinations of external radiotherapy and chemotherapy—actinomycin D or adriamycin—though results even with this multidisciplinary approach are poor. In a recent retrospective report from the M.D. Anderson Hospital of 84 patients with anaplastic carcinoma who were treated by a variety of surgical and adjuvant therapies,[60] a 7.1% five-year survival rate was achieved with a mean survival of 6.2 months. The most important favorable prognostic factor seemed to be a relative paucity of anaplastic elements seen in some of the tumors histologically. Even so, tumors with only traces of spindle cell or giant cell elements are highly malignant and all anaplastic lesions should be treated as if disseminated disease were present.

Future Directions

Given the overall favorable prognosis of well-differentiated thyroid carcinomas, advances in the treatment of these lesions will likely involve early and specific detection of malignant nodules. The avoidance of unnecessary neck explorations by refinement of aspiration and biopsy techniques will be important.

Identification of patients at high risk for recurrence, for example, by DNA analysis of needle aspiration specimens, may provide a means to prevent significant morbidity and mortality. Advances in adjuvant therapy are needed for both well and poorly differentiated lesions, since the prognosis is poor in the face of metastatic disease.

References

1. Thompson NW, Nishiyama RH, Harness JK: Thyroid carcinoma: Current controversies. *Curr Probl Surg* 1979; 25:5–67.
2. Block MA: Surgery of thyroid nodules and malignancy. *Cur Prob Surg* 1983; 3:133–203.
3. American Cancer Society: Cancer statistics 1985. *Ca* 1985; 35:19–35.
4. Nishiyama RH, Ludwig GK, Thompson NW: The prevalence of small papillary thyroid carcinomas in 100 consecutive necropsies in an American population, in DeGroot LJ (ed): *Radiation-Associated Thyroid Carcinoma*. New York, Grune & Stratton, Inc, 1977, pp 123–135.
5. Sampson RJ, Woolner LB, Balin RC, et al: Occult thyroid carcinomas in Olmstead County, Minnesota: Prevalence at autopsy compared with that in Hiroshima and Nagasaki, Japan. *Cancer* 1974; 34:2072–2076.
6. Bell RM: Thyroid carcinoma. *Surg Clin North Am* 1986; 66:13–30.
7. Rossi RL, Cady B, Silverman ML, et al: Current results in conservative surgery for differentiated thyroid carcinoma. *World J Surg* 1986; 10:612–622.
8. Cady B, Rossi R, Silverman M, et al: Further evidence of the validity of risk group definition in differentiated thyroid carcinoma. *Surgery* 1985; 98:1171–1178.
9. LoGerfo P: Evaluation and treatment of solitary thyroid nodule. *Surg Rounds* 1983; pp 39–54.
10. Morteinson JD, Woolner LB, Bennett WA: Gross and microscopic changes in clinically normal thyroid glands. *J Clin Endocrinol Metabol* 1985; 15:1270–1280.
11. Witt TR, Meng RL, Economou SG, et al: The approach to the irradiated thyroid. *Surg Clin North Am* 1979; 59:45–63.
12. Duffy BJ Jr, Fitzgerald PJ: Cancer of the thyroid in children: A report of 28 cases. *J Clin Endocrinol Metabol* 1950; 10:1296–1299.
13. Schneider AB, Favus MJ, Strachurd MF, et al: Incidence, prevalence and characteristics of radiation-induced thyroid tumors. *Am J Med* 1978; 64:243–252.
14. Deaconson TF, Wilson SD, Cerletty JM, et al: Total or near total thyroidectomy versus limited resection for radiation-associated thyroid nodules: A twelve-year follow-up of patients in a thyroid screening program. *Surgery* 1986; 100:1116–1119.
15. Calandra DB, Shah KH, Lawrence AM, et al: Total thyroidectomy in irradiated patients: A twenty-year experience in 206 patients. *Ann Surg* 1985; 202:356–360.
16. Paloyan E, Lawrence AM, Brooks MH, et al: Total thyroidectomy and parathyroid autotransplantation for radiation-associated thyroid cancer. *Surgery* 1976; 80:70–76.
17. Favus MJ, Schneider AB, Stachura MF, et al: Thyroid cancer occurring as a

late consequence of head-and-neck irradiation: Evaluation of 1056 patients. *N Engl J Med* 1976; 294:1019–1025.
18. Behar R, Arganini M, Wu TC, et al: Graves' disease and thyroid cancer. *Surgery* 1986; 100:1121–1126.
19. Farbota LM, Calandra DB, Lawrence AM, et al: Thyroid carcinoma in Graves' disease. *Surgery* 1985; 98:1148–1152.
20. Ott RA, Calandra DB, McCall A, et al: The incidence of thyroid carcinoma in patients with Hashimoto's thyroiditis and solitary cold nodules. *Surgery* 1985; 98:1202–1206.
21. Segal K, Ben-Bassat M, Avraham A, et al: Hashimoto's thyroiditis and carcinoma of the thyroid gland. *Int Surg* 1985; 70:205–209.
22. Rosen IB, Walfish PG: Pregnancy as a predisposing factor of thyroid neoplasia. *Arch Surg* 1986; 121:1287–1290.
23. Cady B, Sedgwick CE, Meissner WA, et al: Risk factor analysis in differentiated thyroid cancer. *Cancer* 1979; 43:810–820.
24. DeGroot MJ, Standburg JB: *The Thyroid and Its Diseases.* New York, John Wiley & Sons, Inc, 1975, p 666.
25. Clark O: *Endocrine Surgery of the Thyroid and Parathyroid Glands.* St Louis, CV Mosby Co, 1985, pp 56–90.
26. Robbins S: *Pathologic Basis of Disease.* Philadelphia, WB Saunders Co, 1974, pp 1320–1345.
27. Wolvos TA, Chong FK, Razvi SA, et al: An unusual thyroid tumor: A comparison to a literature review of thyroid teratomas. *Surgery* 1985; 97:613–616.
28. Rasbuch DA, Mondschein M, Harris NL, et al: Malignant lymphoma of the thyroid gland: A clinical and pathologic study of 20 cases. *Surgery* 1985; 98:1166–1170.
29. Aozasa K, Inoue A, Tajima K, et al: Malignant lymphomas of the thyroid gland: Analysis of 79 patients with emphasis on histologic prognostic factors. *Cancer* 1986; 58:100–104.
30. Thompson NW: Current diagnostic techniques for single thyroid nodules. *Curr Surg* 1983; 40:255–259.
31. Lennquist S: The thyroid nodule: Diagnosis and surgical treatment. *Surg Clin North Am* 1987; 67:213–232.
32. Hoffman GL, Thompson NW, Heffron C: The solitary thyroid nodule: A reassessment. *Arch Surg* 1972; 105:379–385.
33. O'Holleran LW, O'Holleran TP, Mills GQ, et al: Use of thyroid scans in the selection of surgical patients. *Am J Surg* 1982; 144:639–641.
34. Van Herle AJ, Rich P, Ljung BME, et al: The thyroid nodule. *Ann Intern Med* 1982; 96:221–232.
35. Rosen IB, Walfish PG, Miskin M: The application of ultrasound to the study of thyroid enlargement: Management of 450 cases. *Arch Surg* 1975; 110:940–944.
36. Lees WR, Vahl SP, Watson LR, et al: The role of ultrasound scanning in the diagnosis of thyroid swellings. *Br J Surg* 1978; 65:681–684.
37. LoGerfo P, Starker P, Weber C, et al: Incidence of cancer in surgically treated thyroid nodules based on method of selection. *Surgery* 1985; 98:1197–1201.
38. Nishiyama RH, Bigos T, Goldfarb WB, et al: The efficacy of simultaneous fine-needle aspiration and large-needle biopsy of the thyroid gland. *Surgery* 1986; 100:1133–1137.

39. Martin HE, Ellis EB: Biopsy by needle puncture and aspiration. *Ann Surg* 1930; 92:169–181.
40. Esselstyn CB Jr, Crile G Jr: Evaluation of various types of needle biopsies of the thyroid. *World J Surg* 1984; 8:452–457.
41. Wang C, Vickery AL Jr, Maloof F: Needle biopsy of the thyroid. *Surg Gynecol Obstet* 1976; 143:365–368.
42. Broughan TA, Esselstyn CB Jr: Large-needle thyroid biopsy: Still necessary. *Surgery* 1986; 100:1138–1140.
43. Boey J, Hsu C, Collins RJ: False-negative errors in fine-needle aspiration biopsy of dominant thyroid nodules: A prospective follow-up study. *World J Surg* 1986; 10:623–630.
44. Backdahl M, Wallin G, Lowhagen T, et al: Fine-needle biopsy cytology and DNA analysis: Their place in the evaluation and treatment of patients with thyroid neoplasms. *Surg Clin North Am* 1987; 67:197–211.
45. Lowhagen T, Granberg P, Lundell G, et al: Aspiration biopsy cytology (ABC) in nodules of the thyroid gland suspected to be malignant. *Surg Clin North Am* 1979; 59(1):3–18.
46. Christensen SB, Bondeson L, Ericsson UB, et al: Prediction of malignancy in the solitary thyroid nodule by physical examination, thyroid scan, fine-needle biopsy and serum thyroglobulin. *Acta Chir Scand* 1984; 150:433–439.
47. Colacchio TA, LoGerfo P, Feind CR: Fine needle cytologic diagnosis of thyroid nodules. *Am J Surg* 1980; 140:568–571.
48. Silverman JF, West RL, Larkin EW, et al: The role of fine-needle aspiration biopsy in the rapid diagnosis and management of thyroid neoplasm. *Cancer* 1986; 57:1164–1170.
49. Hawkins F, Bellido D, Bernal C, et al: Fine needle aspiration biopsy in the diagnosis of thyroid cancer and thyroid disease. *Cancer* 1987; 59:1206–1209.
50. Mazzaferri EL: Papillary and follicular thyroid cancer: A selective approach to diagnosis and treatment. *Ann Rev Med* 1981; 32:73–91.
51. Woolner LB, Beahrs OH, Black BM, et al: Classification and prognosis of thyroid carcinoma: A study of 885 cases observed in a thirty year period. *Am J Surg* 1961; 102:354–387.
52. Hubert JP Jr, Kiernan PD, Beahrs OH, et al: Occult papillary carcinoma of the thyroid. *Arch Surg* 1980; 115:394–398.
53. Cady B, Sedgwick CE, Meissner WA, et al: Changing clinical, pathologic, therapeutic, and survival patterns in differentiated thyroid carcinoma. *Ann Surg* 1976; 184:541–553.
54. Lennquist S: Surgical strategy in thyroid carcinoma: A clinical review. *Acta Chir Scand* 1986; 152:321–338.
55. van der Sluis RF, Wobbes T: Total thyroidectomy: The treatment of choice in differentiated thyroid carcinoma. *Eur J Surg Oncol* 1985; 11:343–346.
56. Mazzaferri EL, Young RL, Oertel JE, et al: Papillary thyroid carcinoma: A 10 year follow-up report of the impact of therapy in 576 patients. *Am J Med* 1981; 70:511–518.
57. Attie JN, Moskowitz GW, Margouleff D, et al: Feasibility of total thyroidectomy in the treatment of thyroid carcinoma: Postoperative radioactive iodine evaluation of 140 cases. *Am J Surg* 1979; 138:555–560.
58. Jacobs JK, Aland JW Jr, Ballinger JF: Total thyroidectomy: A review of 213 patients. *Ann Surg* 1983; 197:542–549.

59. Katz AD, Bronson D: Total thyroidectomy: The indications and results of 630 cases. *Am J Surg* 1978; 136:450–454.
60. Aldinger KA, Samaan NA, Ibanez M, et al: Anaplastic carcinoma of the thyroid: A review of 84 cases of spindle giant cell carcinoma of the thyroid. *Cancer* 1978; 41:2267–2275.
61. Harness JK, Fung L, Thompson NW, et al: Total thyroidectomy: Complications and technique. *World J Surg* 1986; 10:781–786.
62. Clark OH: Total thyroidectomy: The treatment of choice for patients with differentiated thyroid cancer. *Ann Surg* 1982; 196(3):361–370.
63. Tollefsen HR, Shah JP, Huvos AG: Papillary carcinoma of the thyroid: Recurrence in the thyroid gland after initial surgical treatment. *Am J Surg* 1972; 124:468–472.
64. Noguchi S, Murakami N: The value of lymph-node dissection in patients with differentiated thyroid cancer. *Surg Clin North Am* 1987; 67:251–261.
65. Farrar WB, Cooperman M, James AG: Surgical management of papillary and follicular carcinoma of the thyroid. *Ann Surg* 1980; 192:701–704.
66. Schroder DM, Chambors A, France CJ: Operative strategy for thyroid cancer: Is total thyroidectomy worth the price? *Cancer* 1986; 58:2320–2328.
67. Starnes HF, Brooks DC, Pinkus GS, et al: Surgery for thyroid carcinoma. *Cancer* 1985; 55:1376–1381.
68. Cohn KH, Backdahl M, Forsslund G, et al: Biologic considerations and operative strategy in papillary thyroid carcinoma: Arguments against the routine performance of total thyroidectomy. *Surgery* 1984; 96:957–970.
69. Beahrs OH: Surgical treatment for thyroid cancer. *Br J Surg* 1984; 71:976–979.
70. Wanebo HJ, Andrews W, Kaiser DL: Thyroid cancer: Some basic considerations. *Am J Surg* 1981; 142:474–479.
71. Rosen IB, Maitland A: Changing the operative strategy for thyroid cancer by node sampling. *Am J Surg* 1983; 146:504–508.
72. Cody HS, Shah JP: Locally invasive, well-differentiated thyroid cancer: 22 years experience at Memorial Sloan-Kettering Cancer Center. *Am J Surg* 1981; 142:480–483.
73. Fujimoto Y, Obara T, Ito Y, et al: Aggressive surgical approach for locally invasive papillary carcinoma of the thyroid in patients over forty-five years of age. *Surgery* 1986; 100:1098–1106.
74. Grillo HC, Zannini P: Resectional management of airway invasion by thyroid carcinoma. *Ann Thorac Surg* 1986; 42:287–298.
75. Duh QY, Clark OH: Factors influencing the growth of normal and neoplastic thyroid tissue. *Surg Clin North Am* 1987; 67:281–298.
76. Crile G Jr: The endocrine dependency of certain thyroid cancers and the danger that hyperparathyroidism may stimulate their growth. *Cancer* 1957; 10:1119.
77. Clark OH: TSH suppression in the management of thyroid nodules and thyroid cancer. *World J Surg* 1987; 5:39–47.
78. Cady B, Cohn K, Rossi RL, et al: The effect of thyroid hormone administration upon survival in patients with differentiated thyroid carcinoma. *Surgery* 1983; 94:978–983.
79. Freitas JE: Treatment of thyroid carcinoma with radioiodine. *Curr Concepts Diagn Nucl Med* 1986; 3:8–16.
80. Leeper R: Controversies in the treatment of thyroid cancer: The New York Memorial Hospital approach. *Thyroid Today* 1982; 5:1–4.

81. Beierwaltes WH: Controversies in the treatment of thyroid cancer: The University of Michigan approach. *Thyroid Today* 1983; 6:1–5.
82. Pupi A, Castagnoli A, Morotti A, et al: Prognostic value of the ^{131}I whole-body scan in postsurgical therapy for differentiated thyroid cancer. *Cancer* 1983; 52:439–441.
83. Ashcraft MW, van Herle AJ: The comparative value of serum thyroglobulin measurements and iodine 131 total body scans in the follow-up study of patients with treated differentiated thyroid cancer. *Am J Med* 1981; 71:806–814.
84. McDougall IR, Bayer MF: Follow-up of patients with differentiated thyroid cancer using serum thyroglobulin measured by an immunoradiometric assay: Comparison with I^{131} total body scans. *J Nucl Med* 1980; 21:741–744.
85. LoGerfo P, Colacchio D, Stillman T, et al: Serum thyroglobulin and recurrent thyroid cancer. *Lancet* 1977; 1:881–883.
86. Ericsson UB, Tegler L, Lennquist S, et al: Serum thyroglobulin in differentiated thyroid carcinoma. *Acta Chir Scand* 1984; 150:367–375.
87. Ramanna L, Waxman AD, Brachman MB, et al: Correlation of thyroglobulin measurements and radioiodine scans in the follow-up of patients with differentiated thyroid cancer. *Cancer* 1985; 55:1525–1529.
88. Tubaina M, Haddad E, Schlumberger M, et al: External radiotherapy in thyroid cancers. *Cancer* 1985; 55:2062–2071.
89. Evans HL: Follicular neoplasms of the thyroid: A study of 44 cases followed for a minimum of 10 years, with emphasis on differential diagnosis. *Cancer* 1984; 54:535–540.
90. Schmidt RJ, Wang C: Encapsulated follicular carcinoma of the thyroid: Diagnosis, treatment, and results. *Surgery* 1986; 100:1068–1076.
91. Harness JK, Thompson NW, McLeod MK, et al: Follicular carcinoma of the thyroid gland: Trends and treatment. *Surgery* 1984; 96:972–980.
92. Donohue JH, Goldfien SD, Miller TR, et al: Do the prognoses of papillary and follicular thyroid carcinomas differ? *Am J Surg* 1984; 148:168–173.
93. Crile G Jr, Pontius KI, Hawk WA: Factors influencing the survival of patients with follicular carcinoma of the thyroid gland. *Surg Gynecol Obstet* 1985; 160:409–413.
94. Woolner L: Thyroid carcinoma: Pathologic classification with data on prognosis. *Semin Nucl Med* 1971; 1:481–502.
95. Tollefsen HR, Shah JP, Huvos AG: Follicular carcinoma of the thyroid. *Am J Surg* 1973; 126:523–528.
96. Young RL, Mazzaferri EL, Rahe AT: Pure follicular thyroid carcinoma: Impact of therapy in 214 patients. *J Nucl Med* 1980; 21:733–737.
97. Beierwaltes WH, Nishiyama RH, Thompson NW, et al: Survival time and "cure" in papillary and follicular thyroid carcinoma with distant metastases: Statistics following University of Michigan therapy. *J Nucl Med* 1982; 23:561–568.
98. Tollefsen HR, Shah JP, Huvos AG: Hurthle cell carcinoma of the thyroid. *Am J Surg* 1975; 130:390–394.
99. Bondeson L, Bondeson AG, Ljunberg O, et al: Oxyphil tumors of the thyroid: Follow-up of 42 surgical cases. *Ann Surg* 1981; 194:677–680.
100. Gundry SR, Burney RE, Thompson NW: Total thyroidectomy for Hurthle cell neoplasm of the thyroid. *Arch Surg* 1983; 118:529–532.
101. Caplan RH, Abellera RM, Kisken WA: Hurthle cell tumors of the thyroid

gland: A clinicopathologic review and long-term follow-up. *JAMA* 1984; 251:3114–3117.
102. Heppe H, Armin A, Calandra DB: Hurthle cell tumors of the thyroid gland. *Surgery* 1985; 98:1162–1165.
103. Har-el G, Hadar T, Segal K, et al: Hurthle cell carcinoma of the thyroid gland: A tumor of moderate malignancy. *Cancer* 1986; 57:1613–1617.
104. Rosen IB, Luk S, Katz I: Hurthle cell tumor behavior: Dilemma and resolution. *Surgery* 1985; 98:777–783.
105. Arganini M, Behar R, Wu TC: Hurthle cell tumors: A twenty-five year experience. *Surgery* 1986; 100:1108–1114.
106. Gasain Ak, Clark OH: Hürthle cell neoplasms. *Arch Surg* 1984; 119:515–519.
107. Brunt LM, Wells SA Jr: Advances in the diagnosis and treatment of medullary thyroid carcinoma. *Surg Clin North Am* 1987; 67:263–279.
108. Wells SA Jr, Baylin SB, Johnsrude IS, et al: Thyroid venous catheterization in the early diagnosis of familial medullary thyroid carcinoma. *Ann Surg* 1982; 196:505–511.
109. Russell CF, Van Heerden JA, Sizemore GW, et al: The surgical management of medullary thyroid carcinoma. *Ann Surg* 1983; 197:47–48.
110. Wells SA Jr, Gunnells K, Shelburne JD, et al: Transplantation of the parathyroid glands in man: Clinical indications and results. *Surgery* 1975; 78:34–44.
111. Cance WG, Wells SA Jr: Multiple endocrine neoplasia type IIa. *Curr Prob Surg* 1985; 22(5):1–56.
112. Saad MF, Guido TJ, Samaan NA: Radioactive iodine in the treatment of medullary cancer of the thyroid. *J Clin Endocrinol Metabol* 1983; 57:124–128.

Surgical Aspects of Lymphoma

Michael J. Edwards, M.D.

Senior Surgical Oncology Fellow, Department of General Surgery, The University of Texas, M. D. Anderson Cancer Center, Houston, Texas

Charles M. Balch, M.D., F.A.C.S.

Head, Division of Surgery, Chairman, Department of General Surgery, The University of Texas, M. D. Anderson Cancer Center, Houston, Texas

Progress in histologic classification, clinical and pathological staging, and in effective multimodality therapy has dramatically improved the quality of life and disease-free survival of most patients with lymphoma. To apply advances in treatment originating in a variety of medical specialties, medical oncologists, radiation therapists, pathologists, and surgeons have developed a team approach. Some management decisions are still controversial, however, such as the necessity of staging laparotomy, the extent of radiotherapy, and the use of combination chemotherapy.

Surgeons usually become involved in managing patients with lymphoma when they are consulted about excisional biopsy. Although percutaneous methods of diagnosis such as fine-needle aspiration are currently available in many institutions, surgical excision of suspected lymph nodes is still the most important method of diagnosis. Most patients with lymphoma are first seen with suspicious lymphadenopathy for which the usual diagnostic procedure is an excisional biopsy with local anesthesia. To establish the diagnosis in some patients, however, more invasive procedures such as mediastinoscopy or exploratory laparotomy may be required for diagnosis.

Noninvasive examinations may prove inadequate in determining the extent of disease, and laparotomy may be required so that definitive treatment with radiation or chemotherapy, or both, may be designed specifically according to the patient's stage of disease. Staging laparotomy is most often used for patients with Hodgkin's disease; only rarely do patients with non–Hodgkin's lymphoma benefit from this procedure.

Surgical therapy may also be required for patients with non–Hodgkin's lymphoma who develop splenomegaly resulting in hypersplenism. Splenectomy may be required to treat pancytopenia, and it may in addition facilitate the administration of chemotherapy to pancytopenic patients. For

Adv Surg 22:225–250, 1989

0065-3411/89/22-225–250-$04.00

the occasional patient with non–Hodgkin's lymphoma who suffers from intractable left upper quadrant pain from massive splenomegaly, splenectomy may be required as well. Certainly, the complications of intestinal bleeding, obstruction, and perforation in patients with gastrointestinal (GI) involvement demand the involvement of the surgeon.

To effectively assume his or her role in the multidisciplinary management team, the surgeon must have a firm knowledge of all aspects of lymphoma, including diagnosis, classification, staging, natural history, and management.

Etiology and Epidemiology

In 1832 Thomas Hodgkin established the concept of lymphatic malignancy by describing pathologic lymphadenopathy and splenomegaly associated with lymphomatous disease.

By the 1920s the malignancies of the lymphoreticular system had been separated pathologically into Hodgkin's and non–Hodgkin's lymphomas. Hodgkin's disease is now recognized by the presence of the multinucleated Reed-Sternberg giant cell (Fig 1), but the exact cell of origin has not been conclusively determined. Current theories suggest T lymphocytes, macrophages, or reticulum cells as possible originating cells.

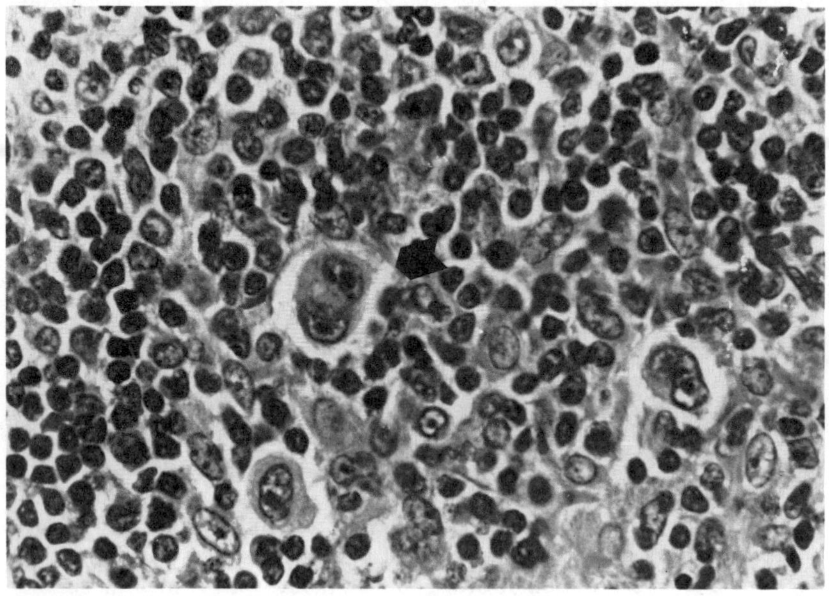

FIG 1.
Photomicrograph showing a typical multinucleated Reed-Sternberg cell.

Most non–Hodgkin's lymphomas derive from monoclonal populations of B lymphocytes; lymphoid malignancies of T-cell origin, such as mycosis fungoides, are less common.[1, 2] Cellular origin may be determined by a number of immunologic techniques, including immunofluorescence staining (Fig 2). Improvements in these diagnostic methods in recent years have provided information for classification of non–Hodgkin's lymphomas according to their cell of origin.

Several epidemiologic factors in lymphoma are known,[3] particularly those of the histologic subtype of nodular sclerosis in Hodgkin's disease. The demographic characteristics of patients with that disease are distinctly different from those who have other histological subtypes. Children of families with above-average incomes, high levels of education, and overall small family size are at slightly higher risk of nodular sclerosis Hodgkin's disease than children of larger, poorer families. Equally common among men and women, the disease has a higher incidence in industrial than in developing countries. Nodular sclerosis Hodgkin's disease is also the only histologic subtype of lymphoma with a distinct peak incidence in young adults.

Other subtypes of Hodgkin's disease share epidemiologic factors with non–Hodgkin's lymphoma in that age-specific rates increase throughout life, incidence has no strong association with socioeconomic status, and the disease subtypes occur more commonly in males.

Clinical Presentation

Usually a patient's first sign of lymphoma is the painless enlargement of peripheral lymph nodes. In most cases, the cervical lymph nodes are the first site, but the disease may first appear as axillary, inguinal, mediastinal, or retroperitoneal adenopathy.

Patients with mediastinal adenopathy are commonly diagnosed by routine chest radiography. Sometimes chronic cough or dyspnea caused by tracheobronchial compression secondary to mediastinal adenopathy is the first sign of malignant lymphoma. In the asymptomatic patient, abdominal lymphoma with splenomegaly or retroperitoneal adenopathy usually presents as a painless palpable abdominal mass. Splenomegaly may give rise to a constant dull ache in the left upper abdominal quadrant, whereas peritoneal adenopathy may cause lumbar back pain.

Unless axillary or inguinal adenopathy is detected early, the patient may develop edema and pain in the extremities. Extranodal abdominal involvement may give rise to intestinal perforation, bleeding, or obstruction requiring emergency surgical intervention.

Fever, night sweats, and weight loss are common when patients are first seen and are used to subclassify the patient's disease. The Pel-Ebstein type of fever is characterized by progressively shortening intervals between fever spikes, giving rise to a continuous fever. Anemia may develop with or

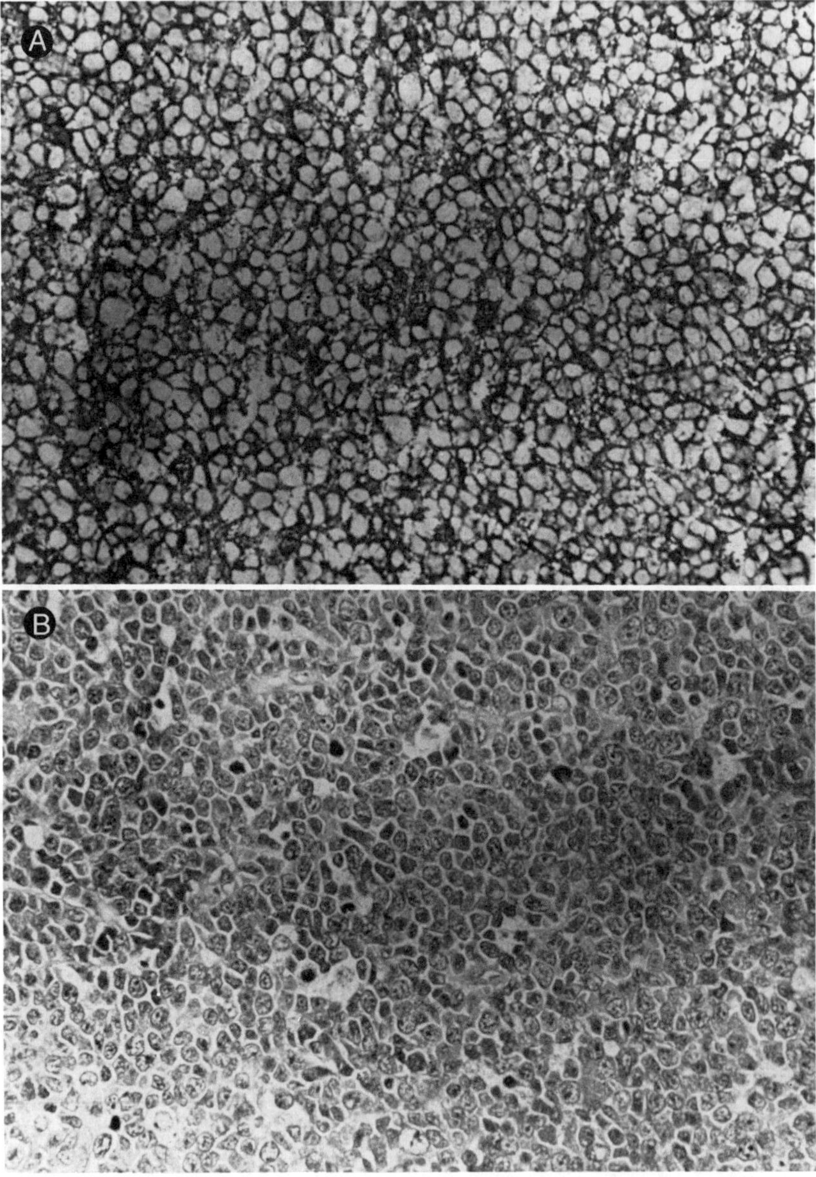

FIG 2.
A, immunofluorescent monotypic staining for the lambda chain of surface immunoglobulin in diffuse large-cell non–Hodgkin's lymphoma of B-cell origin. **B,** diffuse large-cell non–Hodgkin's lymphoma (hematoxylin-eosin ×250).

without the involvement of the bone marrow. Pruritus and malaise are common during the course of the disease.

Disease Characteristics

Some characteristics of the presentation of Hodgkin's disease are distinct from those of the non–Hodgkin's lymphomas. In contrast to the lymphatic involvement that is commonly localized in patients with Hodgkin's disease, those with non–Hodgkin's lymphoma often have widespread nodal disease. In addition, patients with non–Hodgkin's lymphoma commonly have involvement of the epitrochlear nodes and Waldeyer's ring, as well as testicular and GI areas, which are uncommon sites for Hodgkin's lymphoma. Patients with Hodgkin's disease most commonly present with localized cervical and mediastinal disease. Bone marrow involvement is also much more common in non–Hodgkin's than in Hodgkin's lymphoma, and this is true also for extranodal abdominal involvement.

Since Hodgkin's disease spreads by the contiguous involvement of adjacent lymph nodes, direct extension into adjacent visceral organs may occur. Splenic involvement, which is common early in the disease, is believed to be secondary to hematogenous dissemination involving the spleen. Whereas Hodgkin's disease has a propensity to remain confined to a limited area, non–Hodgkin's lymphoma tends to disseminate to extranodal sites.

The increasing incidence of immunodeficiency syndromes has been accompanied by higher incidence of lymphoma, often non–Hodgkin's lymphoma of a high-grade pathologic type and B-cell lymphocytic derivation. Penn[4] first noted that patients who underwent kidney transplantation were at 350-fold higher risk of developing lymphoma than the normal population. Subsequent reports[5, 6] confirmed the development of lymphoma in patients who underwent cardiac and bone marrow transplantations. These B-cell lymphomas have also been noted in patients with congenital immune deficiency disease such as Wiskott-Aldrich syndrome, ataxia-telangiectasia, and Sjögren's syndrome.

The development of high-grade B-cell lymphoma occurs also in patients with acquired immunodeficiency syndrome (AIDS), who commonly present with systemic symptoms and widespread disease. These are, in fact, distinguishing features of AIDS-related lymphoma. Patients with altered immune function more frequently develop lymphomas of the GI tract. A study at the University of Southern California[7] showed that 26% of patients had involvement of the GI tract, and an additional 10% had lymphomatous involvement of the liver. In patients with AIDS-related lymphoma the disease seems to be more aggressive than in the normal host. These immunocompromised patients with high-grade lymphomas of B-cell origin have a median survival of only about six months, and few have lived beyond two years.

Classification and Staging of Lymphoma

Although a consensus was reached with regard to the histologic classification of Hodgkin's disease, the classification of non–Hodgkin's lymphoma continues to be a controversial subject.

The currently accepted histologic classification of Hodgkin's disease is that of Lukes and Butler[8] as modified at the 1965 symposium held at Rye, New York, and therefore known as the Rye classification (Table 1).[8, 9] The classification is based on (1) the characteristics and numbers of Reed-Sternberg cells in relation to the other cellular elements, and (2) the pattern of connective tissue proliferation. Four subclassifications are identified: lymphocyte predominance, nodular sclerosis, mixed cellularity, and lymphocyte depletion. When Butler[10] evaluated the relationship of this histologic subgrouping to patient survival, he noted that patients with the lymphocyte-predominant type of lymphoma generally had the best prognosis. As staging techniques and multimodality therapy have improved, however, survival differences between patients with various histologic subtypes are no longer detectable.[11] Nevertheless, subtyping has allowed a more precise definition of the natural history of subsets of patients with Hodgkin's disease. Potential complications of proposed therapy can therefore be analyzed in the context of defined therapeutic efficacy. Thus, the potential risks and benefits of therapy are more accurately defined by the natural history of individual subsets of patients.

The histologic classification of non–Hodgkin's lymphoma remains a controversial subject, involving at least six different pathologic classifications developed in the last 20 years. Contributing to the controversy is a heter-

TABLE 1.
Histologic Classification of Hodgkin's Disease

Lukes and Butler Classification	Rye Modification
Lymphocyte predominance	Lymphocyte predominance
Diffuse lesion	
Nodular lesion	
Nodular sclerosis	Nodular sclerosis
Mixed cellularity	Mixed cellularity
Lymphocyte depletion	Lymphocyte depletion
Diffuse fibrosis	
Reticular-type fibrosis	

ogeneous population of lymphocytes that give rise to these lymphomas, each having a variety of cellular functions and morphologies. In addition, newer methods of diagnosis and classification (immunohistochemistry, flow cytometry, cytogenetics, and molecular genetics) have created a body of data yet to be effectively incorporated into the classification schema.

The first accepted classification proposed by Rappaport[12] was based primarily on morphologic features. As the immunological characteristics of lymphomas became clearer, Lukes and Collins[13] proposed a new classification system recognizing lymphomas as arising from either subsets of T or B lymphocytes. Lennert and co-workers[14] developed the Kiel system by subclassifying T- and B-cell neoplasms according to histologic grade of malignancy, thus adding a prognostic component to the classification of the system of Lukes and Collins. In view of the obvious difficulty in identifying and comparing treatment results among centers, the National Institutes of Health created the "working formulation."[15] This system divides non–Hodgkin's lymphomas into three major subsets according to degree of aggressiveness: low-grade, intermediate-grade, and high-grade lymphomas. The low-grade lymphomas include small lymphocytic, follicular small cleaved cell, and follicular-mixed cell types. The intermediate group comprises follicular large cell, diffuse small cleaved cell, diffuse mixed cell, and diffuse large cell types. The high-grade group includes lymphoblastic, small noncleaved cell, and immunoblastic lymphomas. In general, patients with the follicular (nodular) patterns and those patients having well-differentiated lymphocytic lymphomas have the better prognoses.

Although histologic classifications of subsets of both Hodgkin's disease and non–Hodgkin's lymphoma allow a better definition of the natural history of the disease, the most important factor in determining treatment is the patient's stage of disease. The most important contribution to staging has been the Ann Arbor classification.[16]

For both Hodgkin's disease and non–Hodgkin's lymphoma, clinical stage describes the findings of history and physical examination, initial laboratory evaluation, radiographic studies, and information obtained from the initial biopsy. Pathologic stage refers to information obtained from additional biopsies such as staging laparotomy. The extent of involvement, with regard to number of involved lymphatic regions, involvement of extralymphatic sites, and the presence or absence of systemic signs of disease (fever, night sweats, and weight loss) are the basis for the pathologic stage classification (Table 2). Patients who have no systemic symptoms or signs of disease are classified as A, and those with signs or symptoms of systemic involvement as B. The development of combination chemotherapy and precisely defined therapeutic strategies targeted to extent of disease as defined by this staging system, has made it possible to achieve ten-year survival rates of up to 90% of patients at stage I Hodgkin's disease and 60 to 70% at stage IV.

Because patients with non–Hodgkin's lymphoma are more likely than Hodgkin's patients to have widespread disease, the Ann Arbor staging sys-

TABLE 2.
Staging of Hodgkin's Disease*

Stage I. Involvement of a single lymph node region (I) or of a single extralymphatic organ or site (IE).

Stage II. Involvement of two or more lymph node regions on the same side of the diaphragm (II) or localized involvement of an extralymphatic organ or site and of one or more lymph node regions on the same side of the diaphragm (IIE).

Stage III. Involvement of lymph node regions on both sides of the diaphragm (III), which may also be accompanied by localized involvement of extralymphatic organs or sites (IIIE) or by involvement of the spleen (IIIS) or both (IIISE).

Stage IV. Diffuse or disseminated involvement of one or more extralymphatic organs or tissues with or without associated lymph node enlargement.

A—no systemic symptoms.
B—fever (>38°C), night sweats, or weight loss.

*From Carbone PP, Kaplan HS, Musshof K, et al: Report of the Committee on Hodgkin's disease staging classification. *Cancer Res* 1971; 31:1860–1861. Used by permission.

tem, although extended to non–Hodgkin's lymphoma, is not nearly as useful for these patients. Moreover, older patients with non–Hodgkin's lymphoma have a higher incidence of systemic involvement and relatively few indications for staging laparotomy. Staging laparotomy in these patients is limited to answering specific management questions concerning individual patients.

Surgical Biopsy of Enlarged Nodes

Certain surgical principles regarding the initial biopsy in patients suspected of having lymphoma are especially important in providing definitive diagnosis. These include: (1) selection of the appropriate biopsy site, (2) of the individual lymph node, (3) complete removal of the suspicious node, and (4) careful surgical technique.

When multiple lymphatic nodal regions are available for excisional biopsy, either a lower cervical or axillary node should be chosen. Lymph nodes in regions of the parotid gland, the submandibular gland, and the inguinal nodal basin are often enlarged by chronic inflammatory processes, and they may be biopsied under the mistaken impression that they represent the patient's disease process. Because large lymph nodes are more likely to be involved with lymphoma than small nodes, the removal of several accessible large nodes is advisable; if there is only one enlarged lymph node, it should be removed for examination.

Removal of a lymph node for detailed pathologic interpretation requires minimal manipulation of the node and maintenance of capsular integrity. Unnecessary distortion or transection of the lymph node disturbs nodal architecture and normal anatomical structures, and it may make pathologic interpretation impossible in some cases (Fig 3). Even the minor trauma of pinching and pulling with tissue forceps introduces artifact. Distortions of this kind may require another biopsy examination, which in turn will delay the beginning of definitive therapy and increase the chance of local wound complications. In the mediastinum or abdominal cavity, a rebiopsy represents a major reoperation.

Meticulous hemostasis is necessary after biopsy to prevent postoperative hematomas and seromas. Afferent and efferent lymphatic vessels should be ligated with sutures to prevent the development of lymphatic fistula and accumulation of chyle. Careful attention to hemostasis obviates the need for drainage catheters.

The frozen section technique should be requested only if the surgeon does not suspect lymphoma. Frozen sections interfere with the pathologic diagnosis of lymphoma (Fig 4). Because they cannot be cut thin enough to allow adequate pathologic interpretation, they do not define cytologic features clearly, and they do not yield satisfactory information by the paraffin-embedded technique after freezing. Thus, the distinction between benign and malignant pathologic entities may be confounded by frozen section.

The need to analyze surface markers should be determined preoperatively to expedite processing of the specimen. Specimens should not be blotted or placed on a dry sponge because dehydration of the surface produces an artifact that interferes with interpretation. The specimen should be placed in a petri dish containing saline and delivered immediately to the pathologist.

An intact node allows for a variety of pathologic examinations. The pathologist bisects the fresh node, and, if infection is a probable cause of adenopathy, sends half the node for appropriate bacterial, fungal, and tuberculus culturing. Imprint preparations, cell suspensions, cryostat sections, and fixative specimens are prepared from the remaining nodal tissue. Slides of imprints showing how the cells look in a cytologic preparation give the pathologist a general idea of the proportions of different types of cells in the node. Cytochemical stains of these imprints may identify particular cell types. Cell suspensions are used for surface marker and chromosome studies. Using specific antibodies to individual cell markers lymphoid and other cells found in lymph reticular tissues may be phenotyped. Cytogenetic studies of cell suspensions may detect chromosome aberrations. Frozen section of a portion of the node may allow rapid diagnosis and is also used for enzyme histochemical and immunohistochemical studies; the

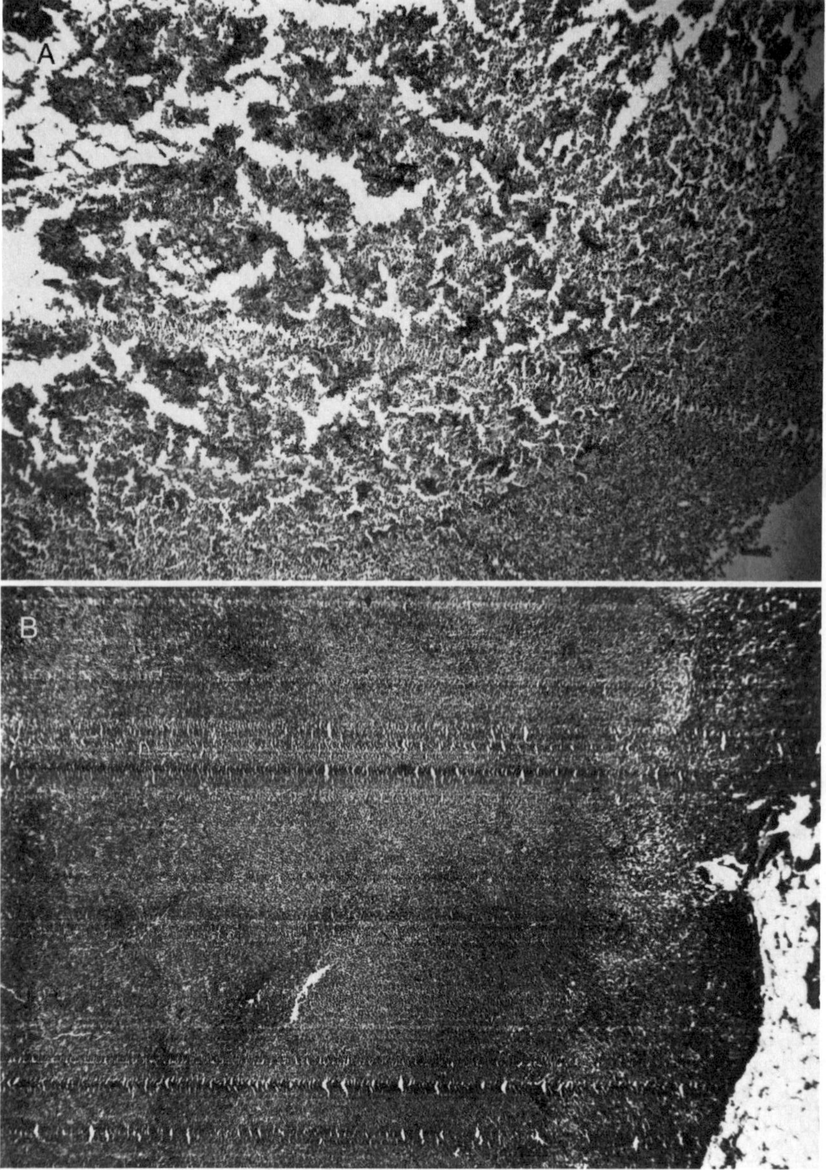

FIG 3.
A, lymph node fragmentation and distortion induced at surgical biopsy; **B,** intact lymph node.

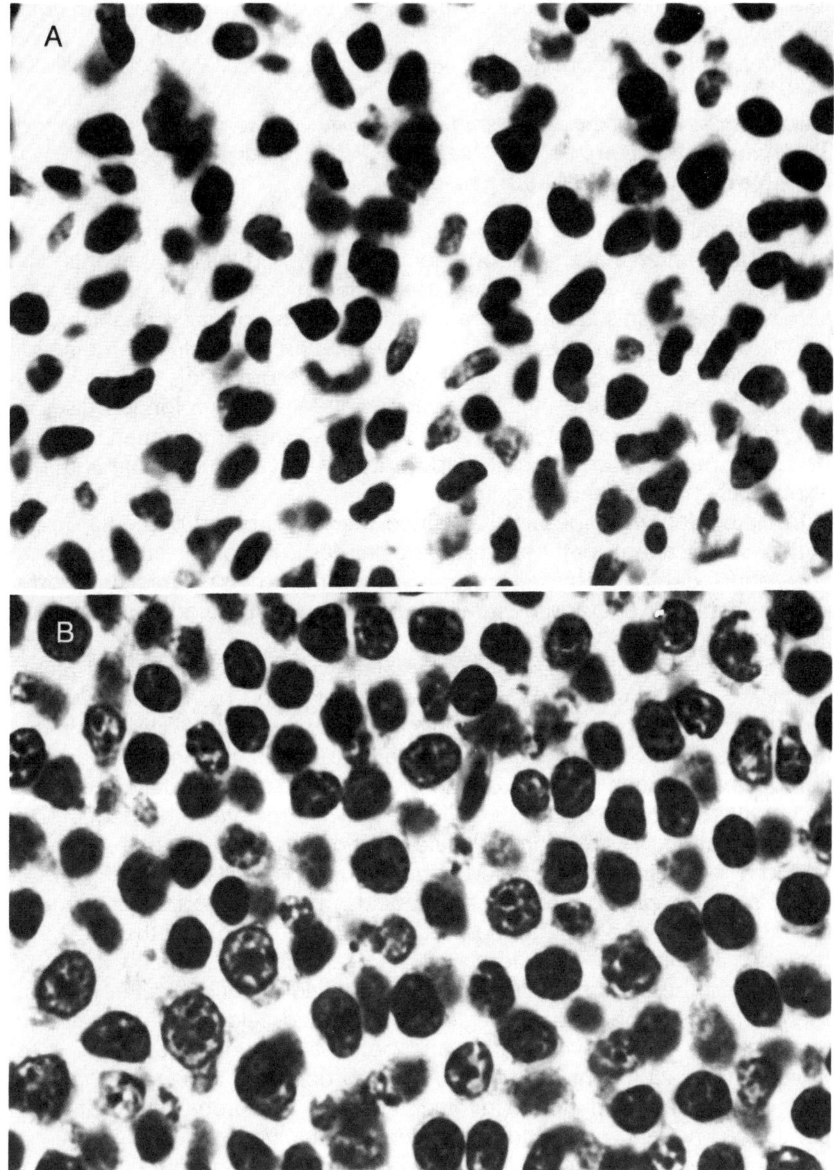

FIG 4.
A, frozen section with distorted nuclear configuration and obscured chromatin pattern; **B,** hematoxylin-eosin, ×250.

remaining nodal tissue is placed in fixative solutions. A small (<2 mm) portion is placed in glutaraldehyde for electron microscopy, and the remainder is placed in formalin for paraffin embedding.

Treatment Strategies for Patients With Hodgkin's and Non–Hodgkin's Lymphoma

The national mortality of Hodgkin's disease has fallen more rapidly than that of any other malignant condition. In 1955, virtually all patients with advanced Hodgkin's disease died. By 1986, about 60% of patients with advanced Hodgkin's disease were being cured. This progress was achieved largely by modern radiotherapy and the evolution of effective combination chemotherapy.[17–19] Even patients developing recurrent disease when radiation therapy was the initial treatment now achieve prolonged disease-free survival with combination chemotherapy. Furthermore, patients who have recurrence after chemotherapy may be salvaged with the same or another chemotherapeutic regimen.

Implementation of specifically defined therapy is based primarily on the patient's clinical and pathologic stage of disease. Histologic subtype, location, and extent of disease, presence or absence of systemic symptoms, and the patient's age and general medical condition are additional factors in choosing therapy.

Patients with limited disease are treated with radiation therapy alone, the doses usually varying between 3,500 and 4,500 rad. "Mantle" refers to radiation therapy given to the neck, chest, and axilla. This technique allows the nodes of the axilla, neck, and mediastinum to be treated in continuity. Although a large volume of normal tissue is irradiated, modern techniques have minimized complications while maintaining adequate tumor irradiation. The abdominal field of radiation may be that of an inverted Y overlying the para-aortic and parailiac vessels, or it may be divided separate para-aortic and pelvic fields. The para-aortic field may be extended laterally to include the portahepatis on the right or the spleen on the left. "Total nodal radiation" refers to radiation delivered to both the mantle and the abdominal fields. "Involved field radiation" refers to treatment of only defined disease regions. "Extended field radiation" refers to treatment of the involved region and potentially involved contiguous regions. The exact extent of radiation therapy delivered depends on the extent of demonstrated nodal involvement and the probability that other contiguous nodal groups and the spleen are involved.

Patients with advanced Hodgkin's disease are treated with combination chemotherapy. In addition, for patients who had a relapse after radiation therapy, combination chemotherapy has been shown to produce prolonged remissions. Targeting therapy specifically to extent of disease is important because more extensive therapy may result in iatrogenic complications.

The most important complications include development of a second neoplasm and loss of fertility.[20–22] Acute nonlymphocytic leukemia is the most common malignancy occurring after treatment for Hodgkin's lymphoma. The combination of chemotherapy and radiation is associated with greater risk of a second neoplasm than either treatment alone. In addition, patients have an increased risk of developing solid tumors within the radiation portals. Both men and women may become infertile as a result of pelvic irradiation or combination chemotherapy. In women who are to be treated with postoperative pelvic irradiation, repositioning of the ovaries to the midline may preserve fertility. In children, in whom radiation may cause growth-related abnormalities in bone and soft tissues, radiation doses may be reduced and combined with chemotherapy to obviate these side effects.

Like Hodgkin's lymphomas, non–Hodgkin's lymphomas are also treated according to stage of disease. They are, however, a much more heterogeneous group of lymphoproliferative malignancies, with a variety of behavior patterns and a spectrum of treatment responses. Histologic subtyping may play a greater role in determining therapy than in Hodgkin's lymphoma. Follicular (nodular) lymphomas are often indolent in nature. They respond to chemotherapy but tend to recur more frequently than other subtypes, such as diffuse lymphoma, which are more aggressive. The indolent follicular lymphomas may eventually convert into a more aggressive subtype.

Although a few patients with localized nodal presentations of non–Hodgkin's lymphoma may be treated with radiation techniques only, patients with unfavorable cell types will require chemotherapy or combined chemotherapy and radiotherapy. The radiation dose usually varies between 3,500 and 4,500 rads. In addition, patients who have indolent forms of extranodal non–Hodgkin's lymphoma (stage IE) may be treated successfully with surgery alone. The use of chemotherapy in patients with early stages of non–Hodgkin's lymphoma is determined by the probability of systemic disease as predicted by stage of disease at presentation, cell type, and anatomic site of origin.

Patients with advanced intermediate-grade non–Hodgkin's lymphoma are best treated with chemotherapy alone, with radiotherapy reserved for those with residual abnormalities after maximal response. All patients with high-grade lymphomas should receive intensive chemotherapy to achieve optimal results.

Clinical Staging of Hodgkin's Disease

After the patient has undergone biopsy to determine the diagnosis of Hodgkin's disease, a detailed evaluation to determine stage of disease is next. As with the staging of any malignancy, history and physical examination is the cornerstone on which accurate clinical staging is based. Particular attention to the patient's symptoms of fever, weight loss, and night sweats is required to determine subclassification.

The physical examination should include all lymph node–bearing areas, including Waldeyer's ring. The adenopathy of Hodgkin's disease is characterized in most patients by a smooth, rubbery, firm nodularity with involvement of multiple contiguous nodes. Potential sites of involvement such as the liver and spleen should be palpated and any enlargement noted. Examining sites of pain for tenderness may help identify metastatic disease. Initial diagnostic laboratory studies should include a complete blood count with a differential and liver function tests (alkaline phosphatase, serum glutamic-oxaloacetic transaminase, serum glutamic-pyruvic transaminase, and bilirubin). All patients should have an initial chest radiograph, including posterior-anterior and lateral projections to assess mediastinal and lung involvement (Fig 5).

The use of lymphangiography and computed tomography (CT) is determined by the patient's stage and site of disease. Lymphangiography has proved particularly reliable in assessing the femoral, inguinal, external iliac, common iliac, and para-aortic nodes to approximately the level of the second lumbar vertebra (Fig 6). Although the false-negative rate of lymphangiography is low, sometimes, however, a patient whose lymphangiogram was negative will be found at surgery to have Hodgkin's disease in nodes. In patients with negative lymphangiograms, therefore, staging laparotomy is used as the definitive diagnostic modality to determine the status of ab-

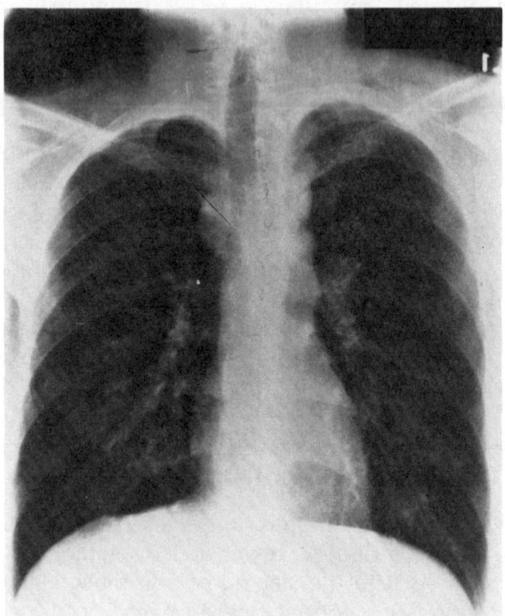

FIG 5.
Mediastinal widening secondary to adenopathy of Hodgkin's lymphoma.

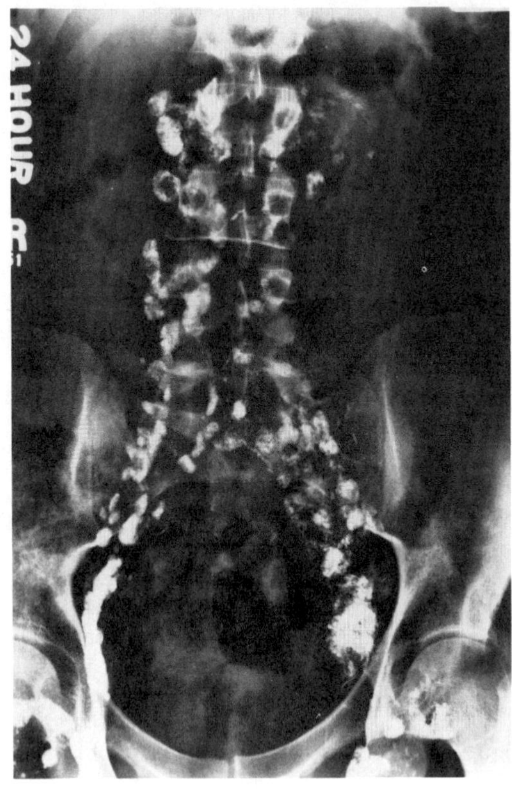

FIG 6.
Lymphangiogram showing foamy appearance of enlarged lymph nodes in Hodgkin's lymphoma.

dominal involvement. A lymphangiogram suggestive of Hodgkin's disease is almost always confirmed by staging laparotomy.

Computed tomography scanning is used also to stage Hodgkin's disease and is especially effective in detecting the presence of mediastinal involvement. In patients who have non–Hodgkin's disease, CT scans are used as an aid in staging the abdomen, because a significant number of patients with non–Hodgkin's lymphoma have extranodal disease outside nodes imaged by lymphangiography. Gallium 67 scans have been used to detect abdominal lymphoma, but their usefulness is controversial.[23] The use of percutaneous bone marrow aspiration, percutaneous liver biopsy, intravenous pyelography, and staging laparotomy is dictated by the patient's disease presentation and initial pattern of disease distribution.

Recent advances in both immunology and molecular biology have found application in the evaluation of lymphoma. Monoclonal antibodies have been used both diagnostically and therapeutically. Monoclonal antibodies that bind Reed-Sternberg cells have been produced and characterized.[24] They may eventually prove useful in diagnosis and staging and also as a potential new therapeutic modality. In addition, this technique may prove useful in determining the exact cell of origin of the Reed-Sternberg cell.

Monoclonal antibodies have been employed diagnostically to detect small numbers of persistent abnormal lymphoid clones in patients in apparent remission. Unique idiotypic determinants expressed by the surface immunoglobulin on the malignant B lymphocytes in patients with nodular lymphoma have been targeted therapeutically by monoclonal antibodies as well.[25]

Staging Laparotomy for Patients With Hodgkin's Lymphoma

Indications

Surgical staging of patients with Hodgkin's lymphoma has been an important component of the pretreatment evaluation. Associated with virtually no mortality and an acceptable morbidity, the procedure has contributed to accurate diagnosis and treatment planning. Glatstein et al.[26] described staging laparotomy almost 20 years ago, yet its potential usefulness is still being debated.[26–29] Scientific reevaluations have generated institutional policies on the use of staging laparotomy that vary from outright proscription to high selectivity. Defined operative risk, degree of probability that the procedure would change the preoperative stage of disease, and the relative toxicities of chemotherapy and radiation are factors evaluated in selecting patients for staging laparotomy.

A multifactorial analysis of factors predicting risk of abdominal disease in Hodgkin's lymphoma in 255 patients at the University of Alabama revealed certain predictors of abdominal disease.[30] These included number of symptoms, histologic subtype, and gender. Patients with more than two symptoms (fever, night sweats, weight loss, and pruritus) were noted to have a higher risk of abdominal involvement. Those with nodular sclerosis and lymphocyte-predominant subtypes had a lower risk than those patients with subtypes characterized by either mixed cellularity or lymphocyte depletion. In addition, women had a lower risk for abdominal disease than men.

With these prognostic factors a statistical approach was designed to estimate probability of abdominal involvement (Table 3). Three groups of patients could be identified. A low-risk group who might be treated with radiation therapy alone and without staging laparotomy included asymptomatic patients with lymphocyte-predominant and nodular sclerosis subsets (especially women) at stage I or stage II disease. The estimated probability of abdominal disease ranged from 6% to 19% in this group. Johnson and colleagues[19] also suggested that, in patients with stage I and stage II disease with nodular sclerosis, the risk of distant disease was suffi-

TABLE 3.
Probability of Abdominal Disease in 194 Lymphoma Patients (Clinical Stage I and II)*†

Disease	No. of Symptoms		One Symptom		> Two Symptoms	
Subtype	Women(%)	Men(%)	Women(%)	Men(%)	Women(%)	Men(%)
NS	6	14	16	33	36	60
LP	8	19	21	41	44	67
MC	20	39	42	66	69	85
LD	36	60	63	82	84	93

*From Trotter MC, Gretchen AC, Davis M, et al: Predicting the risk of abdominal disease in Hodgkin's lymphoma. *Ann Surg* 1985; 201:465–469. Used by permission.
†NS = nodular sclerosis; LP = lymphocyte predominance; MC = mixed cellularity; LD = lymphocyte depletion.

ciently low that they should be treated with radiation and not undergo a staging laparotomy. Thus, the morbidity of staging laparotomy was eliminated in selected patients identified by defined prognostic factors.

A high-risk group, in whom the probability of abdominal disease ranged from 69 to 93%, was identified. These patients could be assumed to have distant disease, and they required more intensive treatment regimens. The group included symptomatic patients with lymphocyte-depletion cellularity (especially men), and patients with two or three symptoms and mixed cellularity, especially males.

In the third subgroup—of intermediate-risk patients—no significant prognostic factors could be determined for abdominal involvement. The recommendation, therefore, was that these patients undergo staging laparotomy to define the presence and exact extent of disease. Accurate staging allows the physician to select minimum curative therapy. Moreover, after staging laparotomy and splenectomy, the portal of radiation can be decreased.

Technique

The technique of staging laparotomy is based on knowledge of the sites of abdominal involvement likely to develop during natural progression of the disease. In patients presenting with mediastinal disease, specific areas of abdominal nodes are more likely to be involved, including the celiac and portal lymphatic groups (Fig 7). Consideration of the probability of abdominal involvement and the assessment and maintenance of adequate hemostasis provide a logical sequence for abdominal exploration and biopsy.

Staging laparotomy is done through a midline incision extending from

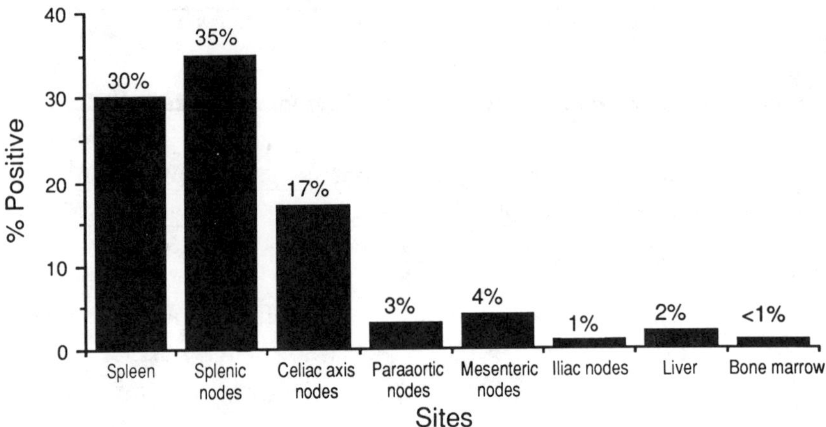

FIG 7.
Positive findings at laparotomy for patients with upper-torso Hodgkin's disease.

immediately below the xyphoid process to immediately below the umbilicus (Fig 8). Abdominal viscera and peritoneal surfaces are explored in a systematic fashion. As a first step, the liver is examined, and obvious, accessible lesions are excised or biopsied along with a rim of normal liver tissue. Needle biopsy samples taken from both lobes of the liver and a wedge biopsy sample of the edge of either lobe are sent for pathologic sectioning. A laparotomy pad is placed over biopsy sites to compress the liver and aid in hemostasis while other potential sites of involvement are assessed.

The spleen and splenic hilar lymph nodes are then removed en bloc. The splenic pedicle is marked with metallic clips after the splenic artery and vein have been ligated. This marking of surgical extent allows radiation therapy to be directed through limited portals, possibly minimizing the complications of radiation-induced nephritis and pneumonitis.

Lymph nodes affected by Hodgkin's disease are often normal in size and appearance, which makes simple palpation inadequate. Histologic examination is the only reliable means of diagnosis and requires excisional biopsy.

Hodgkin's disease usually originates above the diaphragm and extends inferiorly to contiguous lymph nodes. Exploration of potentially involved nodal basins therefore begins in the celiac and portal nodal basin, unless a CT scan or lymphangiogram has shown more inferiorly located suspected nodes.

The gastrohepatic ligament is opened along the superior aspect of the lesser curve of the stomach, and the lesser sac is entered for excision of the nodes along the hepatic artery. Dissection begins at the origin of the gastroduodenal artery, with nodes along the hepatic artery excised en bloc

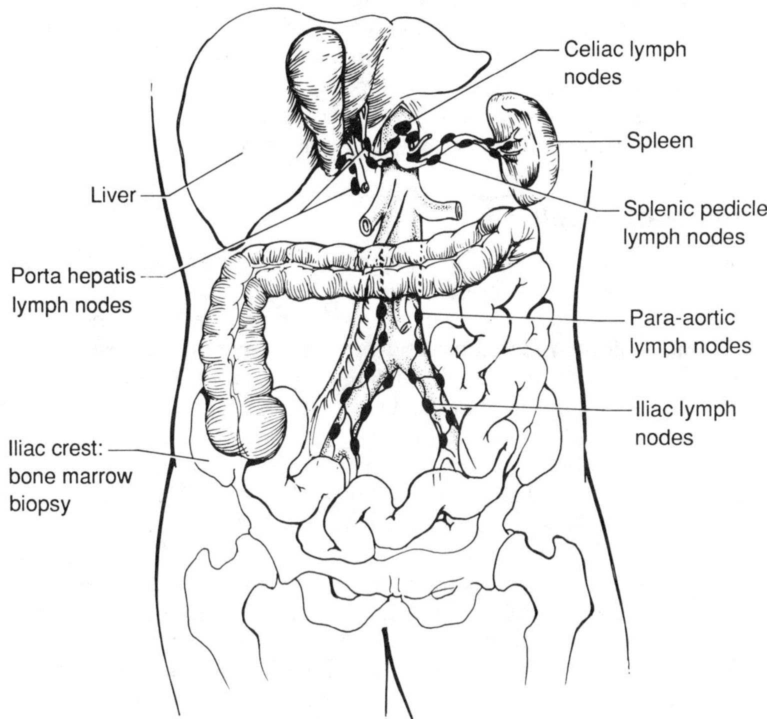

FIG 8.
Sites of biopsy in staging laparotomy.

as the celiac axis is approached. The so-called sentinel cystic duct node, which lies along the distal common bile duct, is then removed, as are other enlarged or suspected nodes of the gastrohepatic ligament.

The transverse colon is then retracted cephalad to approach the para-aortic nodes. The small bowel and its mesentery are reflected to the patient's right, exposing the ligament of Treitz and the retroperitoneum. The peritoneum is incised lateral to the aorta as the inferior mesenteric vein is preserved. Para-aortic nodes from the level of the left renal vein to the origin of the inferior mesenteric artery are excised en bloc. Metallic clips are used for hemostasis at sites of lymph node biopsy and serve as markers for postoperative radiography. Then the parailiac nodes are biopsied. If a bone marrow biopsy examination was not done preoperatively, this type of excision completes the biopsy procedure.

In women of child-bearing age whose fertility would be damaged by the inverted Y abdominal field of radiation, the ovaries are relocated to a low midline position to remove them from the portal of radiation.[31] In patients who have not had an appendectomy, the appendix is removed. This should be considered before the operation and the patient given antibiotics perioperatively to reduce the risk of subcutaneous wound infection. If appendectomy is not expected antibiotic prophylaxis is not necessary. At the end of the operation, packs from the sites of liver biopsy and splenectomy are removed and potential bleeding sites evaluated.

Results and Complications

Staging laparotomy is a valuable diagnostic procedure when its application is limited to patients for whom a minimal risk of morbidity and mortality can be achieved. Taylor and colleagues[29] reported a 9.6% incidence of major complications, most consisting of wound and upper respiratory infections. Only one death occurred in that series of 825 patients who underwent the procedure at Stanford University between 1968 and 1980.[29] Complications included wound infection (21 patients), wound dehiscence (4), pulmonary embolus (1), pneumonia (3), systemic infection (2), subphrenic abscess (2), and small-bowel obstruction (4). Of 371 patients with stage I and II Hodgkin's disease operated on at M. D. Anderson Hospital, 45 patients developed immediate postoperative complications, nine of which were potentially life-threatening.[32] The severe postoperative complications included systemic infection, subphrenic abscess, abdominal hemorrhage, myocardial infarction, and intussusception; one patient died because of myocardial infarction. Delayed complications occurred in four patients who developed bowel obstruction secondary to adhesions and in three patients who developed pneumococcal infections. One patient died from the delayed complication of meningococcal meningitis.

The usefulness of staging laparotomy is determined primarily by the number of patients whose preoperative clinical stage is changed by operative intervention. Evaluating the 12-year Stanford record of 825 staging laparotomies, Taylor and colleagues[29] found that the procedure caused preoperative clinical stage to be changed in 43.2% of patients. At M.D. Anderson Hospital, of 371 patients who underwent staging laparotomy for stage I and II Hodgkin's disease, 33% who had had negative results on lymphangiograms were found to have abdominal involvement, as was true for the Stanford group.

Staging laparotomy identified a subgroup of stage IIIA patients who would benefit from more extensive therapy. Since 1966, M. D. Anderson Hospital patients have received various combinations of multiagent chemotherapy in addition to radiotherapy, with excellent results for all patients with stage III disease. The Stanford group has also reported improved survival rates for patients with stage III disease who received chemotherapy and radiotherapy. The staging laparotomy is, therefore, an important tool for determining therapy in patients who had a negative lymphangiogram but may harbor occult abdominal disease. Because it provides evaluation of the spleen, splenic nodes, and celiac and portal nodes, staging laparotomy may allow patients to be treated with mantle or involved field radiation alone, thus maintaining a low rate of abdominal relapse and avoiding the morbidity of more extensive radiotherapy.

The accuracy of the staging laparotomy depends on the successful sampling of potentially involved nodal groups (see Figs 7 and 8). Most important sites for staging include the spleen, splenic nodes, and celiac and portal nodes. Of 361 patients undergoing staging laparotomy for upper-torso Hodgkin's disease at M. D. Anderson Hospital, 30% were found to have involvement of the spleen. Splenic nodes were found to be involved in 35% of patients whose nodes were biopsied. An additional 17% of patients were found to have involvement of the celiac axis nodes or the nodes of the hepatoduodenal ligament. One of the most useful nodes in terms of abdominal staging is the so-called "sentinel node" at the junction of the distal common bile duct and duodenum. Ease of accessibility makes this particular node a useful site for biopsy. Para-aortic, mesenteric, iliac, liver biopsy, and bone marrow biopsy were all found to be positive in less than 5% of cases. Thus, the celiac-portal complex contains nodes that can be biopsied easily with patients having negative lymphangiograms found to have a much higher incidence of positive findings in these regions. Failure to obtain biopsies from these areas results in false-negative laparotomies and an increased risk of recurrent disease as a result of limited therapy dictated by inaccurate staging.

Restaging Laparotomy

Patients who have persistent or recurrent disease after a course of radiotherapy or chemotherapy may benefit from further treatment. Systematic restaging following therapy should be incorporated, therefore, into the management of all patients with lymphoma. The restaging examination will define remission and identify patients whose disease is either persistent or recurrent and who should undergo further treatment. Repeat chest radiography, lymphangiography, and gallium scans may be helpful. In selected patients with Hodgkin's disease, restaging may identify those with residual lymphoma who require further therapy,[33] and it may also identify those who require no further therapy and will therefore be spared its potential side effects.

The value of posttreatment staging laparotomy remains to be clearly defined in terms of types of patients most likely to benefit from the procedure. Patients who have completed therapy but are suspected of having residual disease seem to be appropriate candidates, whereas asymptomatic patients in apparently complete remission are less likely to benefit from restaging. As it is currently viewed, restaging laparotomy should be done according to research protocols so that subsets of patients benefiting from the procedure may be clearly identified.

Surgical Aspects of Non–Hodgkin's Lymphoma

Staging Laparotomy for Patients With Non–Hodgkin's Lymphoma

Although staging laparotomy was once used to determine the extent of disease in patients with non–Hodgkin's lymphoma, it is seldom done today in these cases. Staging laparotomy has yielded little information for treatment of these patients, and, since most of them are older than patients with Hodgkin's lymphoma, the procedure carries a higher operative risk. At M. D. Anderson Hospital, therefore, staging laparotomy is done only in a few young patients with this disease, those whose lymphangiograms are negative, and have follicular (nodular) lymphomas of the upper torso. Our treatment approach is to give more therapy to patients with abdominal involvement.

Extranodal Lymphoma

The role of surgery for and management of patients with extranodal non–Hodgkin's lymphoma is both diagnostic and therapeutic. For disease at most abdominal sites, surgery and radiotherapy provide satisfactory local control for patients with stage IE tumors. In patients with stage IIE disease, local therapy alone has yielded a five-year survival rate of only 20% to 40%. The diminished survival rate, with death ultimately the result of systemic failure, provides the rationale for adjuvant chemotherapy in patients with locally advanced disease.

In addition, because some anatomic sites—the extrahepatic biliary system, the skin, breast, and testes—are more likely to harbor occult systemic disease, systemic therapy should be considered for patients who present with apparent early disease.[34–36]

Gastric Lymphoma

The most common site of origin of primary GI lymphoma and the site with the best prognosis is the stomach.[37–40] Patients who have gastic lymphoma usually present with vague abdominal pain during their fifth to sixth decade. Diagnostic studies are often inconclusive, although endoscopic examination has improved their accuracy somewhat. Thus it is not uncommon to encounter gastric lymphoma first during an operation. However, because few characteristics at operation distinguish gastric lymphoma from other pathologic conditions, diagnosis is determined postoperatively in many patients.

Primary therapy for gastric lymphoma has been surgical resection. Treatment by radiation alone has yielded poor results in terms of long-term survival. Current surgical therapy consists of partial or total gastrectomy with en-bloc removal of involved nodes. The use of radiation after curative resection is a controversial issue because high-dose radiation with 4,500 to 5,000 rads to the upper abdomen is associated with potentially significant complications and limited therapeutic efficacy. Nevertheless, the low survival rate of patients with locally advanced lymphoma after surgical resection alone requires consideration of postoperative radiation and chemotherapy.

Recently, combination chemotherapy and radiation therapy have been used as primary therapy for stage IE and IIE patients with gastric lymphoma at M. D. Anderson Hospital and Tumor Institute. Treatment results for 35 patients showed disease-free survival equivalent to historical controls treated by surgery.[41]

Primary Lymphomas of the Small Intestine

Extranodal lymphomas arising in the small bowel may cause obstruction, bleeding, and perforation. As in the case of gastric lymphomas, extensive diagnostic evaluations often prove inconclusive. For patients with stage IE disease, which is localized to the bowel wall, surgical resection alone is likely to be sufficient, although adjunctive radiation or combination chemotherapy may be considered and weighed against defined associated risk factors. A number of clinical syndromes have been described in which primary lymphomas of the small intestine are characterized according to clinical, pathologic, geographic, and sociologic features. Subclassifications include "Western" lymphoma, "Mediterranean" lymphoma, and childhood abdominal malignant lymphomas. Consideration of variants in behavior among these subclassifications will influence decisions concerning adjuvant radiation and chemotherapy.

Other Sites

Pancreatic

Lymphoma may occur as a pancreatic mass or with symptoms of biliary tract obstruction.[42] These lesions, arising in the lymph nodes, are therefore not truly extranodal lymphomas. The surgeon considering such pancreatic masses for treatment must consider lymphoma as an etiology because surgery has no role in the definitive therapy of these lesions.

Colonic

Primary colonic lymphomas are rare; typically they are large, bulky ulcerated lesions extending over long segments of colon.[43] As it is for other extranodal abdominal lymphomas, operative extirpation with resection of the involved bowel is the primary therapy. For locally advanced lesions, postoperative radiotherapy and chemotherapy are considered as adjuvant treatment or, if the lesions are unresectable, as primary therapy.

Breast

In a high percentage of patients who present with apparent early disease, primary malignant lymphomas of the breast show evidence of systemic disease.[35] These patients require careful clinical staging. The primary breast lesion may be successfully treated by biopsy and postoperative irradiation. Combination chemotherapy is particularly useful for patients with unfavorable histologic subtypes.

Thyroid

Extranodal lymphomas presenting in the thyroid gland become evident somewhat differently than does thyroid carcinoma. A diffuse enlargement of the gland with or without associated thyroiditis is common at first. The majority of patients with this condition are elderly women, in whom localized thyroid lymphoma may be treated with radiotherapy alone. More extensive disease requires the addition of combination chemotherapy.[44]

Summary

Improvements in histologic classification, staging, and multimodality therapy have dramatically changed the natural history of patients with lymphoma. Systematic staging accurately defines the extent of disease and minimizes the toxic effects of excessive treatment. Surgical diagnosis and staging with laparotomy provide the basis for choosing methods of definitive radiotherapy and chemotherapy for selected patients. Patients with extranodal disease in early stages may be treated effectively by surgical excision.

References

1. Order SE, Hellman S: Pathogenesis of Hodgkin's disease. *Lancet* 1972; 1:571–573.
2. Seligmann M, Brouet JC, Preud'homme JL: The immunological diagnosis of human leukemias and lymphomas: An overview, in Thierfelder S, Rudt H (eds): *Immunobiological Diagnosis of Leukemias and Lymphomas.* New York, Springer-Verlag, 1977.
3. Ross RK, Dworsky RL, Paganini-Hill A, et al: The epidemiology of lymphoma, in Pattengale PK, Lukes RJ, Taylor CR (eds): *Lymphoproliferative Disease: Pathogenesis, Diagnosis.* Dordrecht, Martinus-Nijhoff, 1985, pp 55–71.
4. Penn I: Kaposi's sarcoma in organ transplant recipients: Report of 20 cases. *Transplantation* 1979; 27:8–11.
5. Matas AH, Hertel BF, Rosai J, et al: Post-transplant malignant lymphoma. *Am J Med* 1976; 61:716–720.
6. Gossett TC, Gale RP, Fleischman H, et al: Immunoblastic sarcoma in donor cells after bone-marrow transplantation. *N Engl J Med* 1979; 300:904–907.

7. Ross RK, Dworsky RL, Paganini-Hill A, et al: Non-Hodgkin's lymphomas in never married men in Los Angeles. *Br J Cancer* 1985; 52:785–797.
8. Lukes RJ, Butler J: The pathology and nomenclature of Hodgkin's disease. *Cancer Res* 1966; 26:1063–1081.
9. Lukes RJ, Carver LF, Hall TC, et al: Report of the Nomenclature Committee. *Cancer Res* 1966; 26:1311.
10. Butler JJ: Relationship of histologic findings to survival and Hodgkin's disease. *Cancer Res* 1971; 31:1770–1775.
11. Fuller LM, Madoc-Jones H, Gamble JF, et al: New assessment of the prognostic significance of histopathology in Hodgkin's disease for laparotomy-negative stage I and II patients. *Cancer* 1977; 39:2174–2182.
12. Rappaport H: Tumors of the hemopoietic system, in *Atlas of Tumor Pathology*. Washington, DC, Armed Forces Institute of Pathology, 1966, section 3, pt 8.
13. Lukes RJ, Collins RD: Lukes-Collins classification and its significance. *Cancer Treat Rep* 1977; 61:971–979.
14. Lennert K, Stein H, Kaiserling B: Cytological and functional criteria for the classification of malignant lymphoma. *Br J Cancer* 1975; 31(suppl 2):29–43.
15. National Cancer Institute: The non-Hodgkin's lymphoma pathological classification project: National Cancer Institute-sponsored study of classifications of non-Hodgkin's lymphomas. *Cancer* 1982; 49:2112–2135.
16. Carbone PP, Kaplan HS, Musshof K, et al: Report of the Committee on Hodgkin's disease staging classification. *Cancer Res* 1971; 31:1860–1861.
17. DeVita VT, Serpick AA, Carbone PP: Combination chemotherapy in the treatment of advanced Hodgkin's disease. *Ann Intern Med* 1970; 73(6):881–895.
18. DeVita VT, Simon RM, Hubbard SM, et al: Curability of advanced Hodgkin's disease with chemotherapy: Long-term follow-up of MOPP-treated patients at NCI. *Ann Intern Med* 1980; 92:587–595.
19. Johnson RE, Simber H, Bernard CW, et al: Radiotherapy results for nodular sclerosis Hodgkin's disease after clinical staging. *Cancer* 1977; 39:1439–1444.
20. Valagussa P, Santoro A, Fossati-Bellani F, et al: Second acute leukemia and other malignancies following treatment for Hodgkin's disease. *J Clin Oncol* 1986; 4:830–837.
21. Coleman CN: Secondary malignancy after treatment of Hodgkin's disease: An evolving picture. *J Clin Oncol* 1986; 4:821–824.
22. Horning SJ, Hoppe RT, Kaplan HE, et al: Female reproductive potential after treatment for Hodgkin's disease. *N Engl J Med* 1981; 304:1377–1382.
23. Turner DA, Fordham AA, Slayton RE: Gallium-67 imaging in the management of Hodgkin's disease and other malignant lymphomas. *Semin Nucl Med* 1978; 8:205–218.
24. Hecht TT, Longo DL, Cossman J, et al: Production and characterization of a monoclonal antibody that binds Reed-Sternberg cells. *J Immunol* 1985; 134:4231–4236.
25. Matis LA, Young RC, Longo DL: Nodular lymphomas: Current concepts. *CRC Crit Rev Oncol Hematol* 1986; 5:171–197.
26. Glatstein E, Gurnsey JM, Rosenberg SA, et al: The value of laparotomy and splenectomy in the staging of Hodgkin's disease. *Cancer* 1969; 24:709–718.
27. Johnson RE: Is staging laparotomy routinely indicated in Hodgkin's disease? *Ann Intern Med* 1971; 75:459–462.
28. Kaplan HS, Dorfman RF, Nelson TS, et al: Staging laparotomy and splenec-

tomy in Hodgkin's disease: Analysis of indications in 285 consecutive, unselected patients. *NCI Monogr* 1973; 36:291–301.
29. Taylor MA, Kaplan HS, Nelsen TS: Staging laparotomy with splenectomy for Hodgkin's disease: The Stanford experience. *World J Surg* 1985; 9:449–460.
30. Trotter MC, Gretchen AC, Davis M, et al: Predicting the risk of abdominal disease in Hodgkin's lymphoma. *Ann Surg* 1985; 201:465–469.
31. Gabriel DA, Bernard SA, Lambert J, et al: Oophoropexy and the management of Hodgkin's disease. *Arch Surg* 1986; 121:1083–1085.
32. Fuller L, Hagemeister F: Hodgkin's disease in adults: Stage I and II, in *Hodgkin's Disease and Non-Hodgkin's in Adults and Children.* New York, Raven Press, 1988.
33. Sutcliffe SB, Wrigley PEM, Timothy AR, et al: Post-treatment laparotomy as a guide to management in patients with Hodgkin's disease. *Cancer Treat Rep* 1987; 66:759–766.
34. Evans HL, Winklemann RK, Banks PM: Differential diagnosis of malignant and benign cutaneous lymphoid infiltrates: A study of 57 cases in which malignant lymphoma had been diagnosed or suspected in the skin. *Cancer* 1979; 44:699–717.
35. Wiseman C, Liao KT: Primary lymphoma of the breast. *Cancer* 1972; 29:1705–1712.
36. Paladuqu RR, Bearman RM, Rappaport H: Malignant lymphoma with primary manifestation in the gonad: A clinicopathologic study of 38 patients. *Cancer* 1980; 45:561–571.
37. Contreary K, Nance FC, Becker WE: Primary lymphoma of the gastrointestinal tract. *Ann Surg* 1980; 191:593–598.
38. ReMine SG, Braasch JW: Gastric and small bowel lymphoma. *Surg Clin North Am* 1986; 66:713–722.
39. Hoerr SO, McCormack LS, Hertzer NR: Prognosis of gastric lymphoma. *Arch Surg* 1973; 1097:155–158.
40. Lim FE, Hartman AS, Tan EGC, et al: Factors in the prognosis of gastric lymphoma. *Cancer* 1977; 39:1715–1720.
41. Maor MH, Maddux B, Osborne BM, et al: Stages IE and IIE non-Hodgkin's lymphomas of the stomach. *Cancer* 1984; 54:2330–2337.
42. Boddie AW Jr, Eisenberg BL, Mullins JD, et al: The diagnosis and treatment of obstructive jaundice secondary to malignant lymphoma: A problem in multidisciplinary management. *J Surg Oncol* 1980; 14:111–123.
43. Wychulis AR, Beahrs OH, Woolner LB: Malignant lymphoma of the colon. *Arch Surg* 1966; 93:215–255.
44. Woolner LB, McConahey WM, Beahrs OH, et al: Primary malignant lymphoma of the thyroid: Review of forty-six cases. *Am J Surg* 1966; 111:502–523.

Human Heart and Lung Transplantation

Ishik C. Tuna, M.D.

Resident, Division of Thoracic and Cardiovascular Surgery, Mayo Clinic, Rochester, Minnesota

Stuart W. Jamieson, M.B., F.R.C.S.

Professor and Head, Division of Cardiovascular and Thoracic Surgery, Director, Minnesota Heart and Lung Institute, Minneapolis, Minnesota

Many operations are now performed for congenital and acquired diseases of the heart . . . . There remain, however, many irreversible lesions of the heart in which all existing methods of treatment are unsuccessful, and it is perhaps only by means of homoplastic transplantation of the heart [and lungs] that it will be possible to save a patient's life.

V.P. Demikhov
Moscow, 1940

Heart-lung transplantation has been applied successfully toward the treatment of end-stage cardiopulmonary disease since 1981. Cumulative estimates on the number of patients who have undergone heart-lung transplantation range from 150 to 200 persons worldwide, with primary pulmonary hypertension and end-stage Eisenmenger's disease being the most frequent indications for transplantation. Heart-lung transplantation has been successfully carried out in both pediatric and adult age groups (age range, 10 weeks to 50 years). In experienced hands, approximately 70% one-year survival is possible, with prospects for normal long-term cardiopulmonary function in many of these patients excellent.

While advances in operative technique and immunosuppressive therapy have resulted in immediate benefit from heart-lung transplantation for most patients, significant long-term morbidity may result in some (obstructive airway disease, azotemia, and hypertension).

Recent advances in obviating the undesirable sequelae of heart-lung transplantation through development of new techniques for diagnosis and rejection, improved immunosuppressive protocols, and advances in donor organ procurement are therefore reviewed, within the context of heart-lung transplantation as it is currently performed at the Minnesota Heart and Lung Institute.

Adv Surg 22:251–276, 1989

0065-3411/89/22-251–276-$04.00

Historical Background of Heart-Lung Transplantation

Heart-lung transplantation has emerged as a clinically useful procedure from a background of extensive and prolonged laboratory investigation. The evolution of heart-lung transplantation from an investigational endeavor to one of increasing clinical utility is outlined in Table 1.

The origins of heart-lung transplantation date back to the onset of vascular surgery. Within a few years following the development of techniques for performing vascular anastomoses (Jassinowsky, 1891, Dorfler, 1899), Carrel (1902) predicted the feasibility of organ transplantation utilizing these new techniques.[1–3] Following successful autotransplantation of the hind limb and thyroid gland in laboratory animals (1905), Carrel proceeded to perform heterotopic transplantation of the heart, kidney, ovary, intestine, and lastly the heart and lungs (en bloc).[4–6] Shortly thereafter, Carrel suggested that organ transplantation may have a role in the treatment of the human diseases, and identified (with remarkable foresight) what he considered to be major obstacles facing the clinical implementation of organ transplantation: the presence of poorly understood immunological barriers, imperfect organ preservation techniques, and a long-

TABLE 1.
Historical Milestones in Heart-Lung Transplantation

1905	Carrel performs first experimental heart-lung transplant (heterotopic).
1946	Demikhov initiates epochal series of experimental heart-lung transplants (both heterotopic and orthotopic) without benefit of cardiopulmonary bypass or immunosuppressants.
1952	Marcus performs experimental heart-lung transplantation (heterotopic) utilizing "parabiotic interim perfusion," and introduces use of immunosuppressive agents.
1953	Neptune utilizes profound hypothermia and circulatory arrest to perform experimental orthotopic heart-lung transplantation.
1957	Webb reports use of cardiopulmonary bypass to perform experimental heart-lung transplantation (orthotopic).
1968	Cooley attempts first human heart-lung transplant.
1969	Lillehei (and subsequently Barnard) demonstrate adequate cardiopulmonary function early following human heart-lung transplantation.
1976	Borel introduces cyclosporine as a potent immunosuppressive agent.
1980	Long-term survival in Rhesus and Cynomolgus monkeys demonstrated following heart-lung transplantation by Reitz.
1981	Long-term success following heart-lung transplantation in humans reported (Stanford).

term shortage of suitable human donor organs (for which Carrel suggested the substitution of xenografts).

Laboratory investigation into orthotopic heart-lung transplantation was subsequently initiated by Demikhov in the early 1940s. In a remarkable monogram entitled "Peresadka Zhizneno Vazhnykh Organov V Eksperimente" (Experimental Transplantation of Vital Organs), he described results of extensive laboratory investigations into heart and heart-lung transplantation performed at the Moscow State University.[7] Without the benefit of cardiopulmonary bypass or modern techniques of myocardial protection, Demikhov and colleagues performed 250 heterotopic heart and heart-lung transplants (Fig 1), and 67 orthotopic heart-lung transplants in dogs (Fig 2), with survival up to six days (eight of 67 animals surviving greater than four days, Fig 3). These epochal studies demonstrated for the first time that orthotopic heart-lung transplantation was not only technically feasible, but that the transplanted organs could adequately sustain the life of the recipient (at least acutely). In his extensive series of experiments, Demikhov further described technical refinements for, common complications of, and physiologic characteristics following heart and heart-lung transplantation. Included among Demikhov's contributions were description of the atrial cuff technique for joining the donor to recipient atria during cardiac transplantation; development of an autoperfusing heart-lung preparation specifically for extracorporeal preservation; identification of the potential for recurrent laryngeal nerve damage during combined heart-lung transplantation; and recognition of the inherent weakness of the tracheal

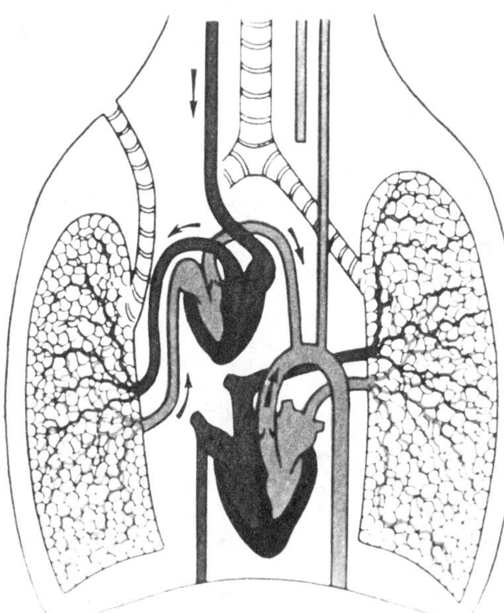

FIG 1.
Technique utilized by Demikhov and colleagues in performing heterotopic heart-lung transplantation. The transplanted heart and lung were placed in the right thorax and the donor bronchus exteriorized. Lightly shaded vessels carry oxygenated blood, while darkly shaded vessels carry desaturated blood. (From Demikhov VP: *Experimental Transplantation of Vital Organs,* Haigh B (trans). New York, Consultants Bureau, 1962. Used by permission.)

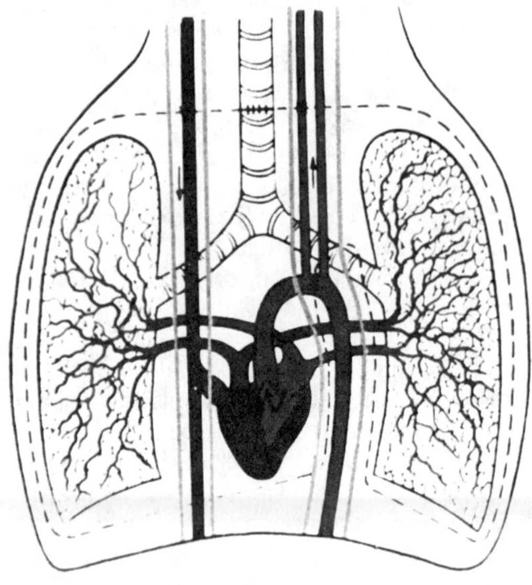

FIG 2.
Illustration of the technique utilized by Demikhov for orthotopic heart-lung transplantation. The *dotted line* encompasses the transplanted organs, with the suture lines indicated. Shading of vessels is similar to that in Fig 1. Phrenic and vagus nerves were preserved. Laryngeal nerve damage (well recognized) was treated with tracheostomy. Transplantation was performed through use of an autoperfusing, ventilated heart-lung bloc, serially connected to recipient vessels to gradually exclude the native heart from the circulation. The tracheal anastomosis was performed last, to exclude the lungs. Native organs were subsequently excised. (From Demikhov VP: *Experimental Transplantation of Vital Organs,* Haigh B (trans). New York, Consultants Bureau, 1962. Used by permission.)

anastomosis following lung transplantation. Demikhov further described (though did not appreciate the significance of) the onset of arrhythmias and decreasing QRS voltage following transplantation (in the absence of immunosuppressive agents). Of interest, Demikhov may be credited with the earliest development and implantation of a biventricular mechanical heart substitute as well (1937).

Demikhov's observations were initially reported in the Russian literature, with English translations becoming available only in the 1960s. Marcus (1952), presumably without knowledge of Demikhov's efforts, performed the first experiments reported in the English literature demonstrating the ability of the transplanted heart and lungs to support a recipient's cardiopulmonary needs.[8] Utilizing a support animal to provide continuous coronary perfusion of the allograft during transplantation ("parabiotic interim perfusion"), Marcus performed heart-lung transplantation into the abdomen of dogs. Through a variety of maneuvers, including insufflation of pure nitrogen into the native lungs, and occlusion of the native pulmonary

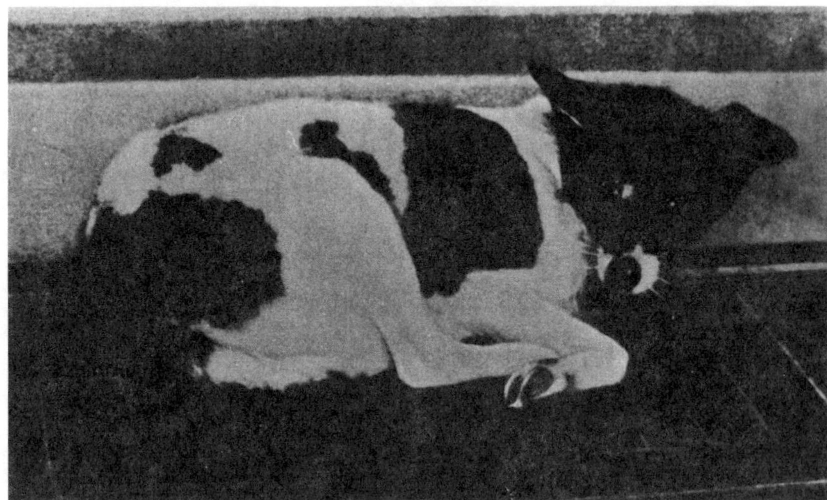

FIG 3.
The longest survivor (six days) of experimental orthotopic heart-lung transplantation performed by Demikhov. The cause of death was thought to be secondary to tracheostomy occlusion (in the presence of vocal cord paralysis) and loss of airway. More likely, rejection was responsible for death, as no immunosuppressive agents were utilized. (From Demikhov VP: *Experimental Transplantation of Vital Organs,* Haigh B (trans). New York, Consultants Bureau, 1962. Used by permission.)

artery, the ability of the heterotopically transplanted organs to provide total cardiopulmonary support of the recipient was demonstrated (Fig 4). Additionally, immunosuppressive therapy (cortisone) was introduced into the postoperative management of animals undergoing transplantation. Neptune (1953) reported on orthotopic heart-lung transplantation performed in dogs, utilizing profound hypothermia and total circulatory arrest.[9] This series of experiments yielded survivors up to six hours following heart-lung transplantation, with adequate cardiopulmonary support provided by the transplanted organs. In 1957, Webb introduced the use of mechanical cardiopulmonary bypass into experimental heart-lung transplantation.[10] In addition, for the first time, myocardial and pulmonary preservation was attempted through flushing of the heart-lung bloc with Ringer's solution and external cooling. While successful at producing acute survivors of transplantation, no long-term survival was attained. Webb subsequently introduced the concept that pulmonary innervation was required in the dog for maintenance of adequate respiratory drive, and suggested in later work that primates differed in this regard, and might provide a more suitable model for evaluating heart-lung transplantation.[11]

The technical feasibility of clinical heart-lung transplantation was subse-

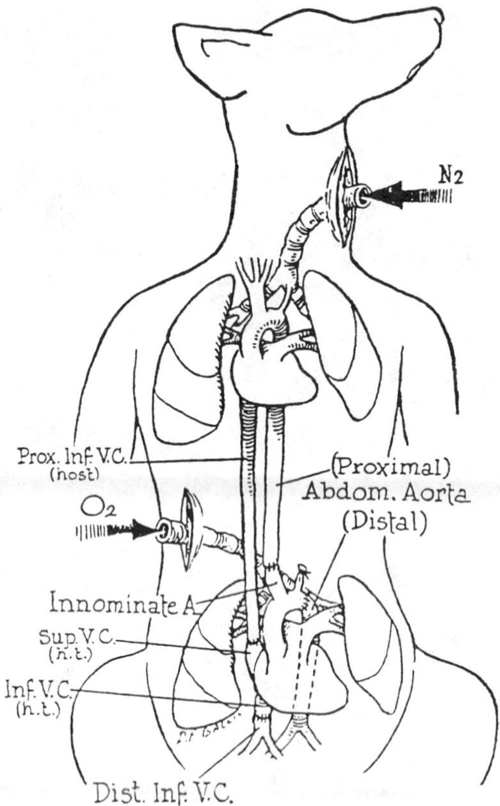

FIG 4.
Technique of intraabdominal heart-lung transplantation employed by Marcus and colleagues. Through insufflation of nitrogen into the native trachea (and intraoperative occlusion of the native pulmonary artery), the ability of the transplanted organs to sustain the circulation of the recipient was demonstrated. (From Marcus E, Wong S, Luisada A: Homologous heart grafts. *Arch Surg* 1952; 66:179. Used by permission.)

quently demonstrated by Cooley in 1968.[12] Combined heart-lung transplantation was performed in a 2-month-old female with a complete atrioventricular (AV) canal defect and concurrent pneumonitis (Fig 5). An anencephalic donor (profoundly hypertensive) was utilized without the benefit of myocardial protection or pulmonary flushing or cooling. Despite these obstacles, the patient survived surgery and demonstrated spontaneous respiratory effort in the immediate postoperative period. Shortly thereafter, the patient developed pulmonary edema and mediastinal hemorrhage (prompting reoperation) and ultimately died (14 hours posttransplantation). Lillehei, in 1969, subsequently carried out heart-lung transplantation in a 43-year-old male with end-stage chronic obstructive pulmonary disease.[13] This patient survived surgery, was extubated, and demonstrated near normal pulmonary function test results. By postoperative day 5, pulmonary infiltrates were noted, and the patient ultimately died on postoperative day 8, presumably from pseudomonas pneumonitis.

In 1971 Barnard had a similar experience, performing combined heart-lung transplantation in a 49-year-old male with obstructive pulmonary dis-

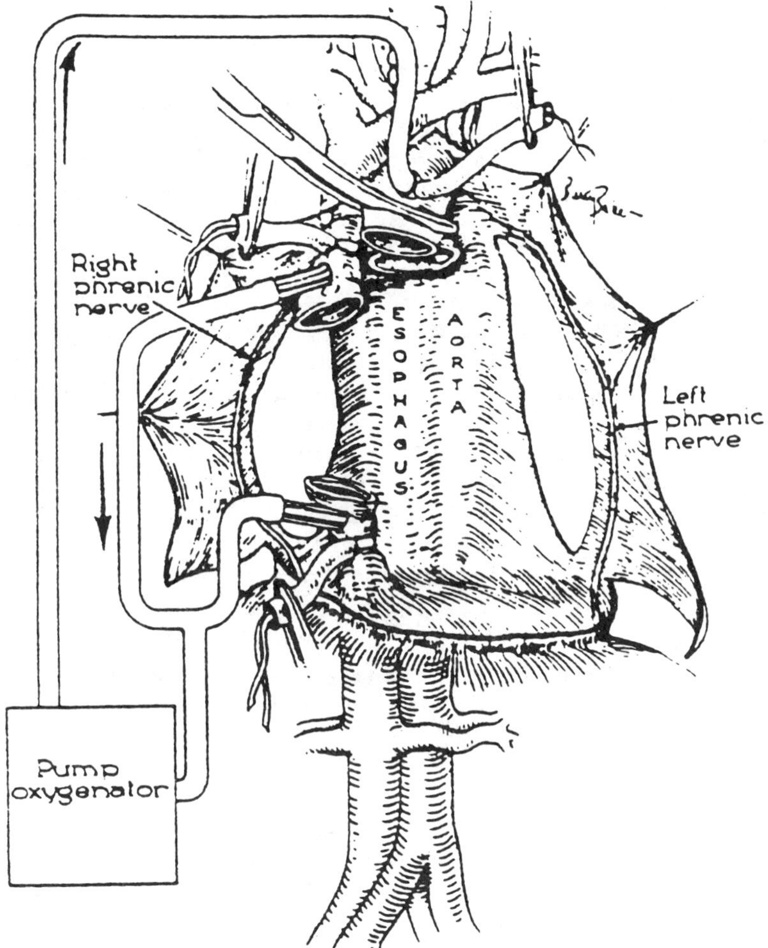

FIG 5.
Technique of heart-lung transplantation employed in the first human heart-lung transplant. Implantation of donor organs was performed through separate anastomosis of SVC and IVC, tracheal anastomosis at the level of the carina, and total excision of the native pulmonary artery. The patient survived transplantation and demonstrated spontaneous respiratory effort (while intubated) postoperatively. (From Cooley D, Bloodwell R, Hallman G, et al: Organ transplantation for advanced cardiopulmonary disease. *Ann Thorac Surg* 1969, 8:30. Used by permission.)

ease.[14] The patient survived surgery, subsequently developed an air leak from a right bronchial anastomosis (prompting a right pneumonectomy), developed pneumonitis in the remaining lung, and died 23 days following transplantation. Experience from these attempts, while confirming the technical feasibility of clinical heart-lung transplantation, primarily served to highlight the inadequacies of available immunosuppressive agents, and inhibited further clinical application of heart-lung transplantation. Finally, with the introduction of cyclosporine in 1976 by Borel (as a potent nonsteroidal immunosuppressive agent), coupled with previous clinical observations, the first successful animal model of the heart-lung transplant patient was developed in primates.[15] Following the demonstration of long-term survival and normal cardiopulmonary function in this model of heart-lung transplantation (1980), renewed clinical application of heart-lung transplantation was initiated by Shumway and colleagues. Subsequently, Jamieson et al. reported early results of human heart-lung transplantation initiated in 1981, and described refinements in operative technique (to its present form), and patient selection criteria to optimize clinical results following combined heart-lung transplantation.[16–19] A partial list of conditions treated by combined heart-lung transplantation is presented in Table 2.[20]

TABLE 2.
Conditions (By Approximate Percent) Treated With Heart-Lung Transplantation

Condition	Percent
Primary pulmonary hypertension	45%
Eisenmenger's syndrome	40%
Other conditions	15%
Valvular heart disease & pulmonary hypertension	
Multiple pulmonary emboli*	
Emphysema	
Alpha$_1$-antitrypsin deficiency	
Cystic fibrosis	
Eosinophilic granuloma	
Fibrosing alveolitis	
Primary pulmonary fibrosis	
Pulmonary asbestosis	
Pulmonary lymphangioleiomyomatosis	
Pulmonary staphylococcus infection*	
Pulmonary sarcoidosis	
Chronic rejection*	

*Conditions not currently treated with heart-lung transplantation.

Clinical Heart-Lung Transplantation (Donor and Recipient Selection Criteria)

The current selection and exclusion criteria utilized in identifying appropriate candidates for heart-lung transplantation are presented in Table 3.

Typically, candidates for heart-lung transplantation should have the general characteristics of cardiac transplant recipients in addition to having terminal pulmonary disease; that is, patients should demonstrate end-stage combined heart and lung disease (New York Heart Association Class III or IV) while being less than 45 years of age. Appropriate candidates should have no concurrent systemic illnesses (sepsis, neoplasia, diabetes, or bleeding diathesis), and have no renal or hepatic dysfunction that is irreversible. A recent history of cerebrovascular accident or recurrent pulmonary embolus additionally contraindicates cardiopulmonary transplantation. Finally, prior major cardiothoracic surgery is a major contraindication to heart-lung transplantation, secondary to an increased risk of life-threatening postoperative hemorrhage. Preoperative evaluation, as listed in Table 4, is therefore aimed at assessing these factors.

Donor availability continues to be a major obstacle in the clinical implementation of heart-lung transplantation. A relative paucity of adequate donors arises primarily from the dual requirements for both pulmonary and cardiac status of the potential donor to be stable and meet certain criteria for suitability. Additionally, the widespread applica-

TABLE 3.
Eligibility Criteria for Heart-Lung Recipient Selection

End-stage heart-lung disease (New York Heart Association Class III or IV)
Age less than 45 years
No prior major cardiothoracic surgery
No evidence of concurrent systemic illness (sepsis, neoplasia, diabetes)
Creatinine clearance >50 ml/minute
Bilirubin <3.0 gm/dl
No evidence of recent cerebrovascular accident
No active ulcer disease or bleeding diathesis
No current tobacco, alcohol, or recreational drug use
No history of recurrent pulmonary emboli
Psychosocially stable

TABLE 4.
Current Evaluation of Potential Heart-Lung Recipients

Consultation and evaluation by:
- Cardiology, cardiovascular surgery, pulmonary medicine, neurology, dental consultation

Laboratory evaluation:
- CBC, platelet count, PT, PTT, TT, fibrinogen, Factor V, serum electrolytes, BUN, creatinine, calcium, magnesium, phosphorous, glucose, cholesterol and triglycerides, serum protein electrophoresis, creatinine clearance, SGOT, alkaline phosphatase, bilirubin, amylase, thyroid index, hepatitis B screen, HIV screen; throat, urine, and blood

Cultures (routine, viral, and fungal); CMV, EBV, VZV, herpes serum titers

Immunologic evaluation:
- ABO typing, HLA typing, anti-leukocyte antibody screen, quantitative serum immunoglobulin determination

Other:
- Chest X-ray; upper GI, barium enema, gallbladder ultrasound (if indicated); fecal occult blood determination, ECG, right and left-sided heart catheterization (if not done), muga or echo of the heart, spine and hip radiographs, pulmonary function tests, ventilation perfusion scan (if indicated), head CT, and PPD

*CBC = complete blood cell; PT = prothrombin time; PTT, partial thromboplastin time; BUN = blood urea nitrogen; CMV = cytomegalovirus; EBV, Epstein-Barr virus; TT, thrombin time; VZV, varicella zoster virus.

tion of cardiac transplantation has further reduced the availability of combined heart-lung donors.

Traditionally, prospective donors have sustained significant traumatic cerebral injury from motor-vehicle accidents, which in many cases may result in concomitant thoracic injury and pulmonary contusion. Prolonged periods of in-hospital, artificial ventilation also predispose potential donors to iatrogenically acquired pulmonary dysfunction, consisting of either infection or barotrauma. Potential donors must therefore be screened for a history of significant chest trauma, ideally should have undergone artificial ventilation for less than five days (to minimize effects of barotrauma), and have no evidence of contaminated pulmonary secretions (acquired pneumonitis). A normal chest radiograph and arterial blood gases demonstrating a PO_2 level more than 100 mm Hg with an inspired oxygen fraction of 40% or less are therefore essential. Once potential suitability as a donor has been determined, matching with a perspective recipient is performed on the basis of ABO blood group compatibility, body size, and a negative crossmatch. HLA typing is only done for retrospective analysis, and does not currently enter into the recipient selection process. Organ size matching is most readily achieved by comparison of PA chest radiographs taken at comparable magnification, an ideal match consisting of donor lung fields slightly smaller than those of the recipient. Serum viral titers should also be evaluated. Donor selection and exclusion criteria are summarized in Table 5.

Technical Considerations in Heart-Lung Transplantation

Donor Organ Procedure

Donor organs have traditionally been harvested in an operating room adjacent to that containing the recipient. Distal organ procurement has been successfully accomplished at our institute (cold ischemia time of up to 4½ hours), and may be considered for routine use. Emerging techniques for donor organ preservation will be discussed below.

Removal of the heart-lung bloc is performed through a median sternotomy. Careful visual examination, particularly of the lung parenchyma, is critical to determine the final suitability of donor organs for transplantation (i.e., lack of pulmonary trauma). Once this has been ascertained, mobilization of the heart-lung bloc is begun. The aorta, pulmonary artery, innominate artery, vena cavae, and trachea are encircled with tapes, utilizing minimal dissection. In particular, the trachea is isolated high in the mediastinum (to preserve carinal collateral blood supply). Infusion catheters are placed directly into the pulmonary artery and into the ascending aorta

TABLE 5.
Selection and Exclusion Criteria for Prospective Heart-Lung Donors

Criteria
Age less than 40 years
Normal examination of pleural cavities and lungs at time of organ harvest
Normal cardiac status (normal ECG, blood pressure)
No significant chest trauma
Normal chest radiograph
PaO_2 greater than 100 mm Hg with fraction of inspired O_2 less than 40%
Normal peak airway pressures
Negative hepatitis B and HIV status

through the innominate artery. Harvesting of the heart-lung bloc is initiated with a ligation of the superior and inferior vena cava, aortic occlusion, and administration of cold, crystalloid cardioplegic solution. The proximal inferior vena cava is divided to vent the right side of the heart. Simultaneously a modified cold Collin's solution (12 mEq $MgSO_4$ and 50% dextrose added per liter) is infused into the pulmonary artery at pressure less than 20 mm Hg to render the lungs asanguinous and aid in pulmonary preservation. Transection of the tip of the left atrial appendage is performed to further vent the left side of the heart. With administration of cardioplegic solution (approximately 10 ml/kg) and Collin's solution (60 ml/kg), the aorta and superior vena cava are divided, the trachea clamped high in the chest (following partial inflation of the lungs) and divided, and the inferior pulmonary ligaments transected bilaterally. Utilizing electrocautery, the posterior mediastinal attachments of the heart-lung bloc are then severed as the organs are elevated out of the chest. With harvesting completed the heart-lung bloc is placed in cold Ringer's solution pending implantation. Minimal manipulation of the lung parenchyma is desirable during harvesting. Techniques are identical whether onsite or distal procurement of organs is utilized.

Heart-Lung Recipient Preparation

Heart-lung recipient preparation begins with median sternotomy. The heart is exposed and both parietal pleurae incised to allow inspection of the right and left chest cavities. Adhesions between the visceral and parietal pleura are divided with electrocautery prior to heparinization and cardiopulmonary bypass (to minimize hemorrhage). The heart is then cannulated for total cardiopulmonary bypass (superior and inferior vena caval cannulation, distal ascending aortic cannulation).

With the institution of cardiopulmonary bypass, the native heart is excised as in isolated cardiac transplantation. The right atrium is opened at the atrioventricular groove. The aorta and pulmonary artery are transected at the level of semilunar valves, the interatrial septum incised, and the left atrium divided circumferentially at the level of the left atrioventricular groove. The left phrenic nerve is then mobilized on a pericardial pedicle. The posterior remnant of the left atrium is incised midway between the right and left pulmonary veins. Electrocautery is used to divide remaining posterior mediastinal attachments of the left pulmonary veins and left atrium. The left vagus nerve, which lays directly beneath on the esophagus, is vulnerable to injury during this maneuver. The left inferior pulmonary ligament is then ligated and divided and the left lung retracted anteriorly. Posterior mobilization of the left hilum is continued with electrocautery, frequently revealing large carinal collateral blood vessels requiring individual ligation. The left pulmonary veins, now completely mobilized, are passed beneath the left phrenic nerve, and the distal left pulmonary artery divided. A TA stapler with 3.5-mm staples is applied to the left main stem bronchus, and the bronchus transected proximally, allowing the left lung to be removed from the chest. Removal of the right lung proceeds in a similar manner. The right phrenic nerve is preserved on a pericardial pedicle. The right inferior pulmonary ligament is ligated and divided. An incision is made in the left atrium posterior to the intraatrial groove. This incision is carried superiorly and inferiorly until the right atrium and posterior left atrium are separated. The posterior mediastinal attachments of the right pulmonary veins are divided with electrocautery, and the right vagus nerve identified and preserved. Any right-sided bronchial collateral arteries are ligated. The right pulmonary veins are passed beneath the right atrium and phrenic nerve, and the right pulmonary artery divided. The TA stapler is applied to the right bronchus, and the proximal right bronchus divided. The right lung is removed from the chest. The posterior mediastinum should be carefully examined, and hemostasis achieved, prior to proceeding with organ implantation. Pulmonary artery remnants are then tailored to leave a small remnant of left pulmonary artery encompassing the attachment of the ligamentum arteriosum (thereby preserving the recurrent laryngeal nerve). A posterior incision immediately to the right of the aorta is employed to visualize the native trachea. The left and right bronchial stumps are mobilized, and the trachea divided at the level of the carina. Minimal dissection of the native trachea should be employed in an attempt to preserve all collateral blood supply. Frequently an enlarged bronchial artery immediately posterior to the trachea is present, requiring ligation. Preparation of the recipient for heart-lung transplantation is now complete (Fig 6).

Implantation of the donor heart and lungs is preceded by culturing and gentle suctioning of the donor trachea. The right and left lungs are passed into their respective thoracic cavities beneath the phrenic nerves. A cold lactate Ringer's infusion is begun in both chest cavities to provide topical cooling of the donor organs.

The donor trachea is tailored at the level of the carina. Utilizing a single continuous monofilament suture (3–0 polypropylene) the recipient and donor trachea are anastomosed (Fig 7). Discrepancies in tracheal diameters may be overcome by differential suturing at the posterior, membranous portion of the trachea prior to anastomosis of the cartilaginous elements. The donor superior vena cava is ligated and tailored. The right atrium is opened utilizing a curvilinear incision extending from the inferior vena cava toward the apex of the right atrial appendage (as in cardiac transplantation). The donor and recipient right atrial cuffs are then anastomosed utilizing a single running monofilament suture (3–0 polypropylene) (Fig 8).

Donor and recipient aorta are next tailored and anastomosed with a continuous 4–0 polypropylene suture (Fig 9). Implantation is complete, and weaning from cardiopulmonary bypass in a standard manner may be initiated.

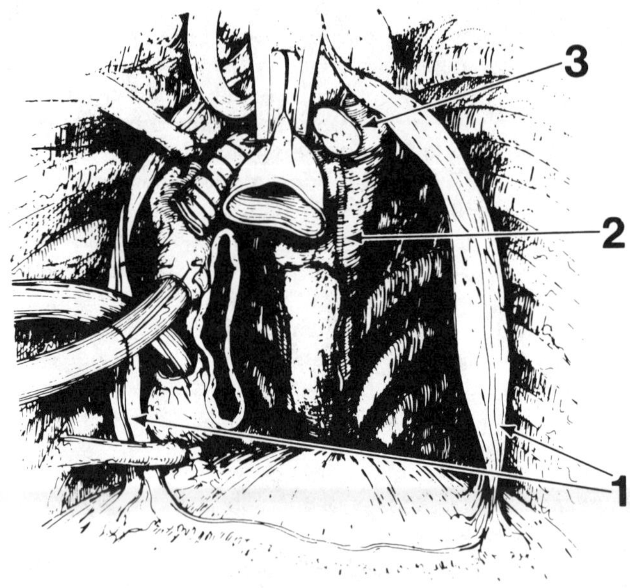

FIG 6.
Illustration of the currently employed technique for preparation of the heart-lung transplant recipient. Through a median sternotomy excision of the native lungs and heart are performed such that: (1) the phrenic nerves are preserved bilaterally on pericardial pedicles; (2) the vagi are preserved; and (3) the recurrent laryngeal nerve is spared through preservation of a small button of left main pulmonary artery which encompasses the origin of the ligamentum arteriosus. The aorta, trachea, and right atrium have been tailored for implantation. (From Jamieson S, Shumway N: *Rob & Smith's Operative Surgery: Cardiac Surgery*. London, Butterworths, 1986. Used by permission.)

Postoperative Management

Early postoperative management of patients undergoing heart-lung transplantation is complex and highly individualized. General medical care and adjustment of immunosuppressive therapy are the primary tasks faced in the immediate postoperative period. Abnormalities in early postoperative lung function provide the most difficult management problems, as these may arise from pulmonary capillary leak, atelectasis, infection, or rejection. Since the diagnosis of lung rejection is one of exclusion, all possible etiologies for deterioration in lung function require evaluation, to guide in selection of appropriate therapy.

Immunosuppressive Therapy

Early postoperative immunosuppressive therapy is aimed at preventing heart and lung rejection while allowing maximal healing of the tracheal

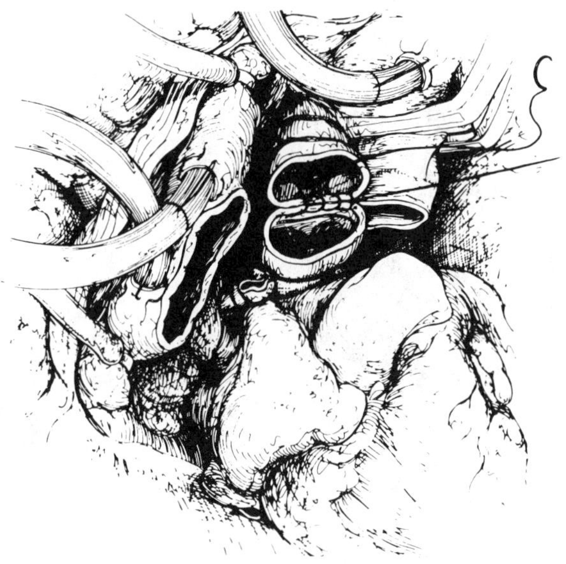

FIG 7.
Following tailoring of the donor trachea just at the level of the carina, implantation of the heart-lung bloc is initiated with anastomosis of the trachea utilizing a single continuous monofilament suture. Discrepancy in tracheal dimensions may be overcome during suturing of the posterior, membranous portion of the trachea. In the illustration the donor lungs have been passed beneath the phrenic nerves into their respective thoracic cavities. (From Jamieson S, Shumway N: *Rob & Smith's Operative Surgery: Cardiac Surgery*. London, Butterworths, 1986. Used by permission.)

anastomosis. This is achieved through the use of high-dose cyclosporine A (12–18 mg/kg/day, to achieve serum levels of 200 mg/ml), and azathioprine (1.5 mg/kg/day). With the exception of parenteral steroids used on the first postoperative day, corticosteroids are avoided for approximately 14 days following transplantation. Azathioprine dosage is subsequently adjusted for leukopenia, and oral prednisone initiated at 0.5 mg/kg/day. Over the next two to four weeks, cyclosporine and prednisone dosages are gradually reduced to their maintenance levels, with cyclosporine tapered until serum trough levels of 100–150 ng/ml are obtained, and prednisone reduced until a dose of 0.2 mg/kg/day is attained. Adequacy of immunosuppressive therapy is assessed by daily determinations of serum cyclosporine trough levels, and weekly endomyocardial biopsies. Additionally, diagnosis of lung rejection (which must ultimately be made clinically) is aided through evaluation of chest radiographs and arterial blood gases.

Evidence of early acute rejection (either heart or lung) is treated with methylprednisone, 1 gm/day IV for three days, supplemented by antithy-

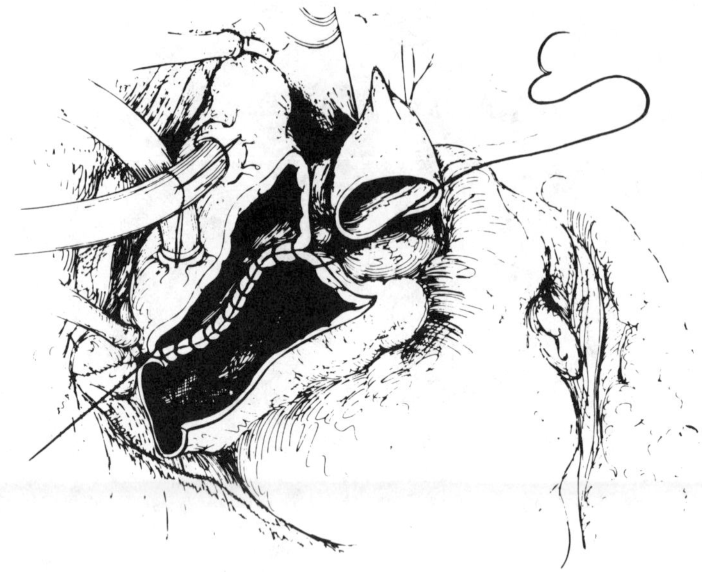

FIG 8.
With completion of the tracheal anastomosis, the superior vena cava is ligated and the right atrium opened with a curvilinear incision extending from the inferior vena cava towards the right atrial appendage (preserving sinoatrial node function). The atria are then anastomosed using a single monofilament suture. (From Jamieson S, Shumway N: *Rob & Smith's Operative Surgery: Cardiac Surgery*. London, Butterworths, 1986. Used by permission.)

mocyte globulin if necessary. Immunosuppressive protocols are summarized in Table 6.

General Medical Care

Early postoperative medical care is focused primarily on preserving and promoting normal lung function. Fluid status is carefully monitored and intentional underhydration maintained. Additionally, emphasis is placed on early extubation (patients typically undergo extubation within 24 to 36 hours following surgery) and the initiation of vigorous chest physiotherapy and breathing exercises.

Careful monitoring of postoperative renal function is mandatory in these patients, due to a 30% incidence of postoperative renal failure that may require transient hemodialysis. Azotemia in the early postoperative period typically results from a combination of factors that may include cyclosporine nephrotoxicity, intentional underhydration (to promote normal lung

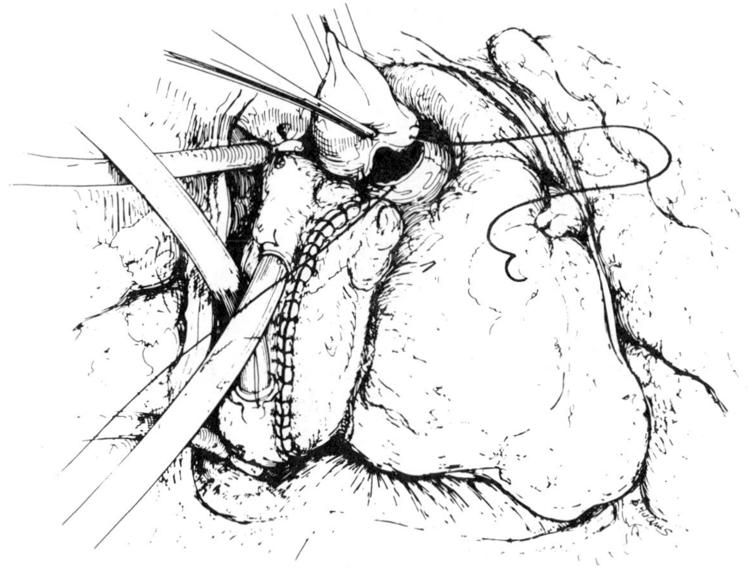

FIG 9.
With completion of the right atrial anastomosis the donor aorta is tailored and anastomosed utilizing a continuous polypropylene suture. Positive pressure ventilation and weaning from cardiopulmonary bypass completes the procedure. (From Jamieson S, Shumway N: *Rob & Smith's Operative Surgery: Cardiac Surgery.* London, Butterworths, 1986. Used by permission.)

function), and exacerbation of preexisting renal failure, typically with an element of each factor being present.

Reverse isolation procedures and room air filtration (to reduce fungal spore and bacterial counts) have also been used in an attempt to decrease the risk of acquired infection, particularly while high levels of immunosuppressive therapy are utilized in the early postoperative period (Table 7).

Late Postoperative Management

The long-term management of heart-lung transplant recipients is directed toward the diagnosis and treatment of acute episodes of heart or lung rejection, and ongoing evaluation for evidence of obliterative bronchiolitis or proliferative coronary atherosclerosis (most likely representing chronic lung and heart rejection, respectively).[21] Hypertension and azotemia may also persist or develop late postoperatively, and require additional medical management.[21] Acquisition of fungal or viral infection (particularly cytomegalovirus) and late development of malignancy additionally accompany chronic immunosuppression and heart-lung transplantation.[23]

In early clinical experience with heart-lung transplantation, allograft re-

TABLE 6.
Immunosuppressive Therapy

Early postoperative therapy:
- High-dose cyclosporine (12–18 mg/kg/day—serum levels 200 ng/ml)
- Moderate-dose azathioprine (1.0–1.5 mg/kg/day—adjusted for leukopenia)
- No corticosteroids

Maintenance therapy:
- Prednisone therapy added (0.2 mg/kg/day)
- Cyclosporine tapered slowly to maintenance levels (trough levels of 100–150 ng/ml)
- Continued therapy with azathioprine (adjusted for leukopenia)

Anti-rejection therapy:
- *Early (within 30 days), acute rejection:*
- Methylprednisone 1 gm IV daily for three days
- Antithymocyte globulin if needed
- *Late, acute, or chronic rejection:*
- High-dose oral prednisone (100 mg/day) gradually tapered and maintained at 30 mg/day for one month

TABLE 7.
General Medical Care: Early Postoperative Management

Early extubation
Hydration minimized
Vigorous chest physiotherapy
Monitoring of renal and hepatic function
Reverse isolation and filtration of room air

jection status (both lung and heart) was monitored solely through endomyocardial biopsy.[24,25] Subsequent clinical and laboratory experience indicated that isolated lung rejection could occur in the presence of normal histological findings on endomyocardial biopsies.[26, 27] Evidence for isolated pulmonary rejection must therefore be additionally monitored through the use of pulmonary function tests, determination of arterial blood gases, and chest radiographs. Lung rejection may be heralded by a decrease in arterial PO_2 from normal to 60 to 70 mm Hg on room air. Pulmonary function tests may additionally show an obstructive ventilatory defect, superimposed on any postoperative restrictive changes, with mean expiratory flow (MEF_{25-75}), and PaO_2 appearing to be the most sensitive indicators of rejection. Forced expiratory volume at one second (FEV_1) and the ratio of FEV_1 to forced vital capacity (FVC), also appear decreased with rejection. A 10% change or more in any of these variables is suspicious for lung rejection. Chest radiograph, while less sensitive, may show nodular infiltrates or parabronchial thickening, further suggestive of rejection.

Late episodes of either heart or lung rejection are treated with high-dose oral prednisone therapy, initiated at 100 mg/day. Dosage is subsequently tapered to approximately 30 mg/day and maintained there for approximately one month.

The usefulness of transbronchial biopsy and bronchial lavage for the diagnosis of acute lung rejection remains to be demonstrated, and is not presently utilized.[28]

The later sequelae of heart-lung transplantation may also include airway obstruction secondary to obstructive bronchiolitis, recurrent pulmonary infection, bronchiectasis, and pulmonary fibrosis.[29] Serial evaluation of pulmonary function (as outlined above in Early Postoperative Management), is therefore essential. Bronchoscopy with transbronchial or endobronchial biopsy, as well as open lung biopsy, are useful in the diagnosis of obliterative bronchiolitis. With early detection of deterioration in pulmonary function (and an infectious etiology excluded), high-dose corticosteroid therapy should be initiated, and may reverse pulmonary abnormalities.[30] Also, for patients not receiving azathioprine, the addition of this agent (1.0–1.5 mg/kg/day) may halt or even reverse the progression of pulmonary dysfunction.[31]

Similarly, concentric coronary atherosclerosis may be a late sequela of heart-lung transplantation, and can result in fatal myocardial infarction.

Postoperative hypertension, a well-recognized consequence of cyclosporine therapy following isolated heart transplantation, may occur following heart-lung transplantation as well. Medical therapy with diuretics and vasodilators may be required, as well as adjustment in salt intake. Progressive renal dysfunction secondary to cyclosporine nephropathy is also common, and may complicate immunosuppressive management with cyclosporine.

The use of low-dose azathioprine, allowing reduction in cyclosporine dosage from that in previous reports, is currently being evaluated as a technique for reducing the incidence of cyclosporine-associated hypertension and nephropathy, while maintaining adequate immunosuppressive therapy. As mentioned previously, the effectiveness of this approach in halting or reversing late decline in airway flow characteristics has already been demonstrated. Further benefits should become apparent from the initiation of azathioprine therapy immediately following transplantation, and this would be our current recommendation.

Clinical Results

Results discussed below are based on the senior author's experience, first at Stanford University Medical Center, and more recently at the University of Minnesota Heart and Lung Institute, in 35 patients operated on over the past six years. Actuarial survival at one, three, and four years for patients has been reported as 65%, 55%, and 40%, respectively. Factors predictive of poor outcome are discussed.

Perioperative Mortality

Thirty-six heart-lung transplants have been performed in 35 patients, with eight patients dying within 30 days of surgery (25% mortality rate). Four deaths were related to hemorrhage, while two patients died of bronchopneumonia, one of multisystem organ failure, and one of adult respiratory distress syndrome. All four patients who died secondary to hemorrhage had massive perioperative bleeding, as a result of adhesions arising from prior major cardiothoracic surgery.

Perioperative Morbidity

Initial experience with heart-lung transplantation was associated with injury to the recurrent laryngeal or vagus nerve in two of the first three recipients. Operative technique was subsequently modified, with heart and lungs removed individually, rather than en bloc, eliminating the problem.

Long-Term Results

Of 26 survivors of combined heart-lung transplantation (a single patient undergoing retransplantation 35 months after original surgery is counted twice), all have demonstrated normal cardiopulmonary function on discharge from hospital. Thirteen patients have subsequently developed evidence of airway obstruction and hypoxemia, with an approximate time of onset of ten months postoperatively (range, 1 to 24 months). Evidence of obliterative bronchiolitis was found at autopsy (in six), or open lung biopsy (in two), transbronchial biopsy (in one), and following retransplantation in a single patient. In the remaining three, a clinical diagnosis was made based on characteristic airway flow parameters. Obstructive bronchiolitis was progressive in nine of 13 affected patients, of whom six have now died. One patient with rapid onset of severe airway obstruction was successfully retransplanted 35 months following initial surgery.

Two patients have become disabled by respiratory distress (NYHA III, IV Class symptoms), with four patients developing asymptomatic moderate airway obstruction. In two patients who developed airway obstruction and hypoxemia, high-dose corticosteroids were implemented early following detection of airway disease, with complete resolution of pulmonary function abnormalities in one patient, and improvement in the second. Eight patients with evidence of obliterative bronchiolitis were additionally treated with the introduction of azathioprine into their immunosuppressive therapy (not initially used). Decline in airway flow characteristics was subsequently demonstrated to improve, and even stabilize among these patients (Fig 10).

In contrast to the 13 patients in whom pulmonary complications developed, the remainder of heart-lung transplant survivors have near normal pulmonary function up to 42 months postoperatively. A minor restrictive ventilatory defect is seen in many patients, with the remainder of pulmonary mechanics essentially normal (Table 8).

Hemodynamic parameters additionally appear normal following transplantation (Table 9).

Finally, in recent experience, distal heart-lung procurement has been initiated, with successful transplantation being performed following up to 4½ hours of cold ischemic time.[32] Simple preservation techniques consisting of flushing of the donor organs with cold perfusate and static storage techniques have resulted in excellent donor organ function postimplant.

This methodology is significantly less complex than utilizing autoperfusing heart-lung preparations, and ultimately may prove suitable for routine use.[33–35]

Discussion

Combined heart-lung transplantation has been demonstrated to be compatible with near-normal cardiopulmonary function in humans, despite the acute loss of innervation, bronchial arterial supply, and lymphatic drainage. With careful recipient selection (previous major thoracic surgery, recurrent pulmonary emboli precluding successful outcome, as a major risk factor for perioperative hemorrhage), a significant reduction in operative mortality has been achieved. With improvements in operative mortality, widened applicability of the procedure to patients with a variety of causes of heart and lung failure is expected.

While long-term survival and maintenance of normal graft function following heart-lung transplantation are possible, the emergence of obliterative bronchiolitis as a significant late complication of transplantation requires ongoing patient surveillance and therapy, and most critically, improvement in techniques for monitoring lung rejection.

In patients with bronchiolitis who have come to necropsy or open lung biopsy, pulmonary arterial vessels frequently demonstrate concentric intimal fibrosis or perivascular lymphocytic cuffing. Concentric coronary atherosclerosis may be seen in these patients at autopsy as well.[36] Perivascu-

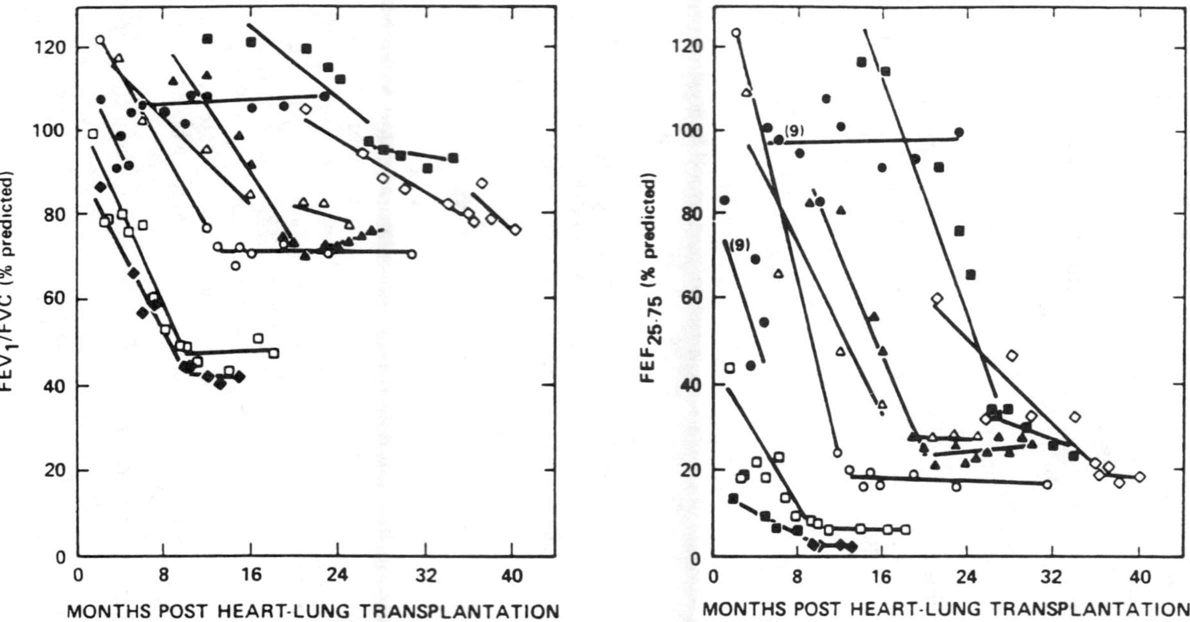

FIG 10.
Effect of augmented immunosuppressive therapy (by introduction of azathioprine) on decline in airway flow characteristics following heart-lung transplantation in patients with obliterative bronchiolitis. *Symbols* represent individual patients. (From Glanville A, Baldwin J, Burke C, et al: Obliterative bronchiolitis after heart-lung transplantation: Apparent arrest by augmented immunosuppression. *Ann Intern Med* 1987; 107:300. Used by permission.)

TABLE 8.
Pulmonary Function in Uncomplicated Heart-Lung Transplant Recipients (% Predicted, Mean ± SD)*†

	Early	Late
FVC	64 ± 17%	66 ± 14%
FEV_1	73 ± 18%	71 ± 14%
FEV_1/FVC	88 ± 8%	84 ± 4%
FEF_{25-75}	84 ± 43%	74 ± 11%
DLCO	77 ± 26%	102 ± 6%
PaO_2 (mm Hg)	89 ± 8%	88 ± 7%

*Adapted from Burke C, Baldwin J, Morris A, et al: Twenty-eight cases of human heart-lung transplants. *Lancet* 1986, vol 517.

†FVC = forced vital capacity; FEV_1 = forced expiratory volume at 1 second; FEF_{25-75} = forced expiratory flow from 25 to 75% of FVC; DLCO = CO diffusion capacity.

lar lymphocytic infiltrates have been associated with pulmonary rejection in animals, while laboratory work in rats suggests that the early stages of lung rejection may involve infiltration of bronchus-associated lymphoid tissues and pulmonary vessels by lymphocytes.[37] Thus, obliterative bronchiolitis may represent the clinical manifestation of chronic low-grade pulmonary rejection, analogous to the chronic vascular rejection seen in cardiac transplant recipients.

Consistent with this interpretation is the demonstrated lack of efficacy in treatment of obliterative bronchiolitis with antibiotics, bronchodilators, or chest physiotherapy. Further, while unsuccessful in reversing congestive pulmonary disease, corticosteroids have proven to be effective in reversing bronchiolitis when diagnosed early in its course. Furthermore, addition of azathioprine to the immunosuppressive therapy of patients developing bronchiolitis receiving prednisone and cyclosporine alone has further been successful in stabilizing pulmonary function tests, which otherwise have been shown to deteriorate relentlessly.

Thus, while abnormalities in mucociliary transport, chronic infection, and cyclosporine toxicity have all been postulated as etiologies for bronchiolitis, chronic rejection appears to be the most likely cause. These findings indicate that immunosuppressive regimens, at least for patients developing this complication, are inadequate.

TABLE 9.
Hemodynamics Pre- and Postoperatively in Heart-Lung Transplant Recipients*†

	Preoperative	Postoperative
Blood pressure (mm HG)	89 ± 11	118 ± 17‡
Cardiac output (L/minute)	4 ± 2	6 ± 2‡
Cardiac index (L/minute/sq m)	3 ± 3	4 ± 1
PAP (mm Hg)	75 ± 19	9 ± 3‡
PACWP (mm Hg)	6 ± 4	3 ± 2
PVR (Wood units)	18 ± 11	1 ± 1‡
PaO_2 (mm Hg)	52 ± 23	88 ± 7‡
$PaCO_2$ (mm Hg)	28 ± 4	36 ± 4‡

*Adapted from Dawkins K, Jamieson S, Hunt S, et al: Long-term results, hemodynamics, and complications after combined heart-lung transplantation. *Circulation* 1985; 71:919. Used by permission.
†PAP = pulmonary artery pressure (mean); PACWP = pulmonary artery capillary wedge pressure; PVR = pulmonary vascular resistance.
‡$P < .05$ preoperative vs. postoperative.

Immunosuppressive therapy may additionally be responsible for significant hypertension and nephrotoxicity following transplantation (with many patients in this series developing impaired renal function).

The implementation of triple drug immunosuppressive therapy, consisting of low-dose cyclosporine, prednisone, and azathioprine, has represented a major advance in ameliorating hypertensive and nephrotoxic side effects of conventional cyclosporine therapy, and is expected to reduce the incidence of posttransplantation obliterative bronchiolitis.

Finally, the development of techniques for distal procurement and prolonged preservation of donor organs is required to expand the availability of suitable donor organs. Heart-lung perfusion ex vivo has been used to prolong donor organ ischemic time for up to 4½ hours with clinical success in our hands. Simple techniques such as flushing of the heart-lung bloc with cold perfusate may ultimately provide donor organ protection for up to six hours following harvest, and will require further evaluation.

In summary, heart-lung transplantation has evolved from a laboratory technique to a clinically applicable procedure for selected patients with terminal heart and lung disease. While advances in operative technique and immunosuppressive therapy now offer patients a reasonable chance for long-term normal cardiopulmonary function, significant morbidity (obstructive bronchiolitis, azotemia, and hypertension) may accompany the procedure for some. Further advances in immunosuppressive therapy, techniques for the diagnosis of lung rejection, and improved heart-lung preservation methods are therefore required before heart-lung transplantation can be made a routine procedure.

References

1. Jassinowsky A: Ein beitrag zur lehre von der gefassnaht. *Arch Klin Chir* 1891; 42:816.
2. Dorfler J: Ueber arterienaht. *Beitr Klin Chir* 1899; 25:781.
3. Carrel A: La technique operatoire des anastamoses vasculaires et la transplantation des visceres. *Lyon Med* 1902; 98:859.
4. Carrel A: Anastomosis and transplantation of blood vessels. *Am Med* 1905; 10(7):284.
5. Carrel A, Guthrie C: The transplantation of veins and organs. *Am Med* 1905; 10(27):1101.
6. Carrel A: The surgery of blood vessels, etc. *Johns Hopkins Hosp Bull* 1907; 18:18.
7. Demikhov V: *Experimental Transplantation of Vital Organs,* Haigh B (trans). New York, Consultants Bureau, 1962.
8. Marcus E, Wong S, Luisada A: Homologous heart grafts. *Arch Surg* 1952; 66:179.
9. Neptune W, Cookson B, Bailey C, et al: Complete homologous heart transplantation. *Arch Surg* 1953; 66:174.
10. Webb W, Howard H: Cardiopulmonary transplantation. *Surg Forum* 1957; 8:313.
11. Nakae S, Webb W, Theodrides T, et al: Respiratory function following cardiopulmonary denervation in dog, cat and monkey. *Surg Gynecol Obstet* 1967; 85:215.
12. Cooley D, Bloodwell R, Hallman G, et al: Organ transplantation for advanced cardiopulmonary disease. *Ann Thorac Surg* 1969; 8:30.
13. Wildevuur C, Benfield J: A review of 23 human lung transplants by 20 surgeons. *Ann Thorac Surg* 1970; 9:489.
14. Barnard C, Cooper D: Clinical transplantation of the heart: A review of 13 year personal experience. *J R Soc Med* 1981; 74:670.
15. Reitz B, Burton N, Jamieson S, et al: Heart and lung transplantation autotransplantation and allotransplantation in primates with extended survival. *J Thorac Cardiovasc Surg* 1980; 80:360.
16. Burke C, Baldwin J, Morris A, et al: Twenty-eight cases of human heart-lung transplants. *Lancet* 1986, vol 517.
17. Theodore J, Jamieson S, Burke C, et al: Physiologic aspects of human heart-lung transplantation: Pulmonary function status of the post-transplanted lung. *Chest* 1984; 86:349–357.
18. Jamieson S, Stinson E, Oyer P, et al: Operative technique for heart-lung transplantation. *J Thorac Cardiovasc Surg* 1984; 87:930.
19. Jamieson S: Heart-lung transplantation, in Jamieson S, Shumway N (ed): *Rob and Smith's Operative Surgery.* St Louis, CV Mosby Co, 1986, pp 594–605.
20. Kaye M, Elcombe S, O'Fallon W: The International Heart Transplant Registry: The 1984 Report. *Heart Transplant* 1985; 4:290.

21. Burke C, Theodore J, Dawkins K, et al: Post-transplant obliterative bronchiolitis and other late lung sequelae in human heart-lung transplantation. *Chest* 1984; 86:824.
22. Myers B, Ross J, Newton L, et al: Cyclosporine A associated chronic nephropathy in potentially irreversible renal injury. *N Engl J Med* 1984; 311:699.
23. Burke C, Glanville A, Macoviak J, et al: The spectrum of cytomegalovirus infection following human heart-lung transplantation. *J Heart Transplant* 1986; 5:267.
24. Reitz B, Wallwork J, Hunt S, et al: Heart-lung transplantation. *N Engl J Med* 1982; 306:557.
25. Reitz B, Gaudiani V, Hunt S, et al: Diagnosis and treatment of allograft rejection in heart-lung transplant patients. *J Thorac Cardiovasc Surg* 1983; 85:354.
26. McGregor C, Baldwin J, Jamieson S: Isolated pulmonary rejection after combined heart and lung transplantation. *J Thorac Cardiovasc Surg* 1985; 90:623.
27. Griffith B, Hardesty R, Trento A, et al: Asynchronous rejection of heart and lungs following cardiopulmonary transplantation. *Ann Thorac Surg* 1985; 40:488.
28. Zeeri A, Fung J, Paradis I, et al: Lymphocytes of bronchoalveolar lavages from heart-lung transplant recipient. *Heart Transplant* 1985; 4:417.
29. Dawkins K, Jamieson S, Hunt S, et al: Long-term results, hemodynamics, and complications after combined heart-lung transplantation. *Circulation* 1985; 71:919.
30. Allen M, Burke C, McGregor C, et al: Steroid-responsive bronchiolitis after human heart-lung transplantation. *J Thorac Cardiovasc Surg* 1986; 92:449–450.
31. Glanville A, Baldwin J, Burke C, et al: Obliterative bronchiolitis after heart-lung transplantation: Apparent arrest by augmented immunosuppression. *Ann Intern Med* 1987; 107:300.
32. Jamieson S, Starkey T, Sakakibara N, et al: Procurement of organs for combined heart-lung transplantation. *Transplant Proc* 1986; 18:616.
33. Starkey T, Sakakibara N, Hagberg R, et al: Successful six hour cardiopulmonary preservation with simple hypothermic crystalloid flush. *Heart Transplant* 1985; 4(6):601.
34. Ladowski J, Kapelanski D, Teodori M, et al: Experimental use of an autoperfusing heart-lung bloc for organ preservation prior to heart-lung transplantation. *Heart Transplant* 1985; 4(2):128.
35. Robicsek F, Tam W, Daugherty H, et al: The stabilized autoperfused heart-lung operation as a vehicle for extracorporeal preservation. *Transplant Proc* 1969; 1:834.
36. Yousem S, Burke C, Billingham M: Pathologic pulmonary alterations in long-term human heart-lung transplantation. *Hum Pathol* 1985; 16:911–923.
37. Prop J, Wildevuur C, Nieuwenhuis P: Lung allograft rejection after combined heart and lung transplantation. *J Thorac Cardiovasc Surg* 1985; 90:623.

What Are Valid Indications for Carotid Endarterectomy?

Denis S. Quill, M.Ch., F.R.C.S.I.

Vascular Research Fellow, Department of Surgery, Section of Peripheral Vascular Surgery, Southern Illinois University School of Medicine, Springfield, Illinois

David S. Sumner, M.D.

Professor of Surgery, Chief, Section of Peripheral Vascular Surgery, Southern Illinois University School of Medicine, Springfield, Illinois

Stroke ranks third as a cause of death in the United States, exceeded only by coronary artery disease and cancer. Each year, there are 200,000 stroke-related deaths and 500,000 new strokes. The prevalence of stroke is 60 per 1,000 persons in the 65- to 74-year age group and 95 per 1,000 in the 75- to 84-year age group. It has been estimated that 1.6 million Americans are affected by stroke, of whom 40% require special services and 10% require total care.[1] These figures underline the immensity of the burden that stroke imposes on the health care facilities of the nation. Many disciplines and individuals are called upon to reduce this burden. The vascular surgeon is just one of these.

The role of vascular surgery is to prevent those strokes that are associated with atheromatous plaques at the carotid bifurcation. Whereas cerebral thrombosis or embolus is said to account for up to 75% of first strokes, the contribution of carotid bifurcation disease to this total is probably much less.[2] In fact, Harrison recorded bifurcation disease or occlusion in only 28% of patients with cerebral infarcts.[3] Since this limits the target population upon which the vascular surgeon can make an impact, the majority of stroke-prone patients will not be candidates for surgical therapy.

Carotid endarterectomy represents one of the more controversial areas of surgery. Even when disease is present at the carotid bifurcation, the majority of patients will not suffer a stroke. To justify surgical intervention, therefore, the risks of surgery must be balanced against its potential benefits. This is not easy. Not only does the risk of stroke vary with the patient's presenting complaints, but also the risk of operation varies with the surgeon. Much of the uncertainty and controversy arises from the lack of controlled trials in well-defined populations and from differing interpretations of the data available in the literature. Some have adopted an aggressive approach—others are almost militantly conservative.

Adv Surg 22:277–300, 1989

0065-3411/89/22-277–300-$04.00

The increasing frequency with which carotid endarterectomy is being performed in the United States is viewed with mounting concern. In 1985, over 100,000 operations were done for carotid bifurcation disease, a figure that represents a 19-fold difference in operation rates over that existing in Great Britain and Ireland.[4] Assuming that the end points are the same and that the populations are similar, it is difficult to reconcile this disparity. One is tempted to conclude that the indications for operation on the western side of the Atlantic may be too liberal. Operations with "soft" indications, those in which surgical judgment is an important determinant, are likely to be responsible for the variation.[5] Consequently, in comparing data, it is important to define the indications for operation as rigidly as possible. The result of such an analysis is a spectrum of presentations, extending from those where the indications are "cast iron" to those where intervention is much more a case of surgical judgment.

In this review, we will first explore the natural history of the various clinical presentations of carotid bifurcation disease and then attempt to compare this information with the published results of surgery in these same circumstances. At present, it is impossible to propose indications for carotid endarterectomy that will remain valid in the future. As more information appears and as the results of clinical trials now underway are reported, it is reasonable to predict that the indications may change. In the meantime, it is hoped that this review will provide working guidelines that will be of some value to the practicing surgeon.

The Pathogenesis of Symptoms Due to Carotid Bifurcation Disease

Early theories postulated that flow reduction was responsible for the symptoms associated with carotid plaque disease. However, this theory was not supported by measurement of cerebral blood flow, which did not increase following endarterectomy. Rather, there appeared to be a redistribution of flow away from collateral channels and back to mainstream routes.[6] These observations were in keeping with certain other features of carotid disease. First, transient ischemic attacks (TIAs) are episodic. To explain how these attacks might occur in the territory supplied by an artery with a constant stenosis required the assumption that cerebral perfusion was sensitive to change in cardiac output; but, experimentally dropping cardiac output did not reproduce symptoms in patients with TIAs.[7,8] Second, it was noticed that when disease progressed to occlusion, symptoms sometimes ceased. Obviously, this was not a result of increased cerebral perfusion. Moreover, anticoagulant treatment was shown to diminish the frequency of TIAs,[9,10] an effect that could not be attributed to increased cerebral blood flow. Finally, it is well known that strokes may develop in the absence of any diminution of carotid blood flow.

As a result of these and other observations, embolization became the preferred hypothesis. It is now recognized that embolic material can vary. Hollenhorst reported the presence of bright plaques in retinal vessels.[11] He proposed that they were embolic in origin and postulated that they were composed of cholesterol. Gunning suggested that mural thrombi were the source of emboli causing transient monocular or hemispheric dysfunction.[12] Moore stressed the importance of plaque ulceration in the genesis of symptoms and documented an increased risk of stroke in those patients with large ulcers,[13, 14] even in the absence of significant stenotic disease. This presumably reflects an increased tendancy for thrombus to form on the ulcer surface with subsequent cerebral embolization.

More recently, Lusby et al. documented the relationship between plaque morphology and the likelihood of symptoms. In particular, they emphasized the importance of recent intraplaque hemorrhage,[15] which they suggest predisposes to plaque ulceration and subsequent embolization of plaque-associated material. This material may be the surface of the plaque, plaque matter such as cholesterol crystals or intraplaque hematoma, or thrombus forming on the surface of the newly created ulcer.

The scanning electron microscope has added a new dimension of understanding to the problems of plaque-induced embolization. When endarterectomy specimens are viewed using this technique, most demonstrate microulceration or microthrombi on their surfaces—even in the absence of gross ulceration or thrombus on light microscopy.[16, 17] This is also true for specimens from asymptomatic patients. Since the asymptomatic patients who were subjected to operation had severe stenoses, it is perhaps not surprising that their plaques also demonstrated these findings.

Emboli may also arise from nonulcerated plaques. Folts reported that smooth stenoses in canine coronary arteries set up areas of flow separation and platelet deposition.[18] When spontaneous reversal to a more laminar type flow pattern occurs, distal embolization may be the result. These findings have to be validated but are consistent with the production of emboli from the carotid stump following internal carotid occlusion. They also support the concept of embolization from a nonulcerated stenosis.

In summary, the major theories regarding the genesis of TIAs involve embolization of material from carotid plaques. The embolic material may consist of platelet or fibrin thrombi or fragments of plaque originating from ulcers. Flow disturbance caused by stenoses or the stumps of occluded vessels may also cause thrombus formation and embolization (Fig 1). Removal of the embolic focus is the rationale underlying carotid endarterectomy.

Natural History: The Justification for Surgery

Patients with carotid stenosis may present to the vascular surgeon in a number of different clinical circumstances, which reflect differing stroke

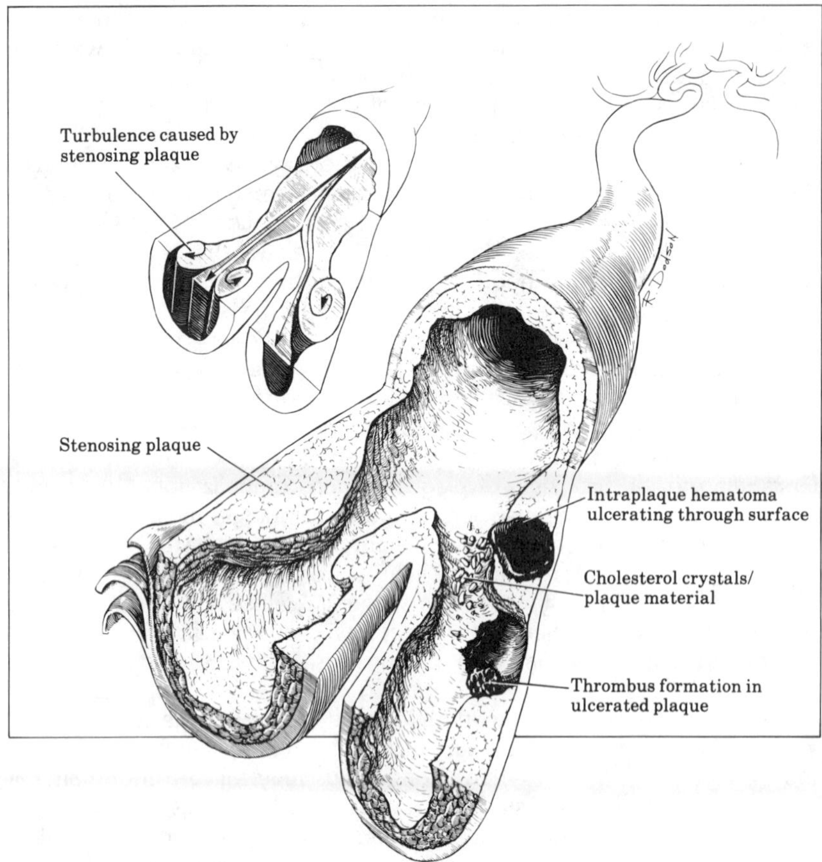

FIG 1.
Illustration of the many pathophysiological mechanisms whereby carotid bifurcation disease may lead to cerebral embolization.

risks. Additional information from noninvasive and radiological investigations will add to or subtract from this sum, to give a working assessment of the chances of serious complications. In this context we are generally speaking of stroke or death.

Transient Ischemic Attacks

Transient ischemic attacks (TIAs) may be defined as focal neurological deficits lasting not more than 24 hours and followed by recovery.[19] When due to carotid bifurcation disease we believe that most of these episodes are embolic. Some patients with TIA will not have significant extracranial arterial disease. In contrast, they may be suffering from heart disease, either valvular or dysrhythmic, hypertension, migraine, or a number of other complaints. This is an important point, as many earlier studies of the natural history of TIA included such patients. For example, studies by Harrison and Ziegler have shown that only 20 to 30% of patients with TIA have significant carotid disease (greater than 30% stenosis).[3, 20] In a later study Harrison stressed that the yield of significant disease can be increased if a patient's symptoms were suggestive of ischemia in a small cortical area.[21]

It is important to remember that many of the early studies that quoted variable stroke risks (between 13 and 30%) contained such mixtures of patients. To illustrate, Acheson and Hutchinson reported a 30% incidence of stroke at almost five years follow-up. This study included all patient subtypes.[22] In contrast, the control group of the joint study survey reported by Fields was restricted to those with symptomatic carotid stenosis.[23] Thirteen percent of the medically managed patients developed strokes within 42 months. This underlines the fact that the natural history of TIA in many studies is not a true representation of the risk in patients whose symptoms are due to significant carotid stenosis. Calculation of a patient's stroke risk can only be made if the data base is appropriate. Table 1 illustrates this variation.

Several studies have shown that increasing carotid stenosis can be related to increasing stroke risk. Ziegler reported a 12% stroke rate in 93 patients with TIA who were followed up for at least three years.[20] This rose to 19% in the subgroup with hemodynamically significant (greater than 50%) lesions. Similarly, there was a 44% stroke rate for those with stenoses greater than 70%. The risk for patients with nonhemodynamically significant disease (less than 50%) was 9.7%.

Moore studied the stroke risk at five years in 46 unoperated patients presenting with TIA.[24] His results showed a 16% incidence of stroke in

TABLE 1.
Stroke Risk Following TIA

Authors	Follow-up	Stroke Rate (%)
Acheson and Hutchinson (1964)[22]	4.8 yr	30
Fields et al. (1970)[23]	42 mo	13
Ziegler and Hassanein (1973)[20]	3 yr	15.6
Toole et al. (1975)[27]	3.8 yr	17
Moore et al. (1985)[24]	5 yr	6.5

those with greater than 50% stenosis. There were no strokes in those with lesser degrees of disease. When the data of Moore and Ziegler are combined the risk of stroke at three to five years is 18% for those with a stenosis greater than 50% (Table 2). Hertzer reported a 31% cumulative stroke rate at 36 months for nonoperated patients with more severe stenoses (greater than 70%), presenting with TIAs.[25] It would appear from these studies that the risk of subsequent stroke parallels the degree of carotid stenosis.

The state of the contralateral carotid artery is another important consideration in risk determination. Hertzer reported a substantially increased risk for patients with bilateral carotid stenoses (greater than 50%) who were nonoperatively managed (23% cumulative stroke rate at four years). This compares with a cumulative stroke rate of 12% for nonoperated patients with unilateral disease; a doubling of stroke risk.[25] Asymptomatic occlusion does not appear to confer the same risk.[26]

In addition to the extent and the degree of the vascular lesion, the pattern of the TIA is probably also important in determining stroke risk. Transient ischemic attacks are traditionally divided into those in the carotid territory, those in the vertebrobasilar territory, and those with mixed-type presentations. Not all studies separate out these groups, but it is probably important as they appear to confer differing risks. Toole demonstrated a 7.6% risk of stroke at 3.8 years of follow-up for symptomatic patients (TIA) with angiographically proven disease restricted to the vertebrobasilar territory.[27] It is unclear from this study whether the clinical pattern of their

TABLE 2.
Stroke Risk (%) Following TIA in Relation to the Degree of Stenosis

	% Diameter Stenosis		
Study	**<50%**	**>50%**	**Total**
Moore[24]			
n	28	18	46
Strokes (%)	0 (0.0)	3 (16.7)	3 (6.5)
Ziegler[20]			
n	72	21	93
Strokes (%)	7 (9.7)	4 (19)	4 (11.8)
Moore & Ziegler combined			
n	100	39	139
Strokes (%)	7 (7)	7 (17.9)	14 (10.07)

symptoms corresponded to their angiographic appearances. Clinical presentation may not parallel the site of angiographic disease. However, there does appear to be a suggestion of lesser risk for this group. Ziegler's study, which did not reveal the angiographic status of patients with vertebrobasilar TIAs, documented a 6.8% stroke rate at three years for this subgroup.[20] These findings are in agreement with Toole's study and suggest that vertebrobasilar symptoms confer a somewhat lesser risk than those arising in the carotid territory.[27]

Amaurosis Fugax

Temporary monocular blindness (amaurosis fugax) has long been associated with increased stroke risk. In this context it is important to realize that there is a whole spectrum of ocular disturbances associated with carotid bifurcation disease. Kirshner reported ocular symptoms in 25% of patients undergoing carotid endarterectomy (amaurosis fugax in 19%, retinal artery occlusion in 4%, ischemic optic neuropathy in 1.5%, homonomous hemianopia in 0.7%.[28] Thirty-three percent of those with amaurosis fugax had associated TIAs and 83% had a high-grade carotid stenosis. It is important to realize that some 6% of patients had permanent visual loss and this was unheralded in 27 of this group of 32 patients.

The risk of stroke has traditionally been regarded as high in this group of patients. Indeed, most classify amaurosis fugax as an example of focal carotid territory TIAs. Pfaffenbach described 208 patients with retinal cholesterol emboli, 27 of whom had amaurosis fugax.[29] Twelve of this group (44%) suffered a stroke during follow-up. Marshall reported a 6% stroke rate and an 11% incidence of monocular blindness during follow-up of 80 patients with amaurosis fugax.[30] This complication rate is almost certainly an underestimate, as it included a number of young female patients. Additionally, only 55% of those who had angiography performed had significant bifurcation disease. Thus we can see that amaurosis fugax is a significant symptom of carotid bifurcation disease and is a herald of stroke or permanent blindness in a substantial proportion of patients.

This series of studies has revealed a number of important features for consideration when assessing the risks of an individual who presents with TIA due to carotid bifurcation disease. Firstly, it must be established that significant carotid stenosis is present. In this respect the more focal the symptoms, and this includes amaurosis fugax, the more likely they are to represent significant carotid disease. Secondly, patients with vertebrobasilar symptoms are probably a group with significantly lower stroke risk. Thirdly, the risks of stroke appear to parallel the severity of bifurcation disease. This is probably the most important feature when assessing risk in this group of patients. Finally, a contralateral severe stenosis or occlusion is an additional risk factor in patients with carotid stenosis and ipsilateral hemispheric TIAs.

Asymptomatic Carotid Disease

A commonly encountered clinical situation is that of the patient who presents with an asymptomatic carotid bruit, discovered incidentally. At the outset one should be certain that the patient is indeed asymptomatic, as a careful history can often reveal significant symptoms. The subsequent strategy is to try to assess the risk of stroke for that individual patient.

The reported incidence of stroke risk in people with asymptomatic carotid stenosis shows striking variation (Table 3).[24, 31–34] Thompson's article is well-quoted as an example of high stroke risk (17%) in medically managed (n = 138) patients with asymptomatic carotid bruits, who were followed up for an average of 45 months.[33] Unfortunately, this was a heterogeneous group of patients and only half of them were assessed with angiography. Also included in this group were patients with other conditions that precluded treatment of their carotid disease (impending gangrene, etc.). Clearly they cannot be taken as representative of patients with asymptomatic carotid stenosis.

Three recent prospective studies have looked at the problem of stroke risk in patients with asymptomatic bifurcation disease. Roederer demonstrated a 2.4% stroke rate in 167 patients with asymptomatic bruits.[32] One should note that follow-up was a little short (17 patients at 36 months). Colgan found a cumulative stroke-free rate at one and three years of 98% and 97%, respectively, in patients with asymptomatic stenosis.[31] Both these studies demonstrated the phenomenon of disease progression (33% and 13%, respectively, over three years). Smoking and diabetes showed significant correlation with progression. Finally, the Toronto asymptomatic cervical bruit study revealed a 1.7% stroke risk at an average follow-up of 23 months.[34] This rose to 3.3% in those with greater than 30% stenosis.

It would seem from these prospective studies, which have to receive greater weighting than the retrospective papers quoted, that this condition

TABLE 3.
Stroke Risk in Patients With Asymptomatic Carotid Disease

Study	Follow-up, mo	Stroke Risk (%)	Total (n)
Roederer[32]	6–36	4 (2.39)	167
Colgan[31]	2–48 (mean, 32)	4 (2.10)	190
Chambers[34]	Up to 48 (mean, 23)	8 (1.6)	500
Thompson[33]	Up to 180	24 (17.4)	138

is a low stroke risk situation. That being the case the next question is whether a high-risk subgroup can be identified. Secondly, what is the natural history of such high-risk subgroups? Do they become symptomatic before developing strokes or are their strokes unheralded?

Taking the second question first, perhaps 35 to 50% of strokes due to extracranial arterial disease will not be heralded by a TIA.[35] This figure cannot be applied to the population of people with asymptomatic carotid stenosis, as it is derived from a population with strokes. However, it does seem to indicate that a proportion of persons will progress to stroke without developing TIA. Unheralded stroke was seen in eight of the 12 patients who suffered this complication in the Toronto asymptomatic bruit study.[34] Similarly, three of the four strokes in Roederer's study occurred without warning.[32] This is an important factor in assessing risk.

There are few studies addressing the problem of the high-grade stenosis in asymptomatic patients (Table 4). Bogousslavsky published a prospective study of 38 patients with internal carotid stenosis greater than 90%, followed up for 48 months.[36] Four of these patients (10.5%) developed an ipsilateral hemispheric defect (three infarcts, one hemorrhage) accompanied by clinical stroke. Overall five patients suffered strokes (one contralateral). In the Toronto asymptomatic cervical bruit study there was a 15% per annum neurological event rate (stroke or TIA) in those with greater than 75% stenosis. The stroke rate at one year in this group was 5.5%.[34] Busattil reported results of a study of 73 patients with asymptomatic bruit followed up for almost three years.[37] Oculoplethysmography was used to determine a hemodynamically significant lesion (greater than 60%). There was a 6.6% incidence of stroke in this group. There were no strokes in the group with a lesser degree of stenosis. Transient ischemic attacks occurred during follow-up in 29% of those with and 7.1% of those without a hemodynamically significant lesion. Hertzer retrospectively studied 290 asymptomatic patients at the Cleveland Clinic with a stenosis greater than 50%.[38] Ninety-five patients were treated operatively; 195 were not. In the

TABLE 4.
Stroke Risk (%) in Asymptomatic Patients With High-Grade Stenoses

Study	Degree of Stenosis	Stroke Risk (%)	Total (n)
Bogousslavsky[36]	>90%	4 (10.5) at 4 yr	38
Chambers[34]	>75%	6 (5.3) at 1 yr	113
Hertzer[38]	>70%	24 (34) at 33–38 mo	70

subset of nonoperated patients with greater than 70% stenosis, 24 (33%) developed completed strokes in the follow-up period (33 to 38 months).

Plaque Morphology

Moore has stressed the importance of plaque ulceration in asymptomatic patients.[19] His group documented an annual stroke rate of 4.5% for large and 7.5% for cavernous plaque ulcers in patients with asymptomatic nonstenotic carotid bifurcation disease.[14] Interestingly, Bernstein's group found a 1% seven-year stroke risk in a similar group of patients.[39] However, their study group did not include any patients with the large type C ulcers. This last mentioned condition, the type C cavernous ulcer, is probably a relatively rare occurrence.

More recently, Lusby has drawn attention to the importance of intraplaque hemorrhage and its diagnosis by noninvasive techniques.[15, 40] His hypothesis is that intraplaque hemorrhage can, by mass effect, change a noncritical stenosis into one that is critical. Alternatively, a recent hemorrhage can ulcerate and thereby embolize. Additionally the resulting ulcer can promote thrombus formation and consequent embolization. He classifies plaque into four subgroups as revealed by duplex scanning. These groupings show a gradation between a heterogenous "eggshell" type lesion (type 1) to a homogenous fibrous plaque (type 4). When removed at endarterectomy the type 1 lesions show a high proportion of recent hemorrhage and are significantly related to the presence of ipsilateral symptoms. These studies may well represent an illustration of how intraplaque hemorrhage, plaque ulceration, and stroke risk can be interrelated. An ongoing prospective study of plaque morphology in unoperated patients will be necessary in order to definitively answer these questions. Ethical considerations make such a study unlikely.

Completed Stroke, Stroke in Evolution, and Crescendo TIA

Previous completed stroke is a significant risk factor for a second stroke. An initial stroke carries a mortality risk of between 15 and 80%, depending on the type of stroke. Intracerebral hemorrhage fares worst.[41] The overall risk of recurrent stroke lies in the region of 20 to 30%, and although estimates of the annual rate of recurrence vary, it has been suggested that for an ischemic stroke, 6 to 12% per year is a realistic range.[42, 43]

The previously quoted figures refer to the overall group, with stroke and ischemic stroke in particular. The majority of those patients will have significant neurological deficits and are clearly not candidates for consideration for surgery. This directs our attention to the natural history of small completed strokes. In this context there are far fewer studies available for guidance. In addition, the terminology and classification of these cerebral ischemic symptoms are somewhat confusing. Patients who have transient deficits that last more than one day but less than 21 days were previously classified as having had a reversible ischemic neurological deficit (RIND).[44] With more experience it has become apparent that TIA, RIND, and small permanent deficits are a spectrum of disease in patients whose symptoms are due to bifurcation atherosclerosis.[45] More recently, it has been shown that RIND and TIA confer similar magnitude risks of subsequent stroke.[45, 46] This has caused some to suggest that the term RIND is confusing and should be disregarded.[47]

Definite small permanent strokes appear to confer a similar stroke risk, as do TIA and RIND. Thus, Humphrey recorded 38%, 38%, and 23% subsequent stroke rates for patients with TIA, RIND, and small completed stroke, respectively.[45] Computed tomographic (CT) scan was obtained selectively in this study and 18%, 52%, and 47% were the respective yields of infarcts in the three groups (TIA, RIND, stroke). Positive CT scan for infarct, in those presenting with TIA, had a high predictive value for subsequent stroke (90%).

The timing of subsequent stroke has important implications for the vascular surgeon. In the previously quoted study, 48% of subsequent strokes in those with RIND or small completed strokes developed within six months. Others have suggested that in patients with small completed strokes, the risk of early subsequent stroke is much higher. Thus, Dosick reported a 21% stroke rate within six weeks or an initial mild stroke, presumed to be due to bifurcation disease.[48] These results require confirmation.

From these studies, it would seem that small stable completed strokes, RIND, and TIA all confer approximately similar stroke risks. In addition, there is a suggestion that for those with small completed strokes, there may be an increased risk of stroke in the early weeks following the first event.

Stroke in evolution and crescendo TIA are far more serious conditions. Due to the great variation in cerebrovascular symptom complexes, it is important to define these conditions precisely. Crescendo TIA refers to a condition characterized by frequent hemispheric or monocular TIAs, usually lasting a few minutes to a few hours, which leave no residual signs between attacks. The attacks abruptly increase in frequency to at least several each day. Stroke in evolution refers to an unstable period of hours or days during which a neurological deficit progresses or waxes and wanes.[49] These are patients with mild to moderate deficits only and do not include patients with altered levels of consciousness.

The natural history of these two conditions is far more severe than for patients with TIA. Millikan described the clinical course of 204 patients with stroke in evolution. Seventy-five percent had suffered a stroke and 14% had died within 14 days.[50] Mentzer's data support this bleak picture: 66% of patients suffering stroke and 15% dying during the acute event.[51]

The natural history of crescendo TIA is somewhat less well-defined but seems to confer similar magnitude risk. In Mentzer's series, four of five untreated patients with this condition either suffered a stroke (three) or died (one).[51] This is the background against which the results of surgery will be judged.

These studies document the natural history of nonoperatively managed carotid bifurcation disease. Despite the conflicting nature of some studies, we can identify certain patient groups with definitely increased stroke risk. Symptomatic (TIA) patients with significant (>50%) stenoses, asymptomatic patients with high-grade stenoses (>75%), and patients with small completed strokes, crescendo TIA, or stroke in evolution are all in this category. The vascular surgeon balances the risks posed by the patients presenting symptom complex, which has just been considered, with the results of surgery, which will be considered next. This enables him or her to make the final decision.

The Results of Carotid Endarterectomy

Lack of modern prospective studies documenting clear benefit following surgery has cast a certain doubt on the efficacy of carotid endarterectomy. Patients with carotid stenosis are a high-risk group with an appreciable mortality from associated disorders (cardiac disease, etc.).[52, 53] This underlines the need to see benefits in as short a time as possible following surgery.

Whereas isolated uncontrolled reports document an apparent improvement in prognosis following endarterectomy, the failure of the one randomized trial, the joint study, to show such a benefit, supports those who criticize surgery (Table 5).[23] Chambers and Norris have stressed the importance of a knowledge of the stroke risk of untreated patients in the

TABLE 5.
Joint Study Data[23]*

	Surgical Treatment (n = 169)	Medical Treatment (n = 147)
Hospital deaths	6	1
Hospital strokes	13	1
Follow-up deaths	23	27
Follow-up strokes	6	18
Total deaths†	29	28
Total strokes†	19	29

*All patients (mean follow-up = 42 months).
†$P > .05$ χ^2.

surgical decision-making process.[54] They suggest that this should be of the order of less than 5% per year in order to justify operation. Using the results of the joint study and the Mayo Clinic, both of which documented a two-third reduction in stroke rate following endarterectomy, they calculated that a 3% combined perioperative stroke and death rate is necessary to justify surgery, on a population with an annual stroke risk of 5% (Fig 2).[23, 55] Hass and Jonas have endorsed this viewpoint and suggested that many units fail to perform to these standards.[56]

The usefulness of these theoretical calculations is that they underline a number of the most important components in the equation of patient benefit analysis. They are: the stroke risk of the condition being treated, the perioperative stroke and death rates, and the late stroke rate—preferably expressed as the cumulative stroke-free survival—of the postoperative survivors. What then of the published results of surgery; do they stand up to these theoretical calculations?

With regard to the natural history and stroke rate of the differing presentations, it has already been seen that high-grade asymptomatic lesions (greater than 75%) and symptomatic (TIA) patients with moderate to severe carotid stenosis (50 to 70%) both provide stroke rates greater than 5% per year. This provides a satisfactory figure for the first variable. Presuming reasonable perioperative performance, which will be dealt with later, a number of studies have documented substantial and significant reduction in the late stroke rate for such patients. Moore compared the late results in 81 operated and 294 unoperated patients who were asympto-

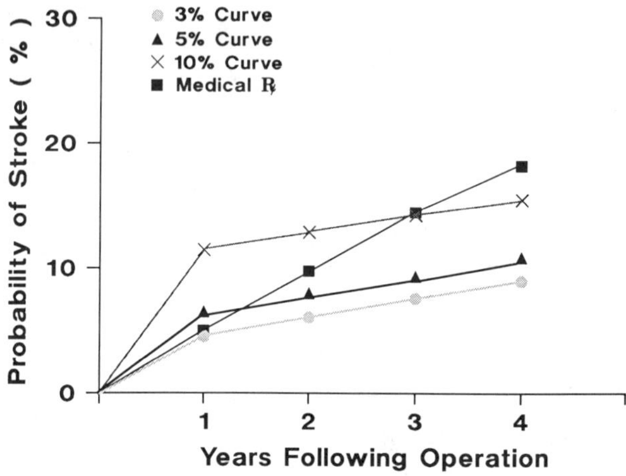

FIG 2.
Graphical illustration of the results of surgical treatment for carotid stenosis (greater than 50%). The different surgical curves reflect perioperative stroke/death rates of 3%, 5%, and 10%. The curve for nonoperative treatment assumes a 5% per-year stroke rate.

matic or who had nonhemispheric symptoms.[57] Using actuarial methods he documented a significant improvement in stroke rate following carotid endarterectomy at five-year follow-up (8% vs. 21%). Hertzer similarly documented significant improvement in the stroke rate of symptomatic patients (TIA) with greater than 70% stenosis when compared with unoperated controls. In this study the unoperated patients had a 31% cumulative stroke rate at four years in comparison to a 7% stroke rate in those treated surgically.[25] Similarly, symptomatic patients with bilateral stenosis or contralateral occlusion demonstrated a benefit from surgery.[25]

A major drawback to many reports of the results of carotid endarterectomy is lack of appropriate control groups. Moore's control group in the study quoted above seems appropriate and also demonstrated an appreciable late stroke rate. In Hertzer's study, however, the control group was not randomly allocated and this probably reduced the risk for these patients, as the surgeons were free to select out those at increased risk and subject them to operation. As the authors themselves commented, this resulted in a predominance of stable lesions in the 50 to 70% range. Consequently it becomes more difficult to show a benefit from surgery, even when one exists. This may account for the fact that no benefit was seen for operated patients with unilateral disease in the 50 to 70% range.

The late stroke rate following endarterectomy might be expected to differ for different patient presentations. This is important, particularly when assessing uncontrolled results. Both Hertzer and Bernstein have reported their units' experiences from this point of view. Both document similar late stroke rates and clinical courses in patients treated for asymptomatic disease and TIA.[58, 59] In contrast, patients who have suffered a previous stroke appear to have a more severe prognosis, as do patients with contralateral symptoms or occlusion, the late stroke rates for these patients being considerably greater. In addition, both Moore and Hertzer have shown that age (greater than 70) and hypertension, but not diabetes, significantly reduce an individual's chances of stroke-free survival—both before and after surgery.[57, 58]

Due to the very different natural history of completed stroke, stroke in evolution, and crescendo TIA, these conditions have to be considered separately. Small completed strokes appear to have the most benign prognosis within this subgroup. The natural history of TIA, RIND, and small completed stroke appears to be similar.[45, 46] The early and late results of surgery, however, appear to be slightly worse for those with small completed strokes and this must be considered when contemplating surgery.[58, 59] Whereas the late stroke rate is difficult to control, the perioperative stroke rate is more variable.

There has been a suggestion that these patients are more at risk of perioperative stroke in the early (within six weeks) poststroke period. Thus Giordano reported an 18% stroke rate in patients operated on within five weeks of a small stroke, as opposed to none in those who had their operations after this time.[60] Because others have suggested that up to 20%

of these patients suffer a second stroke within this six-week time, it has been suggested that CT scan can be used to select those who do not have an infarct. These patients are then operated on promptly, in order to avoid early recurrent stroke. The concept of early recurrent stroke has yet to be validated. Others have produced impressive results from early surgery in this group and have questioned the wisdom of a six-week waiting period.[61]

Crescendo TIA and stroke in evolution are conditions with a much more severe natural history. We have already seen that three quarters of these patients will suffer a stroke if managed along conventional lines.[50, 51] Goldstone and Mentzer both reported small series of these patients, whom they managed operatively. They advocated rapid assessment and operation if a "critical or unstable" lesion was found at angiography.[51, 62] A critical or unstable lesion in this setting was a high-grade stenosis or one associated with intraluminal free-floating thrombus. These two series reported very impressive results following surgery. There were no perioperative strokes in Goldstone's series and over 70% were stroke-free in Mentzer's series, with no patient suffering a deterioration of preoperative neurological status. It must be stated that this is a very controversial and high-risk situation. Such surgery should still be regarded as experimental and be carried out by surgeons with experience with and an interest in these special problems.

Whereas the late stroke rate for patients discharged from the hospital following successful endarterectomy is unlikely to vary greatly between institutions, study of the quoted perioperative stroke and mortality rates reveals a different picture (Table 6).[63–70] This factor is critical with regard to determination of patient benefit following operation. It has already been

TABLE 6.
Perioperative Stroke and Mortality Rates (Percentages) Following Carotid Endarterectomy for TIA

Author	Year	Perioperative Strokes (%)	Perioperative Deaths (%)
DeWeese[63]	1973	5.8	1.9
Takolander[64]	1983	4.9	1.8
Eriksson[65]	1981	2.3	2.3
Till[66]	1987	2.2	1.6
Watson[67]	1981	4.3	0.0
Carmichael[68]	1980	2.1	0.3
Easton[69]	1977	14.0	7.0
Modi[70]	1983	1.6	0.4

seen that this is one of the most important variables in the determination of patient benefit. Perioperative stroke and death rates need to be kept below 5% in order to achieve satisfactory results. The very large variations in surgical performance reported in the literature present a major problem in this respect. Optimization of surgical results involves minimization of perioperative mortality and stroke rates, together with selection of only high-risk patients for surgical treatment.

It would seem from the surgical literature that the stroke and mortality rates following carotid endarterectomy have a bimodal distribution. Naturally, editors will more readily publish results that reflect the extremes of performance. Unfortunately, this tends to produce a very clear-cut distinction between those whose figures do and those whose results do not justify performing these operations. The fact is that the real spectrum of surgical performance is probably a skewed bell-shaped distribution. The point of this argument is that surgical audit is mandatory, for not only will it enable the individual to assess his or her performance, but it has also been shown that feedback can improve a unit's results.[66, 70] Individual surgeons carrying out carotid surgery must know where they lie in the spectrum of performance. This information can then be used to achieve improvement and minimize the risks to their patients.

Two Additional Clinical Problems

Having dealt with the major indications for carotid surgery in isolation, we now turn to two further clinical problems that require consideration. They are: firstly, the problem of combined carotid and coronary artery disease and, secondly, recurrent carotid stenosis.

Carotid and coronary artery stenoses are both manifestations of a widespread disease and their combination in any one patient is not a rarity. Hemodynamically significant carotid disease in a patient scheduled for coronary artery bypass presents the urgent possibility of perioperative stroke. The indications for carotid surgery are the same as when patients present with carotid disease alone. The major question concerns the timing of surgery.

Noninvasive studies by Barnes and Turnipseed revealed that the incidence of perioperative stroke associated with coronary artery bypass is not substantially greater in patients with hemodynamically significant carotid disease.[71, 72] Despite this, others have clearly shown that if this group is intensively studied, it will reveal a substantial proportion of patients who have severe carotid stenosis.[73] These patients will undoubtedly require surgery at some stage; the question remaining is one of timing. Whereas no definite increased perioperative stroke risk can be identified for this group, we must still deal with the individual. Concomitant coronary artery surgery is a definite risk situation.

In the absence of any specific contraindication it is logical to suggest that carotid surgery be carried out as early as possible. Hertzer's group have looked at this problem. They have shown that by performing carotid surgery first, in a staged sequence, there was a 1.5% postoperative stroke rate with none occurring at the time of subsequent coronary artery bypass.[74] The only drawback to this approach is the fact that a certain proportion of patients (up to 20%) will suffer a myocardial infarction in the intervening period.[75, 76] When the operations are performed concomitantly Hertzer reported a much higher combined stroke and myocardial infarction rate (4.5 and 6.3%, respectively).[77] When studied more closely, it became apparent that the poorer results were probably a result of risk weighting in this subgroup. Mean age and the prevalence of prognostically more severe coronary artery disease were both higher in this group. Late survival for this group was not significantly different from the male population at large (life table method).

It would appear from these studies that a certain proportion of patients will require both carotid and coronary artery surgery. The decision regarding staged as opposed to combined operation remains one of surgical judgment. Current studies suggest that either approach may be applied with a reasonable margin of safety.

Recurrent carotid stenosis, although not a primary condition, is another indication for surgery that requires consideration. The incidence of this complication varies greatly between reports and to some extent this appears to be a function of how intensively the condition is sought.[78] Two distinct entities may produce recurrent carotid stenosis. The first is a reaction of the vessel wall, which occurs within the first two years following surgery. This myointimal proliferation produces a relatively smooth stenosis. In contrast, recurrent stenosis occurring after this time is more likely to be due to atherosclerosis. Platelet-derived growth factors have been implicated in the initiation of myointimal hyperplasia, but the mechanisms are incompletely understood.[79] O'Donnell maintains that B-mode ultrasound can distinguish the two processes.[80]

Intervention for recurrent carotid stenosis has generally been limited to patients who develop recurrent symptoms. No individual can present a large enough series to be authoritative, but that appears to be the consensus.[79, 81] As the incidence of symptomatic restenosis (0.5 to 3.6%) is considerably less than the incidence of hemodynamically significant restenosis (12 to 19%), most authors advise a cautious approach rather than early intervention.[79, 81–83] Most series report a higher incidence of myointimal hyperplasia in women. It is uncertain whether this is a real association or merely a reflection of smaller vessels. Operation generally takes the form of re-endarterectomy and vein patch angioplasty.[79] The results of such surgery would appear to be good.

Medical Alternatives to Surgical Treatment

In addition to the natural history of carotid disease, the results of medical therapy must also be considered prior to making a decision regarding the advisability of surgery. It is true that all control groups will have received medical therapy of some form. However, this was probably not standardized and is a poor indicator of its efficacy. As embolism is the mechanism whereby carotid bifurcation disease produces its effects on the brain, it is logical that the main forms of medical treatment are anticoagulant and antiplatelet drugs. In addition, it must be remembered that not all strokes occur due to embolization to the cerebral hemisphere ipsilateral to a carotid stenosis. Consequently, proper control of hypertension, diabetes, and other conditions that contribute to the overall stroke risk will improve the group's outlook.

Before examining the results of medical therapy it should be pointed out that in most trials the carotid bifurcation was not objectively assessed. As a result the study groups included those who were symptomatic due to carotid stenosis in addition to those who had other reasons for their complaints. This is important when interpreting the results of treatment.

A number of studies document a reduction in the incidence of TIAs with warfarin treatment.[84–86] Whereas the stroke rate showed a trend toward reduction, it only achieved significance in one retrospective study.[85] In the last mentioned series the net probability of stroke at five years was considerably less in the treated group (20 vs. 40%). This still constitutes a significant stroke risk.

Antiplatelet therapy has generally employed either aspirin or dipyridamole. A number of large studies have documented significant reduction in the combined stroke and TIA rates with aspirin.[87–89] In contrast, the same studies have shown that dipyridamole adds nothing to the efficacy of aspirin. It must be emphasized that the proportion of patients with significant bifurcation disease varied between these series. In that respect, they cannot be seen as strictly comparable to well-defined candidates for surgical treatment. The stroke risk of some 20% at five years for those treated with aspirin in the American-Canadian cooperative study must be seen in this light.[89]

Analysis of these results forces one to conclude that the available forms of medical treatment can produce a reduction in the incidence of TIA and stroke. The magnitude of this reduction does not appear to be as great as that seen following carotid surgery, although judgment must be reserved as to whether these patient groups are strictly comparable.

Conclusion

Finally, at the end of this review, it must be apparent to the reader that the major problem encountered in the analysis of patient benefit relates to the lack of strong data. There are numerous studies reporting very differing results following surgery. In addition, the natural history of the disease is obtained by careful analysis of subgroups within a number of differing studies. No clear actuarial data exist that might document the extent and degree of disease and relate this to the natural history or, at least, to the results of the "best of medical therapy." Survival and stroke freedom curves following such treatment could then be related to the results of surgery in similarly, clearly documented patients. Such attention to detail might at least enable accurate identification of at-risk groups who would be more likely to benefit from surgery.

Recently, a proposal for a uniform system of recording clinical data in patients with carotid stenosis has come from Browse and Bernstein's group.[90] This system would allow accurate documentation of history, physical findings, full extracranial vascular assessment, hemispheric involvement, and previous neurologic events. The CHAT system, as it is called, is perhaps analogous to the TNM classification of cancer. The adoption of such a system, in scientific papers concerned with extracranial vascular disease, should allow a much more accurate comparison of data. If this were linked to the practice of reporting follow-up results using actuarial methods, we might at last unequivocally identify the relative positions of surgical and medical treatments for extracranial vascular disease.

Despite these problems a number of facts can be established. It is now clear that embolization is the major process whereby carotid bifurcation disease causes symptoms or strokes. Carotid endarterectomy is appropriate treatment provided that a high stroke risk can be established and reasonable perioperative performance can be assured. Patients with high-grade asymptomatic stenosis (greater than 75%), those with symptomatic disease (TIA or small completed stroke) with significant bifurcation pathology (50 to 70% stenosis), or those with symptomatic restenosis are all surgical candidates. Symptomatic patients with significant contralateral disease are also at increased risk. Surgery may be considered even when their ipsilateral carotid stenosis is at the lower end of the usual range for operative intervention. This is an example of a clinical situation where surgical judgment, which must consider the entire spectrum of the patient's presentation and risk factors, is still the order of the day. Stroke in evolution is a complicated problem with a very high mortality and permanent stroke rate. This is best managed, as an emergency, in specialized units with an interest in that problem. Advances in this field will undoubtedly come from further prospective studies of the best of medical vs. the best of surgical treatment. This must be in similar well-defined patient populations. The contentious and grey areas of carotid surgery will finally be elucidated only by such a methodical approach.

References

1. Wolf PA, Dawber TR, Thomas HE, et al: Epidemiology of stroke, in Thompson RA, Green JR (eds): *Advances in Neurology*. New York, Raven Press, 1977, vol 16, pp 5–19.
2. Anderson GL, Whisnant JP: A comparison of trends in mortality from stroke in the United States and Rochester, Minnesota. *Stroke* 1982; 13:804–809.

3. Harrison MJG, Marshall J: Angiographic appearance of carotid bifurcation in patients with completed stroke, transient ischaemic attacks and cerebral tumour. *Br Med J* 1976; 1:205–207.
4. Murie JA, Morris PJ: Carotid endarterectomy in Great Britain and Ireland. *Br J Surg* 1986; 73:867–870.
5. Quill DS, Devlin HB, Plant JA, et al: Surgical operation rates: A twelve year experience in Stockton on Tees. *Ann R Coll Surg Eng* 1983; 65:248–253.
6. Adams JE, Smith MC, Wylie EJ: Cerebral blood flow and haemodynamics in extracranial vascular disease: Effect of endarterectomy. *Surgery* 1963; 53:449–455.
7. Fazekas JF, Alman RW: The role of hypotension in transitory focal cerebral ischaemia. *Am J Med Sci* 1964; 248:567–570.
8. Kendell RE, Marshall J: Role of hypotension in the genesis of transient focal cerebral ischaemic attacks. *Br Med J* 1963; 2:344–348.
9. Fisher CM: The use of anticoagulants in cerebral thrombosis. *Neurology* 1958; 8:311–332.
10. Millikan CH, Siekert RG, Schick RM: Studies in cerebrovascular disease: V. The use of anticoagulant drugs in the treatment of intermittent insufficiency of the internal carotid arterial system. *Proc Mayo Clin* 1955; 30:578–586.
11. Hollenhorst RW: Significance of bright plaques in the retinal arterioles. *JAMA* 1961; 178:23–29.
12. Gunning AJ, Pickering GW, Robb-Smith AHT, et al: Mural thrombosis of the internal carotid artery and subsequent embolism. *Q J Med* 1964; 33:155–195.
13. Moore WS, Boren C, Malone JM, et al: Natural history of non-stenotic asymptomatic ulcerative lesions of the carotid artery. *Arch Surg* 1978; 113:1352–1359.
14. Dixon S, Pais O, Raviola C, et al: Natural history of non-stenotic asymptomatic ulcerative lesions of the carotid artery: A further analysis. *Arch Surg* 1982; 117:1493–1498.
15. Lusby RJ, Ferrell LD, Wylie EJ: The significance of intraplaque haemorrhage in the pathogenesis of carotid atherosclerosis, in Bergan JJ, Yao JST (eds): *Cerebrovascular Insufficiency*. New York, Grune & Stratton Inc, 1983, pp 41–55.
16. Smith RR, Russell WF, Percy MS: Ultrastructure of carotid plaques. *Surg Neurol* 1980; 14:145–153.
17. Hertzer NR, Beven EG, Benjamin SP: Ultramicroscopic ulcerations and thrombi of the carotid bifurcation. *Arch Surg* 1977; 112:1394–1402.
18. Folts JD, Gallagher K, Rowe GG: Blood flow reduction in stenosed canine coronary arteries: Vasospasm or platelet aggregation. *Circulation* 1982; 65:248–255.
19. Moore WS, Quinones-Baldrich WJ: Extracranial cerebrovascular disease, in Moore WS (ed): *Vascular Surgery: A Comprehensive Review*. Orlando, Grune & Stratton Inc, 1986, pp 621–681.
20. Ziegler DK, Hassanein RS: Prognosis in patients with transient ischaemic attacks. *Stroke* 1973; 4:666–673.
21. Harrison MJG, Iansek R, Marshall J: Clinical identification of TIAs due to carotid stenosis. *Stroke* 1986; 17:391–392.
22. Acheson J, Hutchinson EC: Observations of the natural history of transient cerebral ischaemia. *Lancet* 1964; 11:871–874.
23. Fields WS, Maslenikov V, Meyer JS: Joint study of extracranial arterial occlu-

sion: V. Progress report of prognosis following surgery or non-surgical treatment for transient cerebral attacks and cervical carotid artery lesions. *JAMA* 1970; 211:1993–2003.

24. Moore DJ, Sheehan MP, Kolm P, et al: Are strokes predictable with non-invasive methods: A five year follow-up of 303 unoperated patients. *J Vasc Surg* 1985; 2:654–660.
25. Hertzer NR, Flanagan RA, O'Hara PJ, et al: Surgical versus nonoperative treatment of symptomatic carotid stenosis. *Ann Surg* 1986; 204:154–162.
26. Nicholls SC, Kohler TR, Bergelin RO, et al: Carotid artery occlusion: Natural history. *J Vasc Surg* 1986; 4:479–485.
27. Toole JF, Janeway R, Choi K, et al: Transient ischaemic attacks due to atherosclerosis. *Arch Neurol* 1975; 32:5–12.
28. Kirshner RL, Green RM, Searl SS, et al: Ocular manifestations of carotid artery atheroma. *J Vasc Surg* 1985; 2:850–853.
29. Pfaffenbach DD, Hollenhorst RW: Morbidity and survivorship of patients with embolic cholesterol crystals in the ocular fundus. *Am J Ophthalmol* 1973; 75:66–72.
30. Marshall J, Meadows S: The natural history of amaurosis fugax. *Brain* 1968; 91:419–434.
31. Colgan MP, Kingston W, Shanik DG: Asymptomatic carotid stenosis: Is prophylactic endarterectomy justifiable? *Br J Surg* 1985; 72:313–314.
32. Roederer GO, Langlois YE, Jager KA, et al: The natural history of carotid arterial disease in asymptomatic patients with cervical bruits. *Stroke* 1984; 15:605–613.
33. Thompson JE, Patman RD, Talkington CM: Asymptomatic carotid bruit: Long term outcome of patients having endarterectomy compared with unoperated controls. *Ann Surg* 1978; 188:308–316.
34. Chambers BR, Norris JW: Outcome in patients with asymptomatic neck bruits. *N Engl J Med* 1986; 315:860–865.
35. Mohr JP, Kaplan LR, Melski JW, et al: The Harvard cooperative stroke registry: A prospective registry. *Neurology* 1978; 28:754–762.
36. Bogousslavsky J, Despland PA, Regli F: Asymptomatic tight stenosis of the internal carotid artery: Long term prognosis. *Neurology* 1968; 36:861–863.
37. Busattil RW, Baker JD, Davidson RK, et al: Carotid artery stenosis: Haemodynamic significance and clinical course. *JAMA* 1981; 245:1438–1441.
38. Hertzer NR, Flanagan RA, O'Hara PJ, et al: Surgical versus nonoperative treatment of asymptomatic carotid stenosis. *Ann Surg* 1986; 204:163–171.
39. Kroener JM, Dorn PL, Shoor PM, et al: Prognosis of asymptomatic ulcerating carotid lesions. *Arch Surg* 1980; 115:1387–1392.
40. Lusby RJ: Carotid artery disease: Pathophysiology and evaluation of patients with transient cerebral ischaemia. Hunterian Lecture of Royal College of Surgeons of England, London, Charing Cross Hospital, May 1987.
41. Sacco RL, Wolf PA, Kannel WB, et al: Survival and recurrence following stroke: The Framingham study. *Stroke* 1982; 13:290–295.
42. Matsumoto N, Whisnant JP, Kurland LT, et al: Natural history of stroke in Rochester, Minnesota, 1955 through 1969: An extension of a previous study, 1965 through 1954. *Stroke* 1973; 4:20–29.
43. Bernstein EF, Bardin JA: Influence of prior neurological deficit on the benefits of carotid endarterectomy, in Courbier R (ed): *Basis for a Classification of Cerebral Arterial Diseases.* Amsterdam, Excerpta Medica, 1985, pp 246–258.

44. Millikan CH: A classification and outline of cerebrovascular disease II. *Stroke* 1975; 6:564–616.
45. Humphrey PRD, Marshall J: Transient ischemic attacks and strokes with recovery: Prognosis and investigation. *Stroke* 1981; 12:765–769.
46. Wiebers DO, Whisnant JP, O'Fallon WM: Reversible ischemic neurologic deficit (RIND) in a community: Rochester, Minnesota, 1955–1974. *Neurology* 1982; 32:459–465.
47. Caplan LR: Are terms such as completed strokes or RIND of continued usefulness. *Stroke* 1983; 14:431–433.
48. Dosick SM, Whalen RC, Gale SS, et al: Carotid endarterectomy in the stroke patient: Computerized axial tomography to determine timing. *J Vasc Surg* 1985; 2:214–217.
49. McIntyre KE, Goldstone J: Carotid surgery for crescendo TIA and stroke in evolution, in Bergan JJ, Yao JST (eds): *Cerebrovascular Insufficiency.* New York, Grune & Stratton Inc, 1983, pp 213–226.
50. Millikan CH: Discussion, in McDowell FH, Brennan (eds): *Cerebral Vascular Disease.* New York, Grune & Stratton Inc, 1973, p 209.
51. Mentzer RM, Finkelmeier BA, Crosby IK, et al: Emergency carotid endarterectomy for fluctuating neurological deficits. *Surgery* 1981; 89:60–66.
52. DeWeese JA. Longterm results of surgery for carotid artery stenosis, in Bergan JJ, Yao JST (eds): *Cerebrovascular Insufficiency,* ed 1. New York, Grune & Stratton Inc, 1983, pp 507–518.
53. Rob C: Occlusive disease of the extracranial arteries: A review of the past 25 years. *J Cardiovasc Surg* 1978; 19:487–498.
54. Chambers BR, Norris JW: The case against surgery for asymptomatic carotid stenosis. *Stroke* 1984; 15:964–967.
55. Whisnant JP, Sandok BA, Sundt TM. Carotid endarterectomy for unilateral carotid system transient cerebral ischaemia. *Mayo Clin Proc* 1983; 58:171–175.
56. Hass WK: Jonas S: Caution falling rock zone: An analysis of the medical and surgical management of threatened stroke. *Proc Inst Med Chic* 1980; 33:80–84.
57. Moore DJ, Miles RD, Gooley NA, et al: Noninvasive assessment of stroke risk in asymptomatic and nonhemispheric patients with suspected carotid disease. *Ann Surg* 1985; 202:491–504.
58. Hertzer NR: Arison R: Cumulative stroke and survival ten years after carotid endarterectomy. *J Vasc Surg* 1985; 2:661–668.
59. Bernstein EF, Humber PB, Collins GM, et al: Life expectancy and late stroke following carotid endarterectomy. *Ann Surg* 1983; 198:80–86.
60. Giordano JM, Trout HH, Kozloff L, et al: Timing of carotid artery endarterectomy after stroke. *J Vasc Surg* 1985; 2:250–254.
61. Whittemore AD, Ruby ST, Couch NP, et al: Early carotid endarterectomy in patients with small, fixed neurologic deficits. *J Vasc Surg* 1984; 1:795–798.
62. Goldstone J, Moore WS: A new look at emergency carotid artery operations for the treatment of cerebrovascular insufficiency. *Stroke* 1978; 9:599–602.
63. DeWeese JA, Rob CG, Satran R, et al: Results of carotid endarterectomies for transient ischaemic attacks—five years later. *Ann Surg* 1973; 178:258–264.
64. Takolander RJ, Bergentz SE, Ericsson BF: Carotid artery surgery in patients with minor stroke. *Br J Surg* 1983; 70:13–16.
65. Eriksson SE, Link H, Alm A, et al: Results from eighty eight consecutive pro-

phylactic carotid endarterectomies in cerebral infarction and transitory ischaemic attacks. *Acta Neurol Scand* 1981; 63:209–219.

66. Till JS, Toole JF, Howard VJ, et al: Declining morbidity and mortality of carotid endarterectomy: The Wake Forest Medical Center experience. *Stroke* 1987; 18:823–829.
67. Watson MR: Carotid endarterectomy in a small community hospital. *Am J Surg* 1980; 141:543–545.
68. Carmichael JD: Carotid surgery in the community hospital. *Arch Surg* 1980; 115:937–939.
69. Easton JD, Sherman DG: Stroke and mortality rate in carotid endarterectomy: 228 consecutive operations. *Stroke* 1977; 8:565–568.
70. Modi JR, Finch WT, Sumner DS: Update of carotid endarterectomy in two community hospitals: Springfield revisited. *Stroke* 1983; 14:128.
71. Barnes RW, Liebman PR, Marszalek PB: The natural history of asymptomatic carotid disease in patients undergoing cardiovascular surgery. *Surgery* 1981; 90:1075–1083.
72. Turnipseed WD, Berkoff HA, Belzer FO: Perioperative stroke in cardiac and peripheral vascular disease. *Ann Surg* 1980; 192:365–368.
73. Brewster BC, Schlaen HH, Raines JK, et al: Rational management of the asymptomatic carotid bruit. *Arch Surg* 1978; 113:927–930.
74. Hertzer NR, Loop FD, Taylor PC, et al: Staged and combined surgical approach to simultaneous carotid and coronary vascular disease. *Surgery* 1978; 84:803–811.
75. Peterson JJ: Carotid artery stenosis: Association with surgery for coronary artery disease. *Arch Surg* 1972; 105:837–840.
76. Morris CG, Ennix CL, Lawrie GM, et al: Management of coexistent carotid and coronary artery occlusive atherosclerosis. *Cleve Clin Q* 1977; 45:125–127.
77. Hertzer NR, Beven EG, Loop FD, et al: Management of simultaneous carotid and coronary artery disease, in Bergan JJ, Yao JST (eds): *Cerebrovascular Insufficiency*. New York, Grune & Stratton Inc, 1983, pp 417–431.
78. Bandyk DF: Application of duplex scanning for the postoperative evaluation of carotid bifurcation endarterectomy. *J Vasc Tech* 1987; 11:239–243.
79. Callow AD, O'Donnell TF: Recurrent carotid stenosis: Frequency, clinical implications and some suggestions concerning etiology, in Bergan JJ, Yao JST (eds): *Reoperative Arterial Surgery*. Orlando, Fla, Grune & Stratton Inc, 1986, pp 513–535.
80. O'Donnell TF, Callow AD: B mode ultrasound in evaluation of carotid endarterectomy: An anatomic study, in Bergan JJ, Yao JST (eds): *Reoperative Arterial Surgery*. Orlando, Fla, Grune & Stratton Inc, 1986, pp 81–105.
81. Zierler RE, Bandyk DF, Thiele BL, et al: Carotid artery stenosis following endarterectomy. *Arch Surg* 1982; 117:1408–1415.
82. McBride K, Callow AD: Recurrent carotid stenosis after carotid endarterectomy: A limited survey, in Bernhard VM, Towne JB (eds): *Complications in Vascular Surgery*. Orlando, Fla, Grune & Stratton Inc, 1980, pp 259–273.
83. Thompson JE, Austin DJ, Patman RD: Carotid endarterectomy for cerebral vascular insufficiency: Long term results in 592 patients followed up for thirteen years. *Ann Surg* 1970; 172:663–678.
84. Baker RN, Schwartz WS, Rose AS: Transient ischaemic strokes: A report of a study of anticoagulant therapy. *Neurology* 1966; 16:841–847.

85. Whisnant JP, Matsumoto M, Elveback LR: The effects of anticoagulant therapy on the prognosis of patients with transient cerebral ischaemic attacks in a community: Rochester, Minnesota, 1955 through 1969. *Mayo Clin Proc* 1973; 48:194–198.
86. Lind H, Lebram G, Johansson I, et al: Prognosis in patients with infarction and TIA in carotid territory during and after anticoagulant therapy. *Stroke* 1979; 10:529–532.
87. Fields WS, Lemak NA, Frankowski RF, et al: Controlled trial of aspirin in cerebral ischaemia. *Stroke* 1977; 8:301–316.
88. Bousser MG, Eschweg E, Hagenau M, et al: AICLA controlled trial of aspirin and dipyridamole in the secondary prevention of arteriothrombotic cerebral ischaemia. *Stroke* 1983; 14:5–14.
89. The American-Canadian Cooperative Study Group: Persantine-aspirin trial in cerebral ischaemia: II. End point results. *Stroke* 1985; 16:406–415.
90. Hye RJ, Dilley RB, Browse NL, et al: Evaluation of a new classification of cerebrovascular disease: C.H.A.T. *Am J Surg* 1987; 154:104–110.

Prevention of Venous Thrombosis and Pulmonary Embolism

Lazar J. Greenfield, M.D.

Professor and Chairman, Department of Surgery, University of Michigan Hospital, Ann Arbor, Michigan

Thomas W. Wakefield, M.D.

Assistant Professor of Surgery, Section of Vascular Surgery, University of Michigan Hospital, Ann Arbor, Michigan

Major improvements in the understanding and management of most surgical disorders have not been matched by similar advances in the control of venous thrombosis, and patients continue to die of its most serious complication, pulmonary thromboembolism (PE). Although the term *thrombophlebitis* was often used in the past to cover a wide spectrum of venous thromboses, it should more properly be reserved for the superficial inflammatory response that often accompanies venous injury such as by irritating intravenous (IV) fluids. In this chapter we will focus on our present understanding of deep venous thrombosis (DVT), since this is the disorder that leads to PE. The historical basis for our approach to the disorder is based on the work of Virchow,[1] who postulated three fundamental causes of venous thrombosis: venous stasis, hypercoagulability, and endothelial injury.

Disorders Predisposing to Thrombosis

Hereditary Predisposition

The orderly process of conversion of plasma clotting factors from inactive zymogens to active enzymes results in the final conversion by thrombin of fibrinogen to fibrin, which forms the structural framework of the blood clot. Control of the clotting process and its limitation to appropriate sites of injury is the function of the fibrinolytic system. The active enzyme of this system is plasmin that comes from circulating plasminogen and acts to dissolve the fibrin matrix. Defects that either increase the deposition of

Adv Surg 22:301–324, 1989

0065-3411/89/22-301–324-$04.00

fibrin or reduce its enzymatic dissolution can predispose an individual to develop thrombosis. Internal regulation of this complex system involves antithrombin III, a plasma inhibitor protein that blocks the activity of some of the serine protease clotting factors, and proteins C and S, which inhibit clot formation. These natural anticoagulants probably prevent spontaneous intravascular clotting and limit the thrombotic response to vascular injury, thereby preventing the extension of protective thrombi. Assays for these factors are now coming into clinical use and will undoubtedly reveal a larger number of deficiency states responsible for thrombosis that were previously termed idiopathic.

The prevalence of inherited thrombotic syndromes is higher than that of bleeding disorders and estimated to be in the range of 1 in 2,500 to 5,000 persons.[2] These disorders should be considered in the DVT patient under age 40, especially when there is recurrent venous thrombosis or a family history, although absence of the latter does not exclude inherited thrombophilia because the defects have low penetrance.

Laboratory Screening

The intrinsic plasma anticoagulant system includes a number of proteins that have not been associated with inherited thrombophilia. These include $alpha_2$ macroglobulin, $alpha_1$-antitrypsin, and C1 inactivator. The factors that have been associated with thrombotic complications are listed in Table 1[3] along with the estimated frequency of their association with recurrent venous thrombosis. Although antigenic assays are becoming commercially available, they can be misleading due to the presence of possible binding factors or inhibitors. For this reason the functional assays are considered to be more accurate and are currently being developed. For further information concerning the limitations of present assays, the reader should consult the excellent review by Mannucci and Tripodi.[2]

Other Conditions Associated With Venous Thrombosis

Malignancy

The association between venous thrombosis and cancer was first suggested by Trousseau and often has been confirmed in postmortem studies. This should always be considered in the older patient with a history of recent venous thrombosis. In a series reported by Aderka et al.,[4] 34% of otherwise healthy patients with idiopathic DVT were found to have a malignancy diagnosed an average of 24 months later. There was an increased likelihood of cancer in these patients associated with age over 65, anemia, and eosinophilia. The earliest onset malignancies, which were found within one year, tended to occur in the pelvic organs and breasts.

TABLE 1.
Frequency of Protein Deficiencies Predisposing to Recurrent Venous Thrombosis

Protein S	5%–9.5%*
Protein C	7%
Antithrombin III	2%–3%
Plasminogen	2%
Fibrinogen	1%

*Only Type I deficient patients are included in these categories. The overall contribution of functional protein C and protein S deficiencies cannot adequately be determined at this time.

In some cases, however, the malignancies did not appear until after five years.

Platelet Disorders

Abnormal platelet aggregation can also be seen in advanced malignancy, especially involving the lung and uterus. There is also a rare association with carotid endarterectomy, which can be followed by thrombosis due to platelet activation.[5] Accelerated platelet plug formation has been observed with hypercholesterolemia, homocystinuria, vasculitis, and the lupus anticoagulant.[6] Inappropriate platelet aggregation can also be seen with essential thrombocythemia, paroxysmal nocturnal hemoglobulinuria, and heparin-associated thrombocytopenia.

Defects in Control of Thrombus Propagation

In the postoperative and posttrauma patient, stasis and immobilization facilitate propagation of small venous thrombi. This can also be seen in congestive heart failure, the hyperviscosity syndrome, and polycythemia. Defective lysis of fibrin thrombi is seen in the presence of dysfibrinogenemia and decreased plasminogen activity. There is also an association with autoimmune disease, especially in patients who have the lupus anticoagulant, 25% of whom will have severe coagulation problems, moderate thrombocytopenia, increased partial thromboplastin time, and a prolonged prothrombin time.[6]

Prophylaxis of Venous Thrombosis

Pharmacological

Pharmacologic prophylactic agents include subcutaneous heparin, dextran, antiplatelet agents including aspirin and persantin, oral anticoagulants, dihydroergotamine, lidocaine, and ascorbic acid. Low-dose heparin (5,000 units administered subcutaneously) has been studied in great detail, and there are three mechanisms responsible for its antithrombotic action. First, antithrombin III activity with inhibition of Factor Xa is enhanced by only trace amounts of heparin. Second, there may be a decrease in thrombin availability that prevents its activation and thus its fibrin stabilizing role. Finally, small doses of heparin inhibit the second wave of platelet aggregation and the subsequent platelet release reaction. Twenty-seven clinical trials concerning low-dose heparin have documented its effectiveness. The incidence of venous thrombosis in the control groups was found to average 25%, in contrast to only 7% of those receiving low-dose heparin.[7] In addition, thrombi likely to produce major pulmonary embolism were decreased from 6% in the control group to 0.6% in the group treated with low-dose heparin. Also, in a multicentered prospective randomized control trial involving 4,121 patients, low-dose heparin was found to decrease the incidence of massive pulmonary embolism proved at autopsy. However, low-dose heparin does carry an increased risk of wound hematoma and therefore only high-risk patients should be treated with this regimen.[8, 9] The sodium and calcium salts of heparin seem equally effective and the incidence of wound hematoma does not appear to be related to the type of salt used. In addition, there is no advantage to administration of heparin every eight hours as opposed to every 12 hours.

Dextran 70 as an anticoagulant is as effective as heparin in pulmonary embolism prophylaxis but is less effective against labeled fibrinogen-detected deep venous thrombosis.[10, 11] However, it is preferred to heparin for orthopedic procedures, especially hip surgery. With most studies, antiplatelet agents have proved ineffective.[12] Oral anticoagulants are as effective as heparin but carry an increased risk of bleeding.

Recently, 880 patients were randomized into five treatment groups in the United States multicenter trial of the combination of dihydroergotamine and heparin. Dihydroergotamine increases venous smooth-muscle tone without affecting arteriolar tone and should be effective in preventing stasis without increasing blood pressure. It also affects the platelet membrane and prostaglandin synthesis, and complements heparin's effect as a prophylactic agent.[13] In this study, treatment was initiated preoperatively and continued twice daily for five days comparing groups receiving 0.5 mg of dihydroergotamine plus 5,000 IU of heparin, 0.5 mg dihydroergotamine plus 2,500 IU of heparin, 5,000 IU of heparin alone, 0.5 mg dihydroergotamine alone, and placebo. The treatment group with the lowest deep venous thrombosis rate was the dihydroergotamine-5,000 IU heparin group with a rate of 9.4%. Postoperative bleeding occurred in 2 to 3% of cases, injection site hematoma was seen in 6 to 12% of patients, and wound hematoma in 1 to 3% of patients. This combination of dihydroergotamine and heparin has been demonstrated to be effective, although patients who undergo this regimen must be followed up for ergot toxicity, which has been reported.

In an attempt to standardize prophylactic regimens, the National Institutes of Health held a Consensus Conference on venous prophylaxis in 1986.[14] Recommendations were made for a number of different patient groups based on reported clinical trials. For general surgery procedures, patients who are high risk (age greater than 40, obesity, malignancy, prior deep venous thrombosis or pulmonary embolism, or large complicated operations) should receive prophylactic treatment with subcutaneous heparin, 5,000 IU every eight to 12 hours. Dextran in initial doses of 10 ml/kg seems equally effective in decreasing pulmonary embolism but is more expensive. External pneumatic compression and gradient elastic stockings have also been found to be effective for these patients. Dihydroergotamine added to heparin may increase the efficacy of the treatment, but ergot toxicity must be taken into account. Patients less than 40 years of age with no known risk factors undergoing uncomplicated operative procedures most likely do not need prophylaxis.

For high-risk orthopedic patients undergoing hip or knee surgery, low-dose coumadin, dextran, or adjusted dose heparin was recommended. For other orthopedic patients, gradient elastic stockings or external pneumatic compression was recommended. Early mobilization and elevation of the foot of the bed were also recommended. For urology patients over the age of 40 years with a need for prophylaxis, low-dose heparin and mechanical modalities such as external pneumatic compression were recommended. Low-risk gynecologic patients may be managed with early ambulation and gradient compression stockings, while those at moderate or high risk should be managed with low-dose heparin and/or external pneumatic compression. Dextran in this group of patients is also an alternative choice.

Patients with gynecologic malignancy are best treated with dextran and/or external pneumatic compression or a combination of low-dose heparin and external pneumatic compression. Coumadin may also be a useful alternative in this group. Prophylaxis in pregnant patients and in the postpartum period should be provided with low-dose heparin. Postpartum patients at risk should be managed either with low-dose heparin or external pneumatic compression, or both. Neurosurgical patients undergoing craniotomy for tumor, subarachnoid hemorrhage, arteriovenous malformation, aneurysm resection, arterial bypass, shunting procedures, and other intracranial problems should receive external pneumatic compression. For extracranial neurosurgical procedures, either external pneumatic compression or low-dose heparin is effective and was recommended either alone or in combination. Patients who have a nonhemorrhagic stroke should receive low-dose heparin. For all other stroke patients, external pneumatic compression was recommended.

Trauma patients with hip fractures should be protected with either dextran, external pneumatic compression, or pressure gradient elastic stockings. Aspirin and low-dose heparin in this group are of no benefit. Patients with head injury and acute spinal cord injury should receive external pneumatic compression and pressure gradient elastic stockings but not pharmacologic prophylaxis. For severe musculoskeletal trauma, either low-dose heparin prophylaxis or pneumatic compression should be used. For long-term chronic prophylaxis, coumadin is appropriate.

Anesthesia

The association of anesthesia with deep vein thrombosis is usually considered to be causative in view of the stasis resulting from venodilatation and immobilization. To minimize these effects, it has been recognized that there is a significant advantage to the use of regional anesthesia, which lowers the incidence of thromboembolism.[15] Using epidural anesthesia for hip replacement, the incidence of venous thrombosis and pulmonary embolism was reduced 54% and 23%, respectively. The physiological benefits of epidural anesthesia include increased blood flow with less venous stasis and more efficient fibrinolysis.[16] For this reason Raggi et al.[17] have considered the selection of epidural anesthesia for high-risk patients to be a form of prophylaxis for venous thrombosis.

Mechanical Prophylaxis

Mechanical techniques for prevention of DVT are usually directed at reducing venous stasis, but often cause patient discomfort and are associated with poor compliance. In addition, the presence of skin ulceration or severe arterial insufficiency represents a contraindication to their use. Of course, the most innocuous approach is early ambulation postoperatively, which has major benefits for wound healing and prevention of pumonary complications, provided that the patient does not spend more time sitting in a chair at the bedside. Unfortunately, even when combined with leg exercise in bed, it does not reduce the incidence of DVT or PE.[18] Similarly, leg elevation in bed improves venous drainage but does not reduce the incidence of DVT,[19] although some authors continue to recommend it because of its simplicity.[20]

Elastic Stockings

The value of elastic stockings is determined by their ability to provide a pressure gradient to improve venous return in the deep system. Although an increase in venous velocity can be demonstrated, prospective controlled trials have failed to show significant protection.[19, 21]

Calf Muscle Stimulation

Electrical stimulation of calf muscles works to empty soleal veins and appears to reduce the incidence of PE, although the incidence of DVT is unaffected.[22] It can be used while the patient is anesthetized but is less well tolerated when the patient is awake.

Pneumatic Compression

Intermittent pneumatic external compression of the legs is the logical extension of efforts to improve venous drainage and has been documented to be as effective as low-dose heparin in many well-controlled clinical trials.[23–25] It is particularly advantageous in those groups of patients who are not well protected by low-dose heparin, such as after urological and orthopedic procedures.[26] It can also be used effectively when heparin is completely contraindicated, such as in neurosurgical patients.[27]

In addition to the augmentation of venous return, pneumatic compression induces both local and systemic fibrinolysis. The decrease in euglobulin lysis time appears to be proportional to the volume of tissue compressed,[28] and therefore a beneficial effect can be obtained even from compression of the upper extremity.[29] A comparison of effectiveness of pneumatic compression with coumadin for prophylaxis in patients with a history of previous thromboembolism scheduled for hip replacement showed comparable protection except in patients with abnormal preoperative venograms where only coumadin was effective.[30]

The length of time that pneumatic compression should be applied has not been determined conclusively, since there is evidence of some effectiveness when it is used only in the operating and recovery rooms.[31] However, the development of late DVT after pneumatic compression was discontinued suggests that optimal protection requires at least five days' application or longer in the face of prolonged immobilization.[32]

Vena Caval Procedures

Under circumstances where deep venous thrombosis is known to exist, the effectiveness of anticoagulant therapy in preventing thromboembolism was established in the classic trial of Barrett and Jordan,[33] where there was a 26% mortality rate in untreated patients and an equal number of nonfatal emboli. In treated patients, anticoagulation fails to prevent thromboembolism at a rate reported variably from 2%[34] to 18%,[35] but is generally accepted at approximately 10%. In recent studies, we, as well as other authors, have been able to correlate this failure of anticoagulation protection with the presence of a floating tail on the proximal end of the venous thrombosis.[36] Therefore we should recognize the maximal risk of embolism when anticoagulants cannot be used to treat DVT but a continuing lesser risk even when anticoagulation is possible. Under these circumstances there have been a remarkable variety of techniques used to prevent embolism once it was clearly demonstrated that vena caval ligation carried an unacceptable morbidity and mortality rate.[37] There were obviously greater advantages to the concept of filtration over complete occlusion, and DeWeese and Hunter[38] proposed a suture grid, while Spencer et al.[39] developed the technique of suture plication of the IVC in efforts to preserve flow until an embolus was trapped. The plication technique subsequently was modified to utilize a stapling device by Ravitch et al.,[40] but the fact that these procedures violated the intima of the vein and occasionally permitted reopening of a larger channel[41] or further thrombosis[42] led to the development of external clip devices. These were designed to compress the cava into a narrow slot (Moretz et al.[43]), parallel orifices (Miles et al.[44]), or a series of channels to preserve patency after trapping emboli.[45] This approach was successful in reducing the operative mortality and recurrent fatal embolism rates while preserving an overall patency rate of approximately 65%.[46] However, since these procedures required general anesthesia and laparotomy in seriously ill patients, a major conceptual advance was made when a transvenous approach with the patient under local anesthesia was suggested by Eichelter and Schenk[47] in 1968. The Eichelter catheter and the Moser balloon[48] were designed for temporary protection only and subsequent removal, since the catheter remained attached (Fig 1). Concern for the fate of the trapped or attached thrombi, which likely would embolize at the time of removal of the catheter, led to the next advance. This was the use of a transvenous approach to leave a device for permanent caval narrowing (Pate clip),[49] for total occlusion of blood flow (Hunter balloon),[50] or for more gradual occlusion of the vena cava by an umbrella device, as introduced by Mobin-Uddin et al.[51] (see Fig 1). Initially offered only for the more critically ill patients, a generally favorable experience with the latter device led to more widespread application,[52] although complications of migration of the device to the pulmonary artery have led to its withdrawal from the market.

In order to improve the filtering function, we developed a cone-shaped filter to provide a maximal entrapment area while preserving blood flow and reported preliminary results in 1973.[53] The geometry of the cone permits filling of 80% of its depth before the cross-sectional area is reduced by 64%, which would be required before a pressure gradient occurred across it. The filter is made of stainless steel fitted at an angle of 35° to an apical hub and is 46 mm in length and 30 mm at maximal open diameter at the base (Fig 2). Spacing between the wires ranges from less than 2 mm at the apex to 6 mm at the base when inserted, but the principle of axial flow tends to direct a foreign body that contacts one of the struts to stream in to the apex of the cone, ensuring that all emboli larger than 3 mm will be trapped effectively.[54]

Fixation of the device is by means of fine recurved hooks at the end of each of the six limbs, which grasp the wall of the vena cava[55] and prohibit

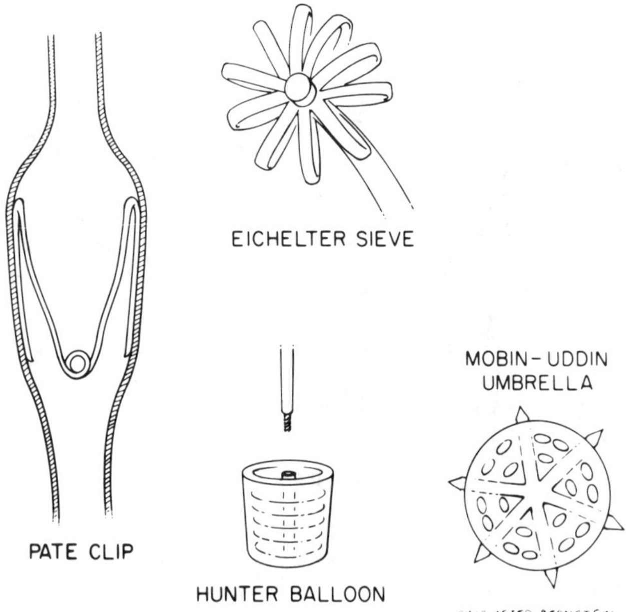

FIG 1.
Early devices used to control thromboembolism were inserted by catheter and designed to be removed later (Eichelter sieve) or to provide permanent caval narrowing (Pate clip). Complete occlusion of the vena cava was accomplished by insertion of a balloon (Hunter) or more gradually by an umbrella device (Mobin-Uddin). (From Brown PO, Elkins RD, Greenfield LJ: Comparison of a new intracaval filter with the Mobin-Uddin device and clinical experience. *Circulation* 1973; 48:(suppl 4):5. Used by permission.)

any tendency for proximal migration regardless of apical or distending vectors of force, which only fix it more securely. Effectiveness of the filter was demonstrated experimentally in comparison with the Mobin-Uddin umbrella, with reduction in morbidity and mortality rates.[56] An unexpected bonus from preservation of flow was demonstrable progressive lysis of trapped thrombus to a varying degree in all animals.

Clinical experience with the Greenfield filter, including long-term follow up, was reported in 1981 in a series of 156 patients with a 23-month average follow-up. Since that time we have extended the experience to 469 patients ranging from 13 to 92 years of age with a mean of 56 years. There were 274 males (60%) and 180 females (40%) with a racial distribution of 298 white (67%) and 147 black or other (33%). Long-term follow up was available on 146 or 61% of the patients alive at one year postoperative for a mean follow up of 43 months (range, .03 to 138 months). The most frequent indication for insertion was a contraindication

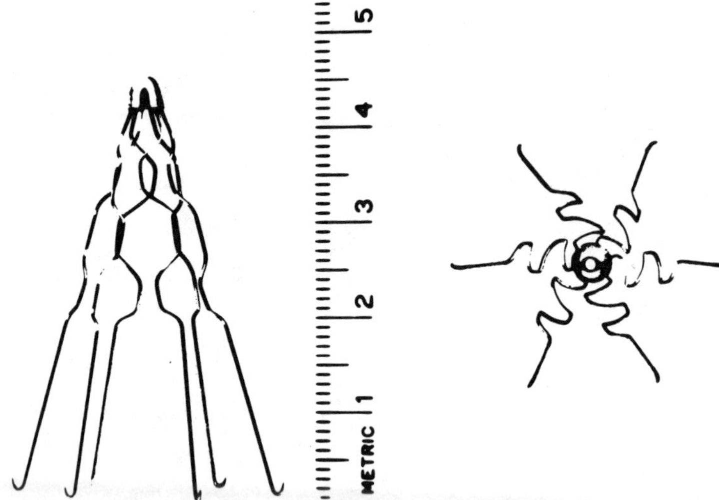

FIG 2.
The Greenfield filter is made of stainless steel in the shape of a cone to trap emboli without interruption of venous flow.

to anticoagulation in 178 patients (38%, Table 2). Evidence of recurrent embolism while receiving anticoagulation was the justification for filter placement in 126 patients (27%). Eighty-one patients (17%) with DVT but without evidence of acute pulmonary embolism received filters prophylactically when they were thought to be at unusually high risk for embolism, i.e., free-floating or poorly adherent proximal thrombus on venogram,

TABLE 2.
Indications for Greenfield Filter Insertion in 469 Patients*

Filter Insertion Indications	Number (%)
Contraindication to anticoagulation	178 (38)
Recurrent PE	126 (27)
Prophylaxis	81 (17)
Complication of anticoagulation	80 (17)
Embolectomy	36 (8)
Previous device failure	10 (2)

*Some patients had more than one indication.

chronic pulmonary hypertension, or respiratory reserve so marginal that the patient could not tolerate any perfusion compromise. A complication of anticoagulation necessitating discontinuance of medical therapy was the indication for filter placement in 80 patients (17%), while pulmonary artery catheter embolectomy and failure of a previous device comprised the remainder of the indications for filter insertion.

Coexisting diagnoses in the patients at the time of their filter insertion are shown in Table 3 in order of decreasing frequency. Not unexpected was the predominance of venous disease, either acute or chronic in 58% of patients. The postoperative state (33%) and preexisting cardiac disease (24%) were also frequently encountered in patients. Several other factors known to predispose to DVT, such as neoplastic disease, obesity, gastrointestinal tract disease, and central nervous system disorders, were also found to be relatively common in this study, while the postpartum state was found to be an associated factor in only a small percentage. Sepsis

TABLE 3.
Coexisting Diagnoses in 469 Patients Who Received Greenfield Vena Caval Filters

Diagnosis	Number (%)
Venous disease	273 (58)
Acute	204 (43)
Chronic	69 (15)
Recent surgery	157 (33)
Cardiac disease	113 (24)
Neurological disorder	90 (19)
Obesity	80 (17)
Malignant neoplasm	78 (17)
Gastrointestinal tract disease	76 (16)
Pulmonary hypertension	61 (13)
Recent trauma	40 (9)
Arterial disease	40 (9)
Pulmonary disease	40 (9)
Renal disease	28 (6)
Psychiatric disease or alcoholism	25 (5)
Diabetes	19 (4)
Hypercoaguable state	18 (4)
Sepsis	18 (4)
Postpartum	4 (1)
Other diagnosis	88 (19)

was not a contraindication to insertion and was documented preoperatively in 18 patients (4%).

The preferred approach to caval filter insertion was via the internal jugular vein in 83% of cases. The right internal jugular route was utilized primarily unless it was known to be obstructed. In four patients in whom this approach failed, placement via a left jugular approach was successful, although technically more difficult. The right femoral vein approach was used in 72 cases (16% of total) while four patients had Greenfield filters placed via the right atrium and one via the left axillary vein. Filter location was confirmed radiographically to be at the level of L-3 in 363 patients, just below L-3 but above the iliac veins in 14 patients, and above L-3 but still in the infrarenal vena cava in another 15 patients for an 89% infrarenal placement.

Thirty-two patients had their filters placed in the suprarenal vena cava but in only five of them was the location classified as misplaced. One filter was placed in the suprarenal cava following misplacement in the right renal vein. The remaining 27 suprarenal filters were placed in patients with renal transplants,[57] renal cell carcinoma with renal vein tumor extension, or infrarenal caval thrombosis. When filters were placed via the right atrium, placement was intentionally in the suprarenal cava in over half the cases. Of these 32 patients, 12 returned for follow-up and ten were found to have a patent vena cava. The two occluded infrarenal cavas were in patients with intentional suprarenal placement because of existing vena caval thrombosis in one and the presence of an umbrella filter in the infrarenal vena cava in the other patient. All suprarenal filters have remained patent. Eleven of the 32 patients died, one of them from pulmonary embolism two days following filter placement via the right atrium during open pulmonary embolectomy. This occurred in a 39-year-old black female who sustained severe head injury from blunt trauma. The remainder of the deaths in this group were attributed to neoplasm in seven, infection in two, and intracranial injury in one.

There were 19 misplaced filters, including one at L-3 and one in the right atrium caught and repositioned in the suprarenal vena cava.[58] The remaining misplaced filters were distributed between the renal vein (2), iliac vein (6), right atrium (2), below L-3 (2), and above L-3 (1). None of the 12 patients with misplaced filters who returned for follow-up had recurrent embolism and all filters were patent.

Patients with misplaced filters who had inadequate caval protection had a second filter placed appropriately within the vena cava. Technical problems with insertion were encountered in 48, or 10% of patients. The largest group constituted those requiring use of a guide wire to facilitate carrier position (4%). Routine use of the guide wire is now recommended to facilitate maneuvering through the right side of the heart rather than waiting until difficulty arises.[59] Another technical adjunct was the Fogarty catheter, which was used for dilitation, guidance, or positioning in 11 cases. The remaining problems included tilted filter, abandonment of the procedure due to a complication, inadequate vein size, or other technical difficulties in 16 patients. In several instances where the initial procedure was abandoned a filter was subsequently placed successfully, usually via the femoral approach. A total of 11 patients underwent multiple insertions, which in five cases was due to misplacement of the filter at first insertion. There were four instances of suspected air embolism during difficult jugular insertion, resulting in abandonment of the procedure and filter placement through the right femoral vein. The remaining two situations requiring multiple insertions were failure of a prior device in one patient, necessitating Greenfield filter placement 15 months after the initial procedure, and the other in a 24-year old woman with renal disease who had a suprarenal filter placed two days following placement at the L-3 level.

Greenfield filter placement was performed with the patient under local anesthesia when the jugular or femoral route was used, except in cases where another surgical procedure requiring general anesthesia was done at the same time. Two patients, one with a psychiatric disorder, could not tolerate local anesthesia and filter placement was done under general anesthesia. There were no intraoperative deaths attributable to filter placement and none of the four patients with presumed air embolism had any residual sequelae.

The total number of deaths for the entire follow-up period was 133, or 28%, with 186 patients lost to follow-up. Of the 133 deaths, 105 (79%) took place within one year of filter insertion and 36 (27%) occurred within two weeks of filter placement, most from associated diseases (Table 4). Pulmonary embolism was listed as the primary cause of death in 16 patients, seven of whom died within 48 hours of filter insertion. A 54-year-

TABLE 4.
Twelve-Year Follow-Up Mortality Rate for Coexisting Disorders at Time of Filter Placement

Disorder	% Died
Malignancy	47
Pulmonary hypertension	36
Cardiac disease	35
Recent surgery	29
Pulmonary disease	22
Obesity	19
Recent trauma	15

old black man who underwent embolectomy for recurrent PE with pulmonary hypertension died two days after filter placement, but had no evidence of recurrent embolism on autopsy. Similarly, a 25-year-old black woman with a history of pulmonary hypertension had no evidence of recurrent embolism on autopsy following filter placement two weeks prior to death. Of the nine deaths from PE in patients surviving for greater than two days after filter placement, five were confirmed by autopsy findings and four were suspected on clinical grounds. A trapped embolus was noted in the filter of only one patient who died of pulmonary embolism. Five patients who died of causes unrelated to embolism were found to have trapped clot within the filter, suggesting a persistent peripheral embolic source. In four patients pulmonary embolism was thought to be a contributing cause of death. In the case of a 67-year-old black man who died of sepsis following surgery for trauma, there was no evidence of recurrent pulmonary embolism at autopsy 20 days after filter insertion.

Review of the preoperative lower extremity status of the patients receiving Greenfield filters showed that 95 patients had right leg edema, 103 left leg edema, and 44 bilateral edema; there were 70 patients in whom there was no evidence of peripheral edema. At the time of operation 283 patients were receiving heparin, with or without additional anticoagulants. Of the patients treated initially with heparin, 25% had complications of bleeding (54), thrombocytopenia (nine), or other complications (eight). Coumadin therapy had a complication rate of 7%, with bleeding most common (ten patients). Venous Doppler evaluation was performed in 144 patients, of whom 129 had abnormal results. One hundred fifty-seven filter patients had venography as part of the diagnostic studies, with abnormal results in 92%, the majority demonstrating either above-knee thrombi or combined above- and below-knee thrombosis.

Pulmonary artery (PA) pressures were measured in 94 patients with the following observations: PA systolic less than 20 mm Hg in 4, 20 to 25 mm Hg in 12, 25 to 30 mm Hg in 14, and over 30 mm Hg in 64. Interestingly, even in the four instances of systolic PA pressure less than 20 mm Hg, three of the angiograms were abnormal, suggesting that significant embolism can occur without elevated PA pressure. Overall, 29% of the patients receiving Greenfield filters underwent angiography, of which 93% were abnormal. Lung scans were performed in 56% of patients prior to filter placement, with 97% showing an abnormality. However, recurrent PE and embolectomy were listed as the indications for filter placement in only 35% of the patients, with the remainder divided between contraindications to and complications of anticoagulation, prophylaxis, and previous device failure. Although this suggests an underestimation of the percentage of people with PE at the time of filter placement, patients with PE and a contraindication to anticoagulation were categorized for the latter indication.

Long-term follow-up was available on 146 patients (391 patient visits) for a mean follow-up time of 43 months. At the time of follow-up, 54 patients were receiving anticoagulant therapy, while 13 others had been treated for greater than four months but had discontinued it at the time of annual follow-up. Elastic support stockings were worn by 45 patients to alleviate symptomatic edema and an additional 19 patients had worn them for several months to years after surgery but no longer required them. Persistent lower extremity edema was present in 44% of those who returned for follow-up, the majority of whom had significant edema preoperatively. Twenty-one patients had either intermittent edema or edema that resolved completely over time. The sequelae of recurrent thrombosis and stasis ulceration were seen in 16 and nine patients, respectively, but in nine and four patients, respectively, these symptoms had resolved completely on subsequent follow-up visits. Of the 16 patients with recurrent thrombosis, 12 were receiving anticoagulant therapy during the time they were symptomatic.

Long-term effects of peripheral deep venous system abnormalities were evaluated by Doppler, venographic, and plethysmographic studies at yearly intervals. Of 106 Doppler examinations, 94% of patients showed improvement or no change with a new abnormality detected in only 5%. Similarly, follow-up plethysmography and venography revealed 93% and 92% improvement or no change, respectively.

Recurrent pulmonary embolism was diagnosed during follow-up in nine patients (4%), by lung scan in four cases, angiogram in two cases, and symptom change in two instances. In no instance of recurrent embolism was the filter malpositioned. During the follow-up period 127 patients had at least one venacavogram, 109 with radionuclide studies and 42 with contrast lower extremity injection and visualization of the venous system. There were ten patients whose vena cava was not patent, for an overall beginning patency rate of 93%. However, in three of the ten cases, the previously occluded cava reestablished patency during follow-up. In one case patency was returned after documented occlusion for seven years. Excluding those patients with restored caval patency, and those who had IVC thrombosis prior to filter insertion, the adjusted patency rate is 96%. In the seven patients whose cava was occluded at the last follow-up visit, four never had documented patency on any follow-up visit, while three patients initially had patent filters that later occluded.

Evidence of a trapped embolus was seen in 18 patients, half of whom had complete dissolution on subsequent annual cavograms. One patient, previously described, had thrombus extending proximally from the filter that was treated successfully by urokinase. Evaluation of plain abdominal radiographs revealed change in filter position in six patients, one of whom had an occluded IVC on follow-up cavogram. In another patient with a patent cava, filter position had been stable for eight years when a change in position was noted. A third person had change in filter position after three years, following which the filter was stable for the following eight years.

Conclusions for Thromboembolism Prophylaxis

Transvenous interruption of the inferior vena cava with the Greenfield filter has become accepted as a safe and effective approach to treatment in those patients who require mechanical protection against pulmonary embolism.[60, 61] Although anticoagulant therapy is still the primary therapy for DVT and pulmonary thromboembolism, this treatment is associated with a mortality rate up to 15%.[62] In addition, thrombus within the IVC is associated with a 35% or greater embolism rate despite full anticoagulation.[63] Failure of medical therapy as documented by recurrent embolism while on therapeutic anticoagulant therapy remains the second most common indication for filter insertion (27%), suggesting that medical therapy alone is inadequate in many cases. In particular, patients with chronic pulmonary hypertension have a high incidence of recurrent thromboembolism with coumadin derivatives having no influence on survival time.[64, 65]

A contraindication to anticoagulation continues to be the most frequent indication for filter placement. Prophylactic filter insertion in patients with free-floating thrombus in the iliac system or above, or those with documented DVT unable to tolerate any pulmonary thromboembolism due to underlying pulmonary disease, is indicated and comprised 17% of our filter patients. The remainder of the filter population was composed of those with complications of anticoagulation, embolectomy patients, and patients with previous device failures.

Venous disease (58%) and in particular acute venous disease (43%) was seen more commonly in this series in comparison with the 52% and 33% incidence, respectively, from a previous study.[66] Since the distribution of indications for filter placement has not changed with time, this may be related to improved accuracy or more frequent usage of radiographic and ultrasonic techniques for the diagnosis of deep venous thrombosis.

The jugular route of insertion continues to be the preferred access (83%), and both right and left internal jugular veins have been successfully used. Routine use of a guide wire facilitates placement,[59] making passage by the eustachian valve of the right side of the heart easier. In cases of failure of internal jugular passage, usually due to a small undilatable vein, the right femoral vein has been used successfully in 16% of patients.

To facilitate proper filter placement, Cimochowski[61] and Wingerd[60] routinely use intraoperative cavography to determine the exact location of the renal veins and to ensure an infrarenal position. Fluoroscopic placement at the L-3 level[67] has allowed accurate positioning in 93% of patients as reported earlier.[66] The corresponding misplacement rate of 7% has declined to a rate of 4% in this study, due primarily to increased use of the guide wire. In cases of caval anomalies as described by Allen et al.,[68] where a filter was discharged in the hepatic vein in a patient with abdominal situs inversus, use of the guide wire is essential for proper placement. Although successful retrieval of misplaced filters has been described by both

Greenfield[69] and Schneider,[70] high patency rates[66, 71] and stability of filter position[72] have eliminated the need for this to all but a few selected cases.

Suprarenal placement of the Greenfield filter has continued to provide long-term protection against recurrent embolism without adverse sequelae on renal function.[58] Its successful use in renal transplant patients[57] and patients with thrombus or occlusion of the infrarenal IVC has been established. Rosenthal et al.[73] described placement of the Greenfield filter in patients with renal vein tumor thrombus at the time of nephrectomy for renal cell carcinoma to shorten operative time and minimize embolism risk. In addition to the above-mentioned indications, Orsini et al.[63] used suprarenal placement in a case of ovarian vein thromboembolism and in a case with recurrent PE after an infrarenal Greenfield filter with proximal thrombus failed streptokinase therapy. Of the 32 patients with suprarenal filters in this series, there was one instance of recurrent PE from a proximal thrombus, which resolved with urokinase therapy.

There was no direct surgical mortality resulting from filter insertion. Four patients suffered air embolism without residual deficit. All of them had filters placed successfully via the femoral route. There were no wound complications noted. Overall mortality was 133 of 469 patients, with 27% of deaths occurring within two weeks of filter placement. Pulmonary embolism was thought to be the cause of death in 3.6% of the patients. However, this probably represents preoperative effect, since 29% of these patients died within 24 hours of filter insertion without evidence of recurrent embolism. Two of the six patients who died within two weeks of filter insertion were thought to have died of pulmonary embolism, but one of them who had embolism listed as a contributing cause of death had no evidence of recurrent PE on autopsy. This discrepancy between death-certificate-presumed cause of death and autopsy findings results from the recognized lack of correlation between clinical signs and both angiographic findings[74] and autopsy results. Because of this, the diagnosis of recurrent pulmonary embolism without radionuclide, angiographic, or autopsy studies may be prone to overestimation, particularly in patients with prior documentation of PE. Seventy-nine percent of the deaths in this series took place within one year of filter insertion, with well over half from cardiac or neoplastic causes. The follow-up mortality rates for coexisting disorders are listed in Table 4.

Elevated pulmonary artery pressures are the usual finding in patients with significant pulmonary embolism.[75] In this series 60 of 64 patients with mean PA pressures above 20 mm Hg had abnormal pulmonary angiography results. However, three patients in whom an angiography result was abnormal had mean PA pressures less than 20 mm Hg. Therefore, normal or slightly elevated PA pressures do not rule out pulmonary embolism, and when embolism is suspected, angiography remains the diagnostic test of choice.[74]

The long-term incidence of lower extremity edema of 44% compares favorably with the incidence of preoperative edema of 52%. The incidence of recurrent thrombosis in the follow-up period was 11%, while 6% developed ulceration. In patients with stasis ulcers 44% healed on subsequent examination after conservative treatment.

The recurrent embolism rate of 4% is consistent with earlier reports.[71, 78] It has been observed that filters with tilted position may have increased likelihood of proximal thrombus propagation of entrapped filter thrombus,[66, 76] but this was not the case in the nine patients in this series with recurrent embolism. Presence of a trapped embolus was diagnosed by radionuclide or contrast cavograms in 18 patients, nine of whom had complete clot dissolution on later follow-up studies. Pasto et al.[77] used Duplex real time and pulsed Doppler ultrasound to assess patency and partial occlusion in patients with Greenfield filters showing good correlation with venography, and 2/41 false-negative results in patients with anechoic thrombus. Long-term patency rates remain high at 96%, consistent with earlier reports by the senior author[66, 71, 77] and several other series.[60, 61, 79] It is worth noting that 30% of those patients with an occluded IVC later reestablished patency, in one case after seven years. Long-term patency is not dependent on anticoagulant therapy. There was no correlation between caval occlusion and venous stasis sequelae of edema, recurrent thrombosis, or ulceration.

Filter migration was noted on plain radiograph in six patients, for an incidence of 4% of follow-up patients. Many filters had been stable for several years. Sixty-nine of these patients were recently reviewed by Messmer and Greenfield[72] in a radiographic study of filter position, span, migration, and angulation. Results showed cephalad migration of 2 to 12 mm in 6% and caudad migration of 3 to 18 mm in 29%. As construction of the hooks results in penetration of the cava wall and subsequent endothelialization of the cava wall over the hooks, dislodgement of the hooks is virtually impossible as a mechanism of migration. It may be that fibrous reaction around the struts or gravity may contribute to the settling of the filter caudally.[72] Filter expansion after strut penetration of the caval wall also may draw the apex of the filter caudally. Conversely, decreased filter span secondary to thrombosis within the filter or occlusion of the IVC may extend the filter tip cranially. Compression by external masses as seen in two instances[72] can also change filter position. Incomplete filter expansion resulting from thrombus formation within the carrier during insertion has been documented[80] and may predispose to filter migration prior to its attachment to the caval wall. This complication is preventable by continuous heparinized saline flush of the catheter. Although penetration of the caval wall by struts has been documented in this and other series,[60, 61, 79] we have seen no resulting complications except hematuria in one woman receiving coumadin therapy that resolved after anticoagulant discontinuation, and a male referred for treatment of a misplaced filter in the iliac vein and chronic pain in the distribution of the obturator nerve who was found to have one of the hooks penetrating the nerve.

Summary

Transvenous Greenfield filter insertion is a safe and efficient mechanical means of protection against recurrent pulmonary thromboembolism both in the infrarenal and suprarenal positions. Long-term follow-up to 12 years has demonstrated a consistently high patency rate of 96%, which is independent of concomitant anticoagulant therapy. The incidence of recurrent embolism in patients with filters has not changed over time, and there has been no significant filter migration over prolonged periods of observation.

References

1. Virchow R: *Gesammalte abhandlungen zur wissenschefflischer, medicine. P. 227.* Frankfurt, Meidinger Suhn, 1956.
2. Mannucci PM, Tripodi A: Laboratory screening of inherited thrombotic syndromes. *Thromb Haematol* 1987; 57:247–251.
3. Comp PC: *Hereditary Disorders Predisposing to Thrombosis: Progress in Hemostasis and Thrombosis.* New York, Grune & Stratton Inc, 1986, pp 71–102.
4. Aderka D, Brown A, et al: Idiopathic deep vein thrombosis in an apparently healthy patient as a premonitary sign of occult cancer. *Cancer* 1986; 57:1846–1849.
5. Korbitz BC, Ramirez G, Mackman S, et al: Coumarin-induced skin necrosis in a sixteen year old girl. *Am J Cardiol* 1969; 24:420–425.
6. Much JR, Herbst KD, Rapaport SI: Thrombosis in patients with the lupus anticoagulant. *Ann Intern Med* 1980; 92:156–159.
7. Kakkar VV: The current status of low dose heparin in the prophylaxis of thrombophlebitis and pulmonary embolism. *World J Surg* 1978; 2:3–18.
8. Ruckley CV: Protection against thromboembolism. *Br J Surg* 1985; 72:421–422.
9. Pachter HL, Riles TS: Low dose heparin: Bleeding and wound complications in the surgical patients: A prospective randomized study. *Ann Surg* 1977; 186:669–674.
10. Kline A, Hughes LF, Campbell H, et al: Dextran 70 in prophylaxis of thromboembolic disease after surgery: A clinically oriented randomized double-blind trial. *Br Med J* 1975; 2:109–112.
11. Gruber UF, Saldeen T, Bishkop T, et al: Incidence of fatal postoperative pulmonary embolism with dextran 70 and low dose heparin: An international multicenter study. *Br Med J* 1980; 280:69–72.
12. Harris WH, Slazman EW, Anthanasoulis CA, et al: Aspirin prophylaxis of venous thromboembolism after total hip replacement. *N Engl J Med* 1977; 297:1246–1249.
13. Comerota AJ, Stewart GJ, White JV: Combined dihydroergotamine and heparin prophylaxis of postoperative deep vein thrombosis: Proposed mechanism of action. *Am J Surg* 1985; 150:39–44.
14. Consensus Conference: Prevention of venous thrombosis and pulmonary embolism. *JAMA* 1986; 256:744–749.

15. Modig J, Borg T: Thromboembolism after total hip replacement: Role of epidural and general anesthesia. *Anesth Analg* 1983; 62:174–180.
16. Arndt J, Hock A: Peridural anesthesia and the distribution of blood in supine humans. *Anesthesiology* 1985; 63:616–623.
17. Raggi R, Dardik H, Mouro AL: Continuous epidural anesthesia and postoperative epidural narcotics in vascular surgery. *Am J Surg* 1987; 154:192–197.
18. Flanc C, Kakkar VV, Clarke MB: Postoperative deep vein thrombosis: Effect of intensive prophylaxis. *Lancet* 1969; 1:477–478.
19. Browse NL, Jackson BT, Mayo ME, et al: The value of mechanical methods of preventing postoperative calf vein thrombosis. *Br J Surg* 1974; 61:219–223.
20. Scholz PM, Jones RH, Wolfe WG, et al: Prophylaxis of pulmonary embolism. *Major Prob Clin Surg* 1980; 25:96–111.
21. Rosengarten DS, Laird J, Jeyasingh K, et al: The failure of compression stockings (Tubigrip) to prevent deep venous thrombosis after operation. *Br J Surg* 1970; 57:296–299.
22. Moloney GE, Morrell MT, Fell RH: The effect of electrical stimulation of the legs on postoperative thrombosis. *Br J Surg* 1972; 59:65–68.
23. Borow M, Goldson H: Postoperative venous thrombosis: Evaluations of five methods of treatment. *Am J Surg* 1981; 141:122–125.
24. McKenna R, Galante J, Bachmann F, et al: Prevention of venous thromboembolism after total knee replacement by high-dose aspirin or intermittent calf and thigh compression. *Br Med J* 1980; 1:514–517.
25. Skillman JJ, Collins REC, Coe NP, et al. Prevention of deep vein thrombosis in neurosurgical patients: A controlled, randomized trial of external preventive compression boots. *Surgery* 1978; 83:354–358.
26. Coe NP, Collings REC, Klein LA, et al: Prevention of deep vein thrombosis in urological patients: A controlled, randomized trial of low dose heparin and external pneumatic compression boots. *Surgery* 1978; 83:230–234.
27. Turpie AGG, Gallus AS, Beattie WS, et al: Prevention of venous thrombosis in patients with intracranial disease but intermittent pneumatic compression of the calf. *Neurology* 1977; 27:435–438.
28. Tarnay TJ, Rohr PR, Davidson AG, et al: Pneumatic calf compression, fibrinolysis and the prevention of deep venous thrombosis. *Surgery* 1980; 88:489–496.
29. Knight MTN, Dawson R: Effect of intermittent compression of the arms on deep venous thrombosis in the legs. *Lancet* 1976; 2:1265–1268.
30. Harris WH, Raines JK, Athanasoulis C, et al: External pneumatic compression versus warfarin in reducing thrombosis in high-risk hip patients, in Madden JL, Hume M (eds): *Venous Thromboembolism: Prevention and Treatment.* New York, Appleton-Century-Crofts Inc, 1976, pp 51–60.
31. Salzman EW, Ploetz J, Bettmann M, et al: Intraoperative external pneumatic calf compression to afford long-term prophylaxis against deep vein thrombosis in urological patients. *Surgery* 1980; 87:239–242.
32. Butson ARC: Intermittent pneumatic calf compression for prevention of deep venous thrombosis in general abdominal surgery. *Am J Surg* 1981; 142:525–527.
33. Barett DW, Jordan SC: Anticoagulant drugs in the treatment of pulmonary embolism: A controlled trial. *Lancet* 1960; 1:1309.
34. Salzman EW, Deykin D, Shapiro RM, et al: Management of heparin therapy: Controlled prospective trial. *N Engl J Med* 1975; 292:1046.

35. Urokinase Pulmonary Embolism Trial: A National Cooperative Study. *Circulation* April 1973, 47(suppl 2).
36. Norris CS, Greenfield LJ, Barnes RW: Free-floating iliofemoral thrombus: A risk of pulmonary embolism. *Arch Surg* 1985; 120:806–808.
37. Piccone VA, Vidal E, Yarnoz M, et al: The late results of caval ligation. *Surgery* 1970; 68:980.
38. DeWeese MS, Hunter DC: A vena caval filter for the prevention of pulmonary emboli. *Bull Soc Int Chir* 1958; 17:17.
39. Spencer FC, Quattlebaum JR, Quattlebaum JK Jr, et al: Plication of the inferior vena cava for pulmonary embolism: A report of 20 cases. *Ann Surg* 1962; 155:827.
40. Ravitch MM, Snodgraff E, McEnany T, et al: Compartmentation of the vena cava with the mechanical stapler. *Surg Gynecol Obstet* 1966; 122:561.
41. Ragins H, Kotler S, Dannis I, et al: Recurrence of pulmonary embolism seven months after inferior vena cava stapling. *N Engl J Med* 1974; 290:668.
42. DeMeester TR, Rutherford RB, Blazek JV, et al: Plication of the inferior vena cava for thromboembolism. *Surgery* 1967; 62:56.
43. Moretz WH, Rhode CM, Shepard MH: Prevention of pulmonary emboli by partial occlusion of the inferior vena cava. *Am Surg* 1959; 25:716.
44. Miles RM, Chappell F, Renner O: A partially occlusing vena caval clip for prevention of pulmonary embolism. *Am Surg* 1964; 30:40.
45. Elkins RC, McCurdy JR, Brown PP, et al: Clinical results with an extracaval prosthesis and description of a new intracaval filter. *J Okla State Med Assoc* 1973; 66:53.
46. Bernstein EF: The place of venous interruption in the treatment of pulmonary thromboembolism, in Moser KM, Stein M (eds): *Pulmonary Thromboembolism.* Chicago, Year Book Medical Publishers Inc, 1973, pp 312–323.
47. Eichelter P, Schenk WG Jr: Prophylaxis of pulmonary embolism: A new experimental approach with initial results. *Arch Surg* 1968; 97:348.
48. Moser KM, Harsany PG, Harvey-Smith W, et al: Reversible interruption of inferior vena cava by means of a balloon catheter: Preliminary report. *J Thorac Cardiovasc Surg* 1971; 62:205.
49. Pate JW, Melvin D, Cheek RC: A new form of vena caval interruption. *Ann Surg* 1969; 169:873.
50. Hunter JA, Sessions R, Buenger R: Experimental balloon obstruction of the inferior vena cava. *Ann Surg* 1970; 171:315.
51. Mobin-Uddin K, McLean R, Bolooki H, et al: Caval interruption for prevention of pulmonary embolism: Long term results of a new method. *Arch Surg* 1969; 99:711.
52. Mobin-Uddin K, Utley JR, Bryant LR: The inferior vena cava umbrella filter. *Prog Cardiovasc Dis* 1975; 17:391.
53. Greenfield LJ, McCurdy JR, Brown PP, et al: A new intracaval filter permitting continued flow and resolution of emboli. *Surgery* 1973; 73:599–606.
54. Elkins RC, Greenfield LJ: Unpublished data, 1974.
55. Greenfield LJ, Kimmel GO, McCurdy WC III: Transvenous removal of pulmonary emboli by vacuum-cup catheter technique. *J Surg Res* 1969; 9:347.
56. Brown PO, Elkins RD, Greenfield LJ: Comparison of a new intracaval filter with the Mobin-Uddin device and clinical experience. *Circulation* 1973; 48(suppl 4):5.

57. Jarrell BB, Szentpetery S, Mendez-Picon G, et al: Greenfield filter in renal transplant patients. *Arch Surg* 1981; 116:930–932.
58. Stewart JR, Peyton JWR, Crute SL, et al: Clinical results of suprarenal placement of the Greenfield vena cava filter. *Surgery* 1982; 92(1):1–4.
59. Greenfield LJ, Stewart JR, Crute S: Improved technique for insertion of Greenfield vena caval filter. *Surg Gynecol Obstet* 1983; 156:217–219.
60. Wingerd M, Bernhard VM, Maddison F, et al: Comparison of caval filters in the management of venous thromboembolism. *Arch Surg* 1978; 113:1264–1271.
61. Cimochowski GE, Evans RH, Zarins CK, et al: Greenfield filter versus Mobin Uddin umbrella: The continuing quest for the ideal method of vena caval interruption. *J Thorac Cardiovasc Surg* 1980; 79:359–365.
62. Silver D, Sabiston DC Jr: The role of vena cava interruption in the management of pulmonary embolism. *Surgery* 1975; 77:1–10.
63. Orsini RA, Jarrell BE: Suprarenal placement of vena caval filters: Indications, techniques, and results. *J Vasc Surg* 1984; 1(1):124–135.
64. Greenfield LJ, Scher LA, Elkins RC: KMA-Greenfield filter placement for chronic pulmonary hypertension. *Ann Surg* 1979; 189:560–565.
65. Walcott C, Burchele HB, Brown AL: Primary pulmonary hypertension. *Am J Med* 1970; 49:70.
66. Greenfield LJ, Peyton R, Crute S, et al: Greenfield vena caval filter experience: Late results in 156 patients. *Arch Surg* 1981; 116:1451–1456.
67. Greenfield LJ: Technical considerations for insertion of vena caval filters. *Surg Gynecol Obstet* 1979; 148:422–426.
68. Allen HA, Cisternino SJ, Ottesen OE, et al: The Kimray-Greenfield vena cava filter: A case of unusual misplacement. *Cardiovasc Intervent Radiol* 1982; 5:82–84.
69. Greenfield LJ, Crute SL: Retrieval of the Greenfield vena caval filter. *Surgery* 1980; 85:719–722.
70. Schneider PA, Bedmarkiewicz V: Percutaneous retrieval of Kimray-Greenfield vena caval filter. *Radiology* 1985; 156(2):547.
71. Greenfield LJ: Current indications for and results of Greenfield filter placement. *J Vasc Surg* 1984; 1(3):502–504.
72. Messmer JM, Greenfield LJ: Greenfield caval filters: Long-term radiographic follow-up study. *Radiology* 1985; 156:613–618.
73. Rosenthal D, Gershon CR, Rudderman R: Renal cell carcinoma invading the inferior vena cava: The use of the Greenfield filter to prevent tumor emboli during nephrectomy. *J Urol* 1985; 134(1):126–127.
74. Goodall RJR, Greenfield LJ: Clinical correlation in the diagnosis of pulmonary embolism. *Ann Surg* 1980; 191(2):219–223.
75. Miller GAH, Sutton GC: Acute massive pulmonary embolism: Clinical and hemodynamic findings in 23 patients studied by cardiac catheterization and pulmonary arteriography. *Br Heart J* 1970; 3.2:518–523.
76. McAuley CE, Webster MW, Jarrett F, et al: The Greenfield intracaval filter as a source of recurrent pulmonary thromboembolism. *Surgery* 1984; 96(3):574–576.
77. Pasto ME, Kurtz AB, Jarrell BE, et al: The Kimray-Greenfield filter: Evaluation by Duplex real-time/pulsed Doppler ultrasound. *Radiology* 1983; 148:223–226.

78. Greenfield LJ, Zocco J, Wilk JD, et al: Clinical experience with the Kim-Ray Greenfield vena cava filter. *Ann Surg* 1977; 185:692–698.
79. Berland LL, Maddison FE, Bernhard VM: Radiologic follow-up of vena cava filter devices. *AJR* 1980; 134:1047–1052.
80. Leiter B, Sequeira J, Wertzma AF, et al: A complication following Kimray-Greenfield filter insertion. *Cardiovasc Intervent Radiol* 1981; 4:215–217.

Index

U

V

Y